Safety Guide for Health Care Institutions

3rd Edition

American Hospital Association
and National Safety Council

This book supersedes the 1972 book entitled *Safety Guide for Health Care Institutions.*

Library of Congress Cataloging in Publication Data
Main entry under title:

Safety guide for health care institutions.

   Bibliography: p.
   Includes index.
   1. Hospitals—Safety measures.   I. American
Hospital Association.   II. National Safety Council.
[DNLM: 1. Accident prevention.   2. Hospital
administration.   WX 185 S128]
RA969.9.S23   1983   363.1'5   83-12265
ISBN 0-87258-302-3

AHA no. 181136
Copyright 1983 by the
American Hospital Association
840 North Lake Shore Drive
Chicago, Illinois 60611

Copying of the figures in this book is permissible if for educational or training purposes.

Marvin Gough, Project Coordinator,
AHA Division of Management and Technology

Dorothy Saxner, Editorial Coordinator,
Karen Downing, Editorial Assistant,
AHA Division of Books and Newsletters

Contents

List of Figures

Recognizing the need for an updated version of *Safety Guide for Health Care Institutions,* the American Hospital Association and the National Safety Council convened an advisory committee to review the 1972 edition and to make specific recommendations for revisions and additions. Their efforts have resulted in this book.

Members of the advisory committee, whose contributions are gratefully acknowledged, were: Edward F. Byrne, Thomas H. Conkling (deceased), Marvin F. Gough, Edwin H. Green, William G. Lawhead, Robert H. Mangold, James A. Morgan, Victor G. Morris, Austin O. Phillips, Paul R. Seidlitz, Raymond S. Stephens, Alvin W. Stewart, and Wallace K. Wileman. In addition, suggestions from Alvin S. Williams and various American Hospital Association staff specialists clarified and improved the text.

The writing and editing were accomplished by Carl V. Boyer, Laura Louise Kuhl, and Joan Pawelski, under the direction of Dorothy Saxner and Rex N. Olsen, American Hospital Association.

Special appreciation is expressed to advisory committee members Marvin Gough, without whose diligence, commitment, and expertise this project would not have been completed, and Paul Seidlitz, who provided substantial review of the book and contributed to chapters 11 and 12.

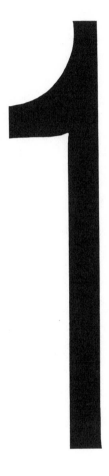

Hospitals, as institutions that exist to improve the quality of life through better health, have a difficult and challenging responsibility to maintain a high standard of safety—a responsibility that in many ways demands more attention than is traditionally associated with good safety practice. With patients, employees, medical staff, volunteers, and visitors, the nation's hospitals have approximately 9 million people—the equivalent of the total population of New York City—passing through their doors daily.

A hospital's safety program is the end product of the hospital's policies and plans as executed by all hospital employees. An effective safety program is unique to the hospital that uses it, as each hospital requires a program appropriate for its particular circumstances and needs.

To the degree that an effective safety program is implemented, the hospitalwide safety consciousness achieved helps avoid the direct and indirect costs associated with unsafe practice, thereby making an important contribution to hospitals' commitment to cost containment. Operating costs are reduced through an effective accident-prevention program.

From the laboratory to surgery and on through to final therapy, today's patient is being given more attention than was possible ever before. But when ultimately put into effect, any medical advance can be limited or even negated by a generally human failure: the accident. A hospital that does not apply vigilance to the total safety of every patient, visitor, and employee is working against its very reason for existence.

Although the essential nature of hospital safety is clear and unquestionable, the means of achieving it are not. For that reason, this book has been written to assist hospitals in developing, implementing, and maintaining policies and programs to meet their individual needs. The book is a guide to good practice. Thus, the guidelines given here are not standards and do not set safety regulations. Rather, they provide an overall view of the requirements for safety and of safety problems and methods.

The book can serve in planning and developing safety programs, in providing a source of safety procedures and safety information, in preparing written and oral in-house safety presentations, in serving as *one* yardstick for measuring existing programs, and in suggesting a source of safety program ideas. Its primary purpose is to be useful to employees in understanding the importance and the place of safety in all hospital procedures. Anticipating all potential hazards, providing information for their elimination, and stimulating staff to improve safety performance require a well-organized and sustained effort.

The book applies specifically to short-term acute-care hospitals—facilities that provide medical services 24 hours a day. With modification, many sections can also be used by special-purpose hospitals, clinics, nursing homes, convalescent homes, skilled-nursing facilities, intermediate-care facilities, and infirmaries in homes for the aged.

The material is presented in a form that optimizes direct use. If pages of the book are reproduced for in-house training or informational purposes, their source should be acknowledged. However, before a chapter is used unchanged for training personnel or for supplying information to personnel, it is advisable to review its content to make sure that all the information is applicable.

The material in this book can be supplemented with the following publications:

■ A complete set of National Fire Protection Association standards, including NFPA no. 56A, *Inhalation Anesthetics*; NFPA no. 70, *National Electric Code*; and NFPA no. 101, *Life Safety Code*

■ Standards promulgated pursuant to the Occupational Safety and Health Act of 1970, including OSHA *General Industry Standards*, Part 1910, and OSHA *Construction Standards*, Part 1926

■ Standards of the National Council on Radiation Protection, including NCRP no. 8, *Control and Removal of Radioactive Contamination in Laboratories*; NCRP no. 21, *Safe Handling of Bodies Containing Radioactive Isotopes*; NCRP no. 26, *Medical X-Ray Protection*; NCRP no. 30, *Safe Handling of Radioactive Material*; and NCRP no. 34, *X-Ray Protection Structural Shielding Design*

■ *Accident Prevention Manual for Industrial Operations*, published by the National Safety Council

■ *Security Programs in Health Care Institutions*, published by the American Hospital Association

■ *Emergency Removal of Patients and First-Aid Fire Fighting in Hospitals*, a joint publication of the American Hospital Association and the National Safety Council

■ Pertinent publications of the Joint Commission on Accreditation of Hospitals, particularly *Accreditation Manual for Hospitals*, revised and published annually

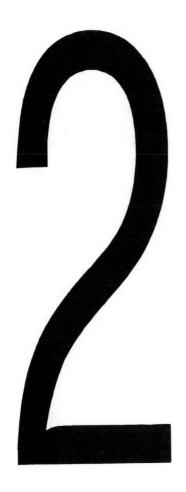

For hospitals and for industrial firms, providing a safe place for employees to work is mandated by law. This requirement is not the only safety responsibility common to hospitals and industries, inasmuch as many safety problems and the methods for handling them are fundamental to both hospitals and industries. Examples of this commonality include general safety information and procedures that are broadly applicable to most work places; specific safety procedures regarding the use of machines and tools in the engineering and maintenance functions; certain building code requirements and specifications; and the handling and disposing of hazardous and chemical wastes, which expand the safety responsibility and accountability beyond the walls of the facility or plant.

Industrial safety methods were formerly the model for hospital safety programs. However, the nature of hospitals, their mission, and their operation make them a unique group characterized by problems that conventional industrial safety programs do not address. In industrial settings, unsafe acts that do not result in employee injury are considered production problems, not safety problems. Damage to equipment or manufactured products is readily visible, and decisions regarding replacement or repair are seldom made under the tension of life-threatening emergency situations and affect only productivity or product quality.

In hospitals, in contrast, few unsafe practices have such limited consequences and few unsafe acts are corrected simply by replacement or repair. Diagnostic errors, improper procedures, and acts of omission have potentially significant consequences for patients. Furthermore, in the case of hospitals' constant fight against infectious microorganisms, the detrimental effects of an unsafe act or act of omission are not readily visible.

Hospitals are responsible for the safety of patients, the on-the-job safety of employees and volunteers, and the on-site safety of visitors, whereas industries are concerned primarily with on-the-job safety of well employees. Patients depend on hospitals for all their needs and may be incapable of contributing to their own safety. Only hospitals and nursing homes face the serious problem of protecting immobile persons in an emergency such as a fire. Care must be tailored to each patient's problems and needs, which change from day to day. As a result, hospital employees, unlike industry employees, must continually make observations and decisions regarding care.

A hospital is unique in that it is many enterprises in one. In addition to providing treatment and care, it includes functions normally associated with hotels, restaurants, and laundries. Support and maintenance systems are numerous and extensive. Many kinds of professional and nonprofessional staff with various levels of training and skill must coordinate and synchronize their functions to provide continuity in patient care and to ensure the delivery of high-quality health care. Because relatively few hospital jobs can be automated, most hospital accidents are the result of human error.

Hospitals must function around the clock. Although activity levels fluctuate, a complete shutdown of services is out of the question. Care is a continuum, with each shift continuing the work of the foregoing shift. Safety in medical procedures usually requires staff to verify that prior work has been completed correctly and safely. This continuity in function from shift to shift, staff to staff, and service to service is critical. An isolation room, for example, must be cleaned before it can be used for another patient. Therefore, hospitals must maintain their equipment hour by hour and day by day, whereas industry uses off hours, downtime, and plant shutdown to inspect and overhaul equipment.

The average hospital uses 5,000 to 10,000 pieces of complex and sensitive equipment and devices that are potentially dangerous to both the patients and the operators. Industrial equipment, although just as complex, sensitive, and potentially dangerous, is not used on patients. Moreover, the dangers associated with complex equipment in industries usually involve mechanically moving parts for which protection can be provided by installing guards and barriers. Such is not the case with most hospital equipment used for direct patient care. Equipment failure in industries is inconvenient and expensive, but in hospitals it can be life threatening.

In hospitals, effective preventive maintenance precludes frequent equipment malfunction. The margin for error or misjudgment is therefore nar-

rower in hospitals than in industries, because the chance of mistakes that endanger life is much greater. Human error may cause an irreparable setback in hard-won public goodwill and community relations; injury to a patient, visitor, or staff member; or, of greatest consequence, permanent disability or loss of life. Recognition of these and other differences has led to the emergence of hospital safety as an independent discipline that requires special knowledge and has its own precepts and practitioners.

Hospital safety has three basic requirements: (1) a structural environment and physical plant in which hazards have been identified and eliminated to the extent possible in compliance with health and safety standards, (2) a work force that functions safely for both self and others, and (3) patient care policies and procedures that ensure safety. Hospital safety requires staff planning and training to handle fire and other disasters. In addition, hospital safety requires a preventive surveillance program that is an integral part of the hospital's comprehensive health services.

Awareness

Increased safety awareness is a result of a number of factors:

■ With the Occupational Safety and Health Act (OSHA) of 1970 (Public Law 91-596), the government enlarged its role in regulating the workplace. The purpose of OSHA is to "assure so far as possible every working man and woman in the nation safe and healthful working conditions." Under OSHA, each employer is required to furnish each employee a workplace free from recognized hazards and to comply with safety and health standards promulgated by OSHA. Employees must be informed of these requirements, OSHA poster "Safety and Health Protection on the Job" must be displayed conspicuously, and annual summaries of occupational injuries and illnesses must be posted. Under OSHA, each employee is required "to comply with occupational safety and health standards and all rules, regulations, and orders issued pursuant to the Act which are applicable to one's own conduct."

■ The Worker's Compensation Act provides for compensation in the event of an occupational injury or illness that causes a loss of more than one

4

scheduled work day, an inability to continue to perform regular job functions, or death. Inasmuch as workers' compensation is regulated by state commissions, procedures vary, but state reporting requirements and compensation schedules are rigid.

■ Litigation resulting from personal injury or illness has increased dramatically. Hospitals have experienced a wave of safety-related and medical malpractice suits in recent years. Many of the precautions used by physicians and hospitals to minimize their liability often necessitate additional diagnostic procedures requiring the more frequent use of new and increasingly more sophisticated equipment, which adds to the potential for safety problems and human error.

As a result of these factors, safety programs have become more structured, and investigation and reporting requirements and procedures stricter and more carefully enforced. Safety is an integral part of performance competency, equipment acceptability, and structural utility. A job done correctly is safe, thorough, and efficient. For equipment to function properly, it also must function safely. Thus, safety is a two-stage process: (1) bringing performance and facilities up to a safe and satisfactory level and (2) maintaining this level.

Many agencies and business organizations can help hospital personnel to implement and ensure adequate safety programs. Important resources are state industrial commissions, hospital workers' compensation insurance carriers and insurance associations, and testing and technical laboratories. The local fire department and the state and local departments of public health and safety are valuable community resources. Publications, educational seminars and materials, and consulting are available from such specialized safety organizations as the American National Standards Institute, Factory Mutual Laboratories, the Health Insurance Association of America, the National Fire Protection Association, Underwriters' Laboratories, state OSHA offices, the National Safety Council, the Joint Commission on Accreditation of Hospitals, and the American Hospital Association.

Risk Management

Increasingly, hospitals approach safety as one aspect of a risk management program. Risk management offers a systematic approach for minimizing all events that increase cost and cause unnecessary diversion of assets away from their intended purpose. Safety, security, and infection control—hospital safety problems that result in substantial loss—are major components of risk management programs, which include risk analysis, record keeping, audits of department activities, investigation and analysis of all incidents, training and education, inspection, and evaluation of all control activities.

Risk management systems have demonstrated the cost-effectiveness of strong safety programs. Most injuries involve the direct costs of medical expense and of compensation, malpractice, and public liability insurance. Although the techniques used in risk management programs and those used in conventional safety programs are basically the same, risk management attempts to centralize, in one administrative point, data from all programs that monitor the safety of patients, employees, visitors, and the physical plant and grounds. This centralization of the hospital's safety performance data in a risk management program accomplishes three purposes: (1) it delineates the risk factors involved in the provision of care in the hospital; (2) it weighs the impact of these factors on the quality of health care delivery in the hospital; and (3) it provides direction for improving the quality of care and for managing the results of unexpected outcomes, whether by arrangements for necessary treatment or for financial compensation through some mode of insurance.

Whether the scope of the hospital's risk management program is broad or narrow, the activities of the hospital safety director, the hospital safety committee, and the infection control officer are crucial to the success of the hospitalwide risk management program.

Infection Control

Infection is a major health risk in hospitals and, as such, is a serious safety problem. Nosocomial (hospital-acquired) infections can result in costs as high as those incurred by injuries.

Infection control is a medical problem and therefore is generally not considered part of the conventional safety program. Infection control is often the responsibility of a committee that reports to the hospital's chief executive officer. The close relationship between safety and infection control should be recognized regardless of how the individual programs are structured. The cooperation and coordination of the safety and infection control committees are therefore important. Proper safety practices and proper infection control procedures intersect in nearly every function performed in the hospital, from replacing filters in air handlers to terminal cleaning of isolation rooms or catheterization of a patient. Many hospitals find it convenient and efficient to present safety and asepsis policies and information together in a staff policy and procedures manual or in in-service training.

Detailed information on infection control programs can be found in *Infection Control in the Hospital,* published by the American Hospital Association, and in *Guidelines for Prevention and Control of Nosocomial Infections,* published in 1981 by the Centers for Disease Control.

Security

Security traditionally has been regarded as protection of people and property. Increasingly, however, the security staff works closely with line management to protect hospital assets. As with infection control, security services should also be closely coordinated with safety functions.

The primary objective of the security department is to ensure the welfare and the safety of patients, visitors, and staff. Other important security functions include protection of the plant, equipment, supplies, and drugs, and control of traffic around, in, and out of the institution.

A major objective of any security program is to educate and motivate hospital employees to recognize the need for protection and to prevent theft, fire, and other incidents. A positive, efficient, courteous, and visible security force is the best deterrent and most effective preventive possible.

Elements of a Safety Program

A structured safety program is essential, whether it is administered as an independent program or as a component of risk management. The basic elements are preventive action, protective measures, training, and motivation:

■ Preventive action includes proper maintenance, monitoring, and inspection of equipment; implementation of safety policies and procedures; elimination of hazards; analysis and correction; and safety audits.

■ Protective measures are primarily mechanical guards, electrical grounding devices and sockets, signal devices, and other physical equipment and apparel to safeguard machines and staff, hazardous areas, and vehicles.

■ Training for health care jobs includes safety training. In-house safety training as part of orientation, periodic in-service education, and job supervision should include safety and emergency drills, instruction in the use of equipment, written materials, demonstrations, review sessions, introductions to new procedures and equipment, and disaster drills. Safety education for all personnel must be a continuing program.

■ Motivation methods can be directed toward groups or individuals. For each, different techniques are required to induce behavioral change and commitment to safe practice. The staff is motivated by the example of superiors and peers and by posters, publications, and promotional campaigns. Individuals are motivated by counseling and discipline.

A safety program in a health care institution is successful when all employees are involved. It must deal with the problems of the entire facility, not with certain trouble areas or with certain people. A successful safety program is built on consistent use and imaginative combination of the four basic elements listed above: preventive action, protective measures, training and motivation.

In developing three of these elements, that is, preventive action, training, and motivation, periodic repetition of information is recommended. One of the difficult aspects of being an effective safety director is to keep a positive and creative approach, yet also maintain an awareness of the need for repetition.

Of the foregoing four elements of a safety program, the first three—preventive action, protection measures, and training—require the resources of the hospital and are successful in proportion to the hospital's effort. Motivation, on the other hand, is a personal force distinctive to each employee and can require a number of different approaches. Although motivation is the most important of the four elements in maintaining a safe hospital, motivation is difficult to elicit successfully. When employees are not motivated to observe safety rules, accidents happen regardless of how well trained the work force is, how well the structure and equipment are maintained, and how much preventive action is taken.

In carrying out safety practices, the use of one technique does not obviate use of another of the same kind. For example, wearing plastic gloves when disinfecting isolation rooms does not eliminate the need for pre-procedure and post-procedure hand washing.

Last, there is a demanding need to transform concern to improve accident statistics into regard for the well-being of real people. The nature of health care delivery involves professionals who have the ability and desire to demonstrate this. Their total concern for patients and co-workers is, in turn, observed by other personnel. Working together for the common cause of safety and relief from suffering, all employees can form a most effective team.

Responsibilities

Every person in a hospital plays a role in maintaining a safe and accident-free environment, although not all of them realize their impact on safety and their influence in bringing about good practice. Members of the safety committee, for example, are more mindful of their safety responsibilities. Nevertheless, all of the following, either directly or indirectly, have responsibility for hospital safety:

■ The governing board, as the group ultimately responsible for policy and for the care provided, must recognize the importance of safety to the successful operation of the hospital and see that safety programs are adequately supported and funded. In addition, it is the responsibility of the governing board to draft and to issue a hospital policy statement.

■ The chief executive officer, as chapter 3 discusses more fully, to a large degree determines the hospitalwide attitude toward safety.

■ Medical staff members should support safety programs and recognize that their support and participation make an important contribution to staff recognition of the importance of safety

measures. The hospital policy statement on safety should state that medical staff members are required to follow the hospital's safety programs to ensure the support of all medical staff members.

■ Line supervisors have direct responsibility for the safe day-to-day job performance of employees.

■ The safety committee recommends policy, and its competence is reflected in the safety program.

■ The safety director works with management and staff to develop and maintain proper practice. This person must know and understand safe methods and practice.

■ The engineering staff is responsible for the safety of the structure, equipment, and grounds through preventive and corrective maintenance.

■ The nursing staff has the major responsibility for patient safety.

■ The in-service training staff advances safety by emphasizing safe practices through in-service educational programs.

■ The materials manager and staff, who are responsible for supply and engineering purchases, can raise the level of product safety through prudent selection.

■ The personnel department, through its hiring practices, contributes to staff safety.

■ Staff members play important roles in specific safety situations. For example, in an emergency operations plan, each employee has a specific essential role.

A number of groups outside the hospital also are important to the safety program. The Joint Commission on Accreditation of Hospitals specifies safety requirements as a condition of accreditation. Local and state fire authorities, public health departments, building inspection authorities, the Nuclear Regulatory Commission, and the Environmental Protection Agency also promulgate guidelines and regulations that recommend or mandate safety precautions and procedures for various hospital functions.

The American Hospital Association, its affiliate the American Society for Hospital Engineering, the National Safety Council, and state, metropolitan, and regional hospital associations are professional groups that promote hospital safety and conduct extensive training programs. Insurance carriers develop programs and are excellent sources of counsel and advice.

Others who by the nature of their work are secondarily responsible for hospital safety include architects, builders, manufacturers, equipment installers, servicers of equipment and machinery, and suppliers of materials.

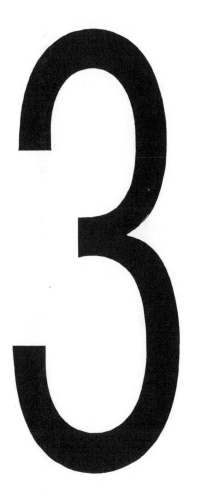

The care of human beings is the primary factor that distinguishes hospitals from other institutions. Also, the fact that hospitals are large and diverse service institutions adds significantly to the complexity of safety management functions in them. Each department within the hospital requires a specific set of safety standards; each piece of equipment requires periodic and, very often, special maintenance. Because a hospital is continually in operation, it cannot suspend operation while its equipment is inspected and repaired under any circumstances other than a disabling disaster. The hospital must provide its occupants with *all* services necessary for personal maintenance and comfort. It can never have a meeting of the full staff; training programs must be scheduled at various times so that all staff can attend.

Most important, in addition to providing a safe environment for its employees, medical staff, and volunteers, the hospital is charged with the safety of its patients, many of whom are not able to take any positive role in maintaining their own safety, are completely dependent on others, or may even endanger their safety and that of others.

Establishing a Hospital Policy

The hospital's policy on safety provides the foundation on which safety programs and procedures are built. No policy should be enacted unless there is a positive intent to put it into effect by providing staff with the motivation and training to apply it. The level of safe practice required by hospitals cannot be based on a vague set of traditional ways and means already generally familiar to most of the work force, but should emanate from a clear understanding of the function and specific tasks performed by the employees in each department.

The policy statement is the responsibility of the chief executive officer; it should be prepared carefully and presented under the CEO's signature. The members of the safety committee, the safety director, the personnel director, and legal counsel should study the policy statement before it is endorsed. A clearly and concisely expressed policy statement reflecting the hospital's prevailing attitudes, practices, and procedures will enhance the statement's usefulness.

The policy statement should begin with a general introduction setting forth the principles of the safety program: the hospital considers of prime importance the safety of patients, employees, volunteers, and visitors; requires compliance with safety rules; endeavors to prevent accidents; maintains its plant and equipment in safe operating condition; and complies with all appropriate safety codes and standards.

The responsibilities of management, employees, volunteers, the safety director, and the safety committee should follow the statement of goals. The Occupational Safety and Health Act (OSHA) of 1970 can be cited in this section of the policy statement. Under this law, an employer is required to furnish a place of employment free from recognized hazards that might cause serious injury or death and to comply with specific safety and health standards established by the U.S. Department of Labor. Each employee is required to comply with safety and health standards and with rules and regulations that apply to his or her job responsibilities.

The policy should clearly state the authority and duties of the safety director and the organization, composition, and duties of the safety committee. The *Accreditation Manual for Hospitals,* published annually by the Joint Commission on Accreditation for Hospitals, provides basic guidance regarding these requirements. Safety program procedures such as inspections, follow-up, and documentation should be outlined, and training and orientation programs should be described.

The policy statement should be posted so that the entire work force can take note of it, and it should be included in the hospital and departmental safety manuals.

Implementing a Safety Program

When the hospital policy statement has been disseminated to all employees, outlining clearly their responsibilities in delivering safe, high-quality patient care, the hospital administrative staff and the safety committee must transform the words of the policy statement into an active safety program understood and practiced by all employees.

The Role of Management

The key to a safe hospital is the total support of management for the goal of providing a safe environment for all. For a safety program to be effective, management must be convinced that safety is a major factor in preventing loss to the individual and institution and is integral to the quality of care. Management can lead the safety campaign by participation, demonstrating its commitment to safety in a number of ways:

■ High-profile participation in safety training and in fire and other disaster drills is leadership activity visible to rank-and-file employees.

■ Management must carefully observe all in-house safety rules. In places where protective equipment is required, managers must use it even though they may be in the area only for a few minutes.

■ Important safety memorandums should go out under the name of the chief executive officer or the appropriate senior member of the administrative staff. Departmental managers should regularly communicate safety information pertinent to their department staffs.

■ All levels of management should work to ensure that the safety surveillance program is followed.

■ Smoking regulations are difficult to enforce, so management should set an example by consistent adherence to smoking regulations.

In addition to highly visible means of leading the safety endeavor, management can demonstrate its commitment to safety in a number of more subtle ways that can affect not only employees' behavior but employees' attitudes as well. When management considers safety an integral part of performance, its outlook is reflected in criteria for performance reviews and job promotion.

Management must also understand the objectives of the hospital safety program. The administrative staff and department managers should be in agreement with the hospital safety policy and all the rules of the safety program. If they are not, the reasons should be determined.

Chief executive officer

The CEO, in addition to understanding the fundamentals of hospital safety, should be familiar with and supportive of all safety programs and should also be aware of the programs' limitations.

The CEO establishes hospital safety policy, appoints the head of the safety committee, and selects the safety director. These delegations of authority do not, however, relieve the CEO of the responsibility to monitor the hospital's safety standards. By reviewing such indicators as inspection reports, minutes of safety committee meetings, and incident reports, the CEO can be kept informed of safety conditions in the hospital. Safety awareness and a commitment to safe practices in the hospital start with top management recognizing safety as a vital but routine part of the institution's operation, to be interwoven with daily work procedures.

The duties of the hospital administrator are extremely broad. Apart from the medical aspects, they enter into areas of law, finance, construction, governmental relations, purchasing, accounting, personnel, housekeeping, inspecting, and family counseling. Although no hospital administrator can possess expertise in each of these diverse areas, he or she must be familiar with each departmental function if the hospital as a whole is to perform efficiently. Likewise, an administrator cannot be expert in all phases of safety but must be familiar with all of its standards and ramifications.

Because some aspects of safety are highly technical, the administrator must depend upon the safety director, the safety committee, and department managers, all of whose specialized expertise is essential to administering an effective safety program. The administrator's primary responsibility in this area lies in overseeing department managers in their discharge of all their specific duties and helping them recognize that safety is an integral part of each of these duties.

Line management

Line managers and supervisors—those persons who directly supervise the work of others—have major responsibility in ensuring on-the-job safety. The safety committee and the safety director can advise, counsel, and support; but only those directly supervising activity can ensure that safe work practices are routine and that carelessness, apathy, and incorrect procedures are not permitted.

Managers should have a clear understanding of all safety regulations that apply to their departments and should keep abreast of pertinent safety-related information. In addition to familiarity with

OSHA regulations, managers should know the safety precautions that the equipment and materials used in the department necessitate, the devices and clothing required for protection, and the procedures to be followed in case of an accident. They should know how department equipment operates and the signs of malfunction. They should know the hospital's safety programs as well as the procedures for coping with fire and other disasters. In departments that include any work directly involved with patient care, managers should be trained in and always be conscious of the safest way to deal with patients.

Staffing a Safety Program

The major resources for development of a hospital safety program are the safety committee and the safety director. The safety committee recommends policy and works with the safety director to determine effective means of prevention and enforcement. The safety director is the staff person charged with organization, coordination, and implementation of the safety program and is the committee's resource person. The functions of the director and the committee, and the relationship between them, vary in each hospital.

According to the *Accreditation Manual for Hospitals*, the safety committee and the safety director are responsible for the following:

■ Developing written policies and procedures designed to enhance safety within the hospital and on its grounds to the maximum degree possible

■ Coordinating and cooperating in the development of department/service safety rules and practices

■ Establishing an incident reporting system that includes a mechanism for investigating and evaluating all incidents reported and for documenting the review of all such reports and actions taken

■ Maintaining liaison with the infection control committee and assuring a mutual exchange of information

■ Providing safety-related information to be used in the orientation of all new employees and in the continuing education of all hospital employees

■ Conducting a hazard surveillance program at specifically defined intervals

■ Establishing methods of measuring results of the safety program and periodically analyzing the

program, including a review of all pertinent records and reports, to determine its effectiveness
■ Being familiar with local, state, and federal safety regulations applicable to the hospital
■ Being familiar with major safety-oriented agencies, both governmental and nongovernmental
■ Developing a reference library of pertinent documents and publications dealing with all facets of hospital safety, including copies of all applicable building and safety codes and standards

Safety committee

The safety committee, an in-house group composed of representatives from each major department, is charged with the responsibility of developing and implementing the hospital's safety program according to the hospital's safety policy.

The size and the composition of the safety committee will vary according to the individual facility. However, the committee's membership should include representatives from hospital administration, the medical staff, nursing service, the engineering and maintenance department, the housekeeping department, and the dietary department. The second and third shifts should be represented. In-house specialists such as the radiation physicist, clinical engineer, or biomedical engineering technician should also participate, at least in a consultative capacity. In some hospitals, departments that have the greatest work force, such as nursing, have the most representatives. This arrangement permits more complete coverage of complex functions and equalizes voting power when controversial matters are put to the ballot.

In hospitals where employees are unionized, a union representative provides a useful communication channel. A union representative can promote safety by identifying the need for safe practice and encouraging compliance. In hospitals that employ many minority workers, representation from these groups is important, particularly when language and cultural differences are a factor. In some hospitals, volunteers serve on the safety committee. Participation of outside agencies, such as the local fire department and civil defense group, is also useful.

To be effective, committee members must work actively, using their professional expertise and authority to further a safe environment. Each must know all the hospital's safety rules and set an example for the rest of the staff. It is a disservice to the hospital when the committee consists of persons already overburdened, who do not have the time or the commitment to make a significant contribution to safety.

Periodic rotation of committee members, particularly employee members, broadens and strengthens the committee's educational value. At the time of rotation, however, care must be taken to make members understand that they are not being replaced, but succeeded. To ensure smooth operation of the committee, rotations should be staggered rather than concurrent.

A large committee often does not function efficiently; the greater the number of members, the more difficult it is to assemble them in a set place at a set time and to have a quorum. In general, a committee of about 15 or fewer committed and informed members can provide the information and advice necessary.

In large and complex hospitals, subcommittees are an effective means of dealing with the specific safety problems of various departments. These subcommittees are structured in a manner similar to the safety committee, meet periodically, and perform the same functions. They are also represented on the safety committee. The safety director attends their meetings. Under this arrangement, the safety committee devotes its time to problems that affect all hospital activities, referring specific problems to a subcommittee for solution.

Safety committee meetings should be regularly scheduled by the chairperson and held at least monthly. An agenda for every meeting should be prepared in advance and distributed to members to apprise them of business to be handled. The duration of the meeting should be established in advance, and, in planning the agenda, realistic time should be allotted to each item. Formal minutes of each meeting should be taken and distributed; they provide useful information and help to avoid duplicative and overlapping efforts.

The effectiveness of the committee is determined in large measure by the chairperson, who is selected by the CEO. The choice of committee chairperson is especially consequential in hospitals that have limited safety resources and have a safety director who has other duties besides safety. The person appointed should be familiar with the hospital, understand how it operates, and know its policies and politics. The person should understand the concepts of safety and have both the interest and the time to keep abreast of developments in this field. Enthusiasm and creativity in the chairperson's approach to safety programs contribute to their success. He or she should recognize the value of the safety director and other in-house resources, taking full advantage of their counsel.

The chairperson requires on-the-job time for handling committee affairs. Many of its activities, such as conducting inspections and reviewing incident reports, are repetitive, so it is essential that these tasks be managed effectively to retain members' interest and conserve their time, as well as to obtain useful data. The duties and expectations of the position should be explained to the appointee, and the length of term stated. If possible, the appointee should be told the amount of time to be committed to this activity.

Announcement of this appointment should be handled in the same manner that the hospital handles other important appointments, for example, in a staff memorandum, a newsletter item, or a newspaper item. In the announcement, the chairperson's authority and the support of the safety department should be made clear.

Safety director

Directing the safety program may require anywhere from partial time of one employee who also has another staff position to more than one full-time person. Staffing depends on the size and location of the hospital and its safety policy and practices.

In some instances the safety director serves as chairperson of the safety committee, but this two-hat arrangement may not always be the best approach. In any event, because the safety director's and the safety committee chairperson's efforts are directed toward the same goal, that of a safe hospital, both positions should work together to establish common priorities and the same basic safety approach.

Although the services of a full-time safety director and staff would appear to be a major budgetary item, proponents of this system point out that it is not necessarily more expensive than the total time required of all members of the committee to effectively execute the safety program. An assertive, energetic safety director can expedite program elements that too often are lost in paper shuffling, committee meetings, or lack of knowhow. The safety director is a professional whose experience is acknowledged and can justify the cost of the position by preventing one major disaster or lawsuit.

The concept of safety as a professional discipline requiring specific education and experience is somewhat new, and only recently has the safety director become a recognized job category in the health care field. In some hospitals, the safety responsibility is delegated to the engineering department, and hospital engineers supplement their technical training so that they are proficient in all aspects of safety administration. The areas in which the safety staff can work effectively to optimize safety in the hospital environment have increased substantially.

The safety director should be qualified by training or experience, or both, to develop programs and to educate and motivate hospital personnel on safety matters. Safety has evolved into a field requiring particular knowledge that may be obtained through college or other training programs.

The duties of the safety director differ from hospital to hospital, but they generally include advising the CEO on safety matters; reviewing all incident reports and maintaining records and statistics on all injuries; analyzing injury, trend, and inspection reports and recommending preventive action; initiating and participating in safety motivation programs; directing the fire safety program; and conducting fire drills and other disaster preparedness programs.

Management should provide the safety director with the authority to perform the job, with access to the persons necessary for counsel, with the resources to provide a safe environment, and with cooperation at all levels. The safety director should be considered by all staff as a knowledgeable resource willing to assist.

Administering a Safety Program

The safety director should report to top-level administrative staff and may have staff reporting to him or her. The director should work closely with line supervisors, functioning as an adviser. A potential problem in achieving strong, adequately enforced safety programs is the lack of a clearly defined scope of authority for the safety director consistent with the broad responsibilities of the position. The safety director must have access to top management and the authority to act in hazardous situations, but always in cooperation with line management.

Working together, the safety director and department supervisors can achieve the goals of the safety program. Although the safety director holds hospitalwide responsibility for the success of the safety program, line managers have responsibility for safety in their particular departments. Where the work and responsibility of each begins and ends should be clearly defined, and any disagreement that arises should be immediately resolved.

For the hospital safety program to be effective, its findings must be made known to all personnel. Physicians will be aware of their responsibilities to the hospital safety program if communication with medical staff is maintained through physician representation on the safety committee, through the CEO, and through the chief of the medical staff. The primary function of the safety program must be to engender, stimulate, and maintain interest in the safety and fire prevention program among all personnel, including department directors, supervisors, line employees, students, patients, and visitors.

Motivating employees

The supervisor is the motivating force in safe practices. Managerial personnel who understand the importance of safety and advocate safety programs convey their attitude to those who report to them, and they are responsible for the successful performance of these people. When employees realize they are part of the safety effort and that they share its success, their enthusiasm increases. Commendation and participation in the development of department safety goals motivate employees. Conversely, managers and supervisors who are negative or ambivalent about safety programs or consider them a hindrance to production cannot motivate others to employ safe work habits.

Supervisors should circulate all safety material issued by the hospital or post it prominently. They should acquire or develop safety information specific to the department and make it available to staff. They should be trained in principles of first aid.

Because supervisors are familiar with their department's activities, they are in the best position to determine areas in need of improvement. Using available resources such as the safety committee, the safety director, engineering personnel, and the in-service training department, supervisors can initiate new safety measures, such as modification of equipment, alteration of surroundings, or modified presentation of information.

Training employees

All employees should be adequately trained, preferably on a one-to-one basis, in the correct and safe way of doing their individual jobs. In giving training for each job in the hospital, the department director should:

■ **Prepare.** Provide sufficient background information to ensure that the rationale and practicality of the instruction are clearly understood. Relate the project to other aspects of the total job, and attempt to create in the new employee a sense of ease and confidence.

■ **Present.** Explain how the task is done, demonstrate how the task is done, and explain why it is done that way. A step-by-step approach is recommended even for the simplest of procedures. Then repeat; make the key points clear. Be patient and go slowly; clear up one point at a time. Then repeat again.

■ **Try it out.** Have the employee perform the task and observe him or her doing it. Emphasize correct procedure and that proficiency will come with practice, especially for the new employee who feels compelled to complete tasks quickly. If the employee tends to skip a process, learn why; he or she may have a justifiable reason. Have the new employee repeat the task, and then explain what is being done each time and why. In that way, the department director can determine whether the employee is grasping the point or merely imitating the department director. Correct the employee's errors, but in an encouraging manner.

■ **Follow up.** Have the worker perform the task alone, making sure that he or she is followed up to keep from developing bad habits. If the new employee is put under the immediate direction of another person, make sure that person does not undo the prior teaching by the department director or supervisor. Insist that correct, safe procedures be followed in the future.

No one should be permitted to work unassisted until he or she has demonstrated proficiency and understanding. The safe and correct performance of each job by each staff member is critical to the overall safe and successful operation of the hospital. Pride in work leads to job satisfaction and helps to create a safe environment.

The hospital regularly uses potentially dangerous supplies and equipment, so an understanding of how machines work and knowledge of the properties of materials is important. Most managers can determine the extent of a person's knowledge and perception of materials or equipment during a one-to-one training session.

Language is often a barrier to training. When English is the employee's second language, training techniques may require some adjustment. In such cases, the supervisor should tell how, show how, observe, correct, and monitor. Managers and others responsible for in-service training should be aware of such problems and understand how to cope with them.

Safety, including fire safety and other disaster preparedness training, (chapters 11 and 12), should be carefully planned and presented in a manner that maximizes comprehension and enthusiasm and minimizes boredom. The choice of speaker is important, and visual aids and handouts should be planned to enhance the presentation.

At the end of a training session, there should be some provision for review, such as a test or question period. The most important test of the effectiveness of a training program is how well the instructions are put to use. If a disaster does occur, the functioning of all departments should be carefully recorded and analyzed with a view to improving teaching methods.

Formalization of safety training is in itself important; it tells the staff that this activity is important enough to take up valuable work time. If the hospital takes training seriously and invests its resources in a good program, the staff will respond.

Orientation

When a new employee joins the staff, safety training should be part of his or her orientation.

The hospital's policy on safety, the underlying reasons for it, and the strict and serious enforcement of it should be expanded. Safety orientation usually considers overall hospital safety, not department safety requirements. Fire safety requires perhaps an initial half-day of instruction by the hospital fire marshal or by a member of the safety committee.

Staff safety meetings

Safety requires continuous reinforcement, which can be achieved through a continuing training program. All staff and volunteers should attend quarterly or semiannual safety updates. As a minimum, the following areas should be covered in separate programs: patient safety, fire safety, electrical safety, and the body mechanics of lifting. When incident reports indicate a problem or when the safety staff thinks a subject should be reviewed, a presentation should be prepared and a meeting called. Individual departments should have departmental safety review meetings.

To save time, meetings should be tightly constructed. To make maximum attendance possible, they should be held at the beginning or end of a shift. Flexible scheduling is necessary. The challenge to the safety director to make meetings interesting can be accomplished in part by concentrating on hospital-specific safety concerns; the obligation of hospital administration and department directors is to ensure attendance.

Eleven steps to safety

Under the direction of the CEO, the following steps should be taken in administering a comprehensive and effective hospital safety program:

1. **Uncover the problems.** Records should be reviewed to determine who was involved in previous incidents, where, and why. A comprehensive inspection should be conducted that includes an assessment of safe or unsafe practices as well as safe or unsafe conditions.

2. **Present the problem to the department directors.** Supervisory staff should be involved in planning all efforts to reduce accidents and to increase safety. Without their understanding, agreement, and cooperation, the safety effort will not succeed.

3. **Set up a committee organization and an executive head.** A safety committee that has the

CEO's authorization and a responsible chairman can implement an effective safety program.

4. **Establish safety records.** A reporting form for individual injury cases should be adopted that includes a description of the cause of each incident.

5. **Set up inspection routines.** Safety conditions and work practices should be monitored regularly, and the types of inspections to be made, how often, and by whom should be determined. Inspection reports should be filled out completely, and their recommendations followed.

6. **Study work procedures.** Jobs that seem to cause frequent injury should be studied, and ways to reduce the risk of job tasks should be devised and implemented.

7. **Give job instruction.** All employees should be taught to do their work properly. Jobs requiring minimal skills or in which there is rapid employee turnover necessitate constant, specific job instruction to avoid injury. Refresher sessions, including fire safety training, should be held regularly for all employees.

8. **Motivate employees.** Employees should be persuaded to emphasize safe practice in their job duties in order to be committed to the hospital's whole safety effort.

9. **Investigate, analyze, and cure.** The causes and circumstances for each incident should be examined, and remedies to prevent recurrence should be implemented.

10. **Follow up.** Unless periodic checking is undertaken to be sure that fire and accident prevention programs are consistently followed, the goals of the safety program will not be achieved.

11. **Assess the elements of the safety program.** In order for the safety and fire protection programs to be effective for all patients, visitors, and employees, the entire program must be reviewed periodically. Additional effort in any area of the program should be applied when needed.

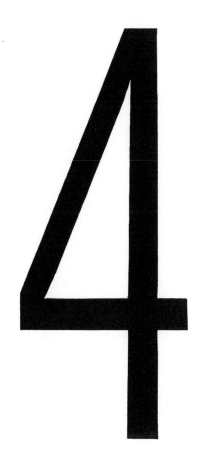

Members of the hospital safety surveillance team must cope with many of the same problems that their counterparts in industry face: maintenance and housekeeping; materials handling and storage; operation of power equipment; utilization of gases and chemicals; possible exposure to electronic, radiation, and nuclear devices; and handling and disposal of hazardous wastes.

The hospital team has the added problem of possible contraction of communicable diseases. This ever-present threat of contagion may come from direct contact with the patient or from fomites in the laundry, linen exchange, laboratory, kitchen, or waste disposal process.

Advances in medical science can be applied safely only if exacting rules, proper procedures, and engineering controls are observed. An effective, comprehensive safety program can minimize or eliminate employees' and patients' exposure to the potential hazards that are posed by the wide spectrum of instruments, devices, and other technical equipment used daily within the hospital.

The *Accreditation Manual for Hospitals,* published annually by the Joint Commission on Accreditation of Hospitals, is a valuable resource in organizing and executing a comprehensive safety program. JCAH standards provide specific guidelines that can be used to measure and improve the safety performance of the hospital. The most practical framework for an extensive program of compliance with the JCAH's standards is departmental safety inspections and surveillance. Safety inspections are one of the principal methods of locating hazards and help to determine what safeguards are necessary to promote on-the-job safety for employees and to assure patients and visitors of optimal protection. Inspections should include the observation of unsafe conditions and unsafe acts.

Management's Role in Inspections

Finding unsafe conditions and work practices and promptly correcting them constitute basic ways for management to prevent accidents; to safeguard employees, patients, and visitors; and to demonstrate to those groups and to the public its sincere interest in accident prevention. Inspections demonstrate management's commitment to the well-being of each employee, especially in departments not generally visited by upper management. They provide the opportunity to build rapport with employees and to increase motivation. In addition, inspections serve as a visible indication of management's concern for safety as an important aspect of the hospital's primary mission.

Safety inspections provide a key link in employee/management communication, which facilitates policies that are realistic and actually result in improved safety. Because hospital safety policy cannot be based strictly on the accident record of the facility, it is important for those who recommend and enforce safety policy to understand the operating environment in which the policies are being applied.

Inspections are an important means of documenting hospital safety initiatives in the event of litigation and for insurance reasons.

Inspections help management to plan, organize, and execute the safety program. They justify budgetary expenditures within each department. Also, they may indicate a need for revised purchasing criteria, more training, improved departmental or facility work-flow patterns, or modifications in current or future building design. Inspections by management also provide insight into the impact of one department's operation upon another, which may lead to revisions in practice or procedures.

Informal Inspections

Informal inspections are rounds generally made by the safety director, the chairperson of the safety committee, or the chief executive officer using a tape recorder or a note pad for comments. Informal safety inspections by the administrative representative on call can shed light on safety practices and problems on weekends and night shifts. Such inspections are useful in eliminating conditions that could cause accidents. For example, equipment left in a heavy-traffic corridor can be noted during an informal inspection and moved before an incident occurs.

Regular informal inspections provide insight into recurring safety problems unique to certain departments or to the hospital in general that would not be detected through periodic formal inspections. Informal inspections are less intimidating than formal inspections and therefore provide an excellent opportunity to discuss with employees and supervisors specific safety needs and conditions in detail that would not be possible or appropriate during formal inspections.

Formal Inspections

Formal inspections are those made at regular, scheduled intervals. They should be scheduled for the entire hospital, for certain operations, or as preventive maintenance for certain types of equipment. They should be made by a specified group, usually members of the safety committee, accompanied by an individual within the department being surveyed, at intervals of 1, 3, 6, or 12 months, as the situation demands.

Every area of the health care facility should be given a general inspection at least once a year. Included should be those places where "no one ever visits" and "no one ever gets hurt" and areas that are not the specific responsibility of any one department. Many of these out-of-the-way places are overhead or underground, where the maintenance employees may work alone. Some types of equipment, such as elevators, boilers, unfired pressure vessels, and fire extinguishers, are subject by law to inspection regularly. All formal inspections must be planned so that they can be made systematically and efficiently. A report of the inspections should be prepared by the safety director or the safety committee representative, reviewed by the department director involved, and then forwarded to the hospital administrator.

In preparing for an inspection, all accidents reported from the previous several years, including noninjury accidents and near-misses, should be analyzed so that special attention can be given to those conditions and locations known to be accident producers. Tables and charts that show the types and numbers of accidents by department, the causative factors, and the remedial action taken or recommended are helpful. To facilitate the inspection routine, lists of hazard spots should be compiled for each department. Insurance companies often have appropriate inspection forms available; the National Safety Council is another source of such material.

Departmental inspections

The most practical framework for an extensive program of compliance with the JCAH's standards is departmental safety inspections and surveillance. Although formal institutionwide inspections should be based on a prepared checklist covering all departments and all personnel, some overlapping of inspection areas will ensure 100 percent correction of conditions and practices that are potential hazards.

An effective safety inspection depends on several factors. The individual or safety surveillance team should:

■ **Be selective.** Coverage of all safety aspects in one tour of a department is difficult, if not impossible. Therefore, an inspector might check for basic safety the first time, for improvement of operations the second time, for training needs the third, and so forth.

■ **Know what to look for.** The more a supervisor or safety committee member knows about a job and each worker's responsibilities, the better an observer he or she will be.

■ **Practice observing.** The more often a person makes a conscious effort to observe, the more will be seen each time.

■ **Keep an open mind.** The inspector must avoid judging facts in advance and should act only when all the facts have been gathered.

■ **Go beyond general impressions.** A clean laboratory or careful routine may still contain hidden hazards.

■ **Guard against habit and familiarity.** Asking the basic questions who, what, where, when, why, and how often will uncover the real meaning of a situation.

■ **Record observations systematically.** All notes should be dated, with space for comments on the action taken and its results. The notebook can serve both as a reminder and as a record of progress.

■ **Prepare a checklist.** To streamline the inspection process and the paper work, the health care facility should develop a checklist for each area to be surveyed by any one person or group. Thus, the chief engineer would have his own checklist of equipment for which he is responsible, as would the nursing supervisor, the dietitian, and so forth. Checklists must be constantly updated to include new or changed equipment and facilities. A

merely mechanical follow-through with an outdated checklist will not be effective.

■ **Set a good example.** No matter what planned routine of inspection may be established, it cannot replace the day-to-day, hour-by-hour alertness of supervisors and employees.

Periodic inspections

Many types of equipment and processes require periodic inspections if they are to be used safely and efficiently. A number of maintenance departments require that all hand tools and appliances be returned to a central storeroom after use each day; there they are carefully checked and repaired before they are reissued. Often this excellent practice is extended to the central service department. In some hospitals, inspections of all electrical equipment are scheduled and include a thorough "knockdown" inspection periodically.

An adequate periodic inspection will call attention to the following items and conditions:

■ **Electrical equipment.** All electrical devices, power tools, and equipment should be checked daily for defective wiring or improper grounding. The physical plant survey should include a periodic inspection of all wiring, outlets, transformers, and switchboards.

■ **Housekeeping.** General housekeeping throughout the health care facility should be checked. A comprehensive list of checkpoints appears in chapter 9. Housekeeping is a continuous element of the safety program and is not limited to periodic inspections.

■ **Floors.** Regardless of construction, floors should be carefully inspected, especially in areas subject to heavy traffic. Slipperiness of floors should receive special study and treatment. Floors should be checked for rapid surface wear; shrinking flooring material; decayed, worn, curling, or slippery surfaces; and holes, unguarded openings, or cracks that present hazards to walking and trucking. Inclined ramps, which present a special problem for many hospitals, require the surface application and frequent inspection of nonskid material or tape. The hazard of overloading floors should be checked, especially in frame structures. Storage of books and records in frame buildings constitutes a hazard; such materials are unusually heavy and require firm flooring.

■ **Storage areas.** Almost every department has a frequently used and often neglected area for storing equipment, records, supplies, and other items. These areas may contain materials that are subject to spontaneous combustion, as is the case with photographic film and x-ray negatives, which must be stored in covered fireproof containers in accordance with the requirements of the local fire marshal. Compressed medical gases require a specified fire-resistance-rated construction for the storage area, continuous ventilation, and a means for securing freestanding cylinders. Storage areas often become depositories for equipment in disrepair, which, if not properly labeled and separated from usable equipment, can result in a serious accident.

■ **Elevators.** State laws usually govern periodic inspections of elevators. However, these are minimal codes; more frequent inspections are desirable to prevent cable slippage and intercommunication system failures.

■ **Pressure vessels.** State and local laws require periodic inspections of boilers and unfired pressure vessels. Such equipment is usually inspected by the insurance carrier rather than the hospital employees. A predetermined schedule of inspections, as required by law, should be established well in advance, so that arrangements can be made to put the vessels out of service during the check.

■ **Loading and shipping platforms.** These get severe use from trucks and heavy machinery. Bumper strips are needed to prevent damage from trucks and from deterioration of concrete due to inclement weather and use of salt or other chemicals for snow and ice removal.

■ **Grounds.** Parking lots, roadways, and sidewalks need frequent inspection for cracks, holes, breaks, and tripping hazards. Proper types of snow removal equipment are necessary for these and other areas traveled by visitors and staff, and the equipment should be safely maintained. Special attention to paths usually traveled by handicapped persons is important, especially during the winter season.

■ **Roofs.** Monthly inspections of roofs for storm damage or damage from tree branches is advisable. In winter months during heavy snowfall, it may be advisable to check the weight limits of the roof. Gutters should be checked for clogging by leaves. Roof anchorage of signs, hoisting anchors for window cleaning, and other structural elements should be inspected with special care.

■ **Chimneys and stacks.** These should be checked for clogging from soot and effluents, the need for tuckpointing of brick mortar, and anchorage of guy wires and cables.

■ **Outside structures.** Small, isolated buildings should be inspected in the same way as the main building. Fencing, lighting fixtures, and other structures attached to or separate from the main buildings should be inspected for damage or corrosion.

■ **Catastrophe hazards.** These include foundation failure, structural deterioration (including that of window frames), overloading, and conditions that cause fire and explosion.

Night Inspections

It is desirable to conduct department safety inspections occasionally during night shifts, instead of limiting them to daylight hours. Work routines within a department may vary with the supervisory shifts. Safety conditions also can change considerably after dark, because of artificial illumination or lack of proper lighting.

Using a light meter, the surveillance team should make sure that adequate illumination is provided, especially in outdoor areas. Because security becomes a greater problem after dusk, proper floodlighting should be installed in areas surrounded by trees, shrubs, and bushes, as well as near steps, reflecting pools, and pathways. To keep outdoor lighting from creating a glare in pedestrians' eyes and to keep electrical cables from forming a tripping hazard, low-voltage lighting installations with automatic timers are recommended.

Special Inspections

Special inspections sometimes are necessary because of new equipment or procedures, construction of new buildings or remodeling of old ones, or discovery of new hazards. Accident investigations require special inspections by the safety committee and the safety director. Special inspections are also made wherever there is a suspected health hazard. Emphasis should be directed toward determining the extent of the hazard and the precautions or mechanical safeguards needed to eliminate it. The inspections usually require sampling of air for toxic fumes, gases, and dust, and testing of ventilation and exhaust systems for efficiency.

Many other types of special inspections frequently are necessary, including inspection of scaffolds, window-washing platforms and cables, personal protective equipment, machinery guards, lighting facilities, ventilation equipment, disposal facilities, excavations, and construction work. Such inspections may be made at the request of supervisors or groups of employees or because of a special need indicated by accident trends.

Reports and Report Forms

The basis of an effective hospital safety program lies in the incident reporting system. Detailed record keeping can point out to the hospital administrator accident trends, high-hazard areas, and the frequency and severity of incidents involving personnel and equipment.

Separate but coordinated records on accidents involving employees, patients, and visitors must be maintained. A thorough and complete system for reporting incidents and inspections can usually provide information on trouble areas before a serious accident occurs and provides vital protection by serving as court evidence when a hospital is involved in litigation.

Reporting individual injury cases is indispensable to the hospital's accident and fire control program. Simple addition of cases is not enough to provide a base of operations against hospital hazards. There also must be an understanding of causes and their related frequency and severity. Insurance records or similar records are not adequate for this purpose, although special reports or records may be required by the hospital's insurance carrier.

Each report should be on a separate sheet. A hospital may work out its own reporting form, giving emphasis to factors it considers most important for recording injuries to employees, patients, or visitors. Such a form should call for specified indispensable data on unsafe conditions and unsafe acts involved in the reported case. Before using any form exclusively, a hospital should determine that the form will be acceptable to its legal counsel and insurance carrier for their respective purposes. These records will not be an acceptable substitute for the records that hospitals subject to the Occupational Safety and Health Act of 1970 are required to maintain.

Although some health care facilities require that individual injury reports be computed only for disabling injuries to employees, it is recommended that near-incident reports also be a part of the hospital's reporting procedure. Reports of all employee mishaps that have significant causes, regardless of whether they result in disabling injury, provide another means for the administrator and the safety director to find areas that may need correction. Such reports, which include incidents when an accident has been averted before it started or in which injury is minor but could have been serious, also afford an excellent means of keeping all personnel alerted to potential hazards.

The report of injury should be completed by or under the direction of the department director or supervisor in whose jurisdiction the accident occurred. It should be read carefully by the administrator and studied by the safety committee. Full, detailed reporting, particularly of the incident's reasons or causes, should be insisted upon. Loose explanations such as "carelessness," "don't know what employee was doing," "couldn't be helped," or "disobeyed orders" should be avoided. Such answers shift responsibility to the injured person and repudiate the essential premise that management is responsible for what happens on the job.

The National Safety Council (NSC) has published an accident report form (see figure 1 at the end of this chapter) that can provide information about factors leading to an accident.

NSC also has published an investigator's cost data sheet (see figure 2) that provides for a cost study of an accident. Although such a study may be time-consuming and laborious, by determining costs for each case and then compiling them into a semiannual or annual summary, the hospital can obtain results that amply justify the time, money, and effort expended.

Another recommended NSC form (see figure 3) compiles a running tabulation of cases. This form, the Accident Analysis Chart, can be readily adapted for use by hospitals. Such a summary can give the administrator and safety committee a quick picture of the safety program's overall progress. Ample material for diagnosis and eventual correction is provided by simple classification of the listed cases according to departments, groups of persons involved, types of causes, kinds of equipment involved, unsafe behavior found, and other causal factors.

Pertinent information

Every accident report form used in the hospital should contain the following pertinent information:

■ Identification of the injured person, including statistics on height, weight, and mention of eyeglasses or any physical impairment. These particulars are important. A person over six feet tall, for instance, may find low-hanging steam pipes in the boiler room a personal hazard, whereas other workers may not. In short, a hazard may lie within an individual and not be inherent in a given practice or aspect of the physical plant.

■ A detailed description of the incident scene.

■ A statement of what caused the incident, including any contributory negligence on the part of the injured. For instance, an employee walking down a maintenance department corridor may encounter at a blind corner an employee carrying an extension ladder, which cuts the first person's eye. The injured victim committed no unsafe act; the careless worker is not injured. These points should be brought out in the report.

■ Names and addresses of witnesses to the incident.

■ A physician's statement on the extent of the injuries and the treatment prescribed.

■ Steps taken later to prevent the recurrence of such an incident.

■ The possible cost sustained or time lost because of the incident.

The administrator has the responsibility for ensuring proper preparation of accident forms and maintenance of complete records of incidents and actual injuries to employees, patients, and visitors. However, both the administrator and the hospital must recognize that records are not an end in themselves but only a means to an end. An integral part of the work of the safety function is to determine where hazards exist.

Benefits of accurate reporting

In summary, systematized records on incidents and accidents provide these benefits:

■ A basis for improving the hospital environment and job routines and thus the safety of the visitor, the patient, and the employee

■ A basis for improving and continuing the education of all employees

■ A valuable record admissible as evidence in court in the event of a personal injury or damage suit

It bears restating that the function of a record system is to determine where the hazards lie and that follow-up education, engineering, and enactment are needed to eliminate such hazards.

Figure 1. This accident report, if completed immediately after an accident occurs, can provide pertinent information about factors contributing to the accident and steps that should be taken to prevent its recurrence. Published by the National Safety Council.

Department Director's Accident Report

1. ACCIDENT CATEGORY   ☐ Injury   ☐ Illness   ☐ Property Damage   ☐ Fire   ☐ Other

   Company name and address _____

   Plant location (if different from above) _____
2. Name and address of injured (or ill) person _____
   _____ SSN _____ 3. Age _____
4. Sex _____ 5. Years of service _____ 6. Time on present job _____
7. Title/occupation (at time of occurrence) _____
8. Department _____ 9. Date of incident _____
10. Time of incident _____ a.m.-p.m.
11. SEVERITY OF INJURY OR ILLNESS   ☐ First-aid   ☐ Medical treatment   ☐ Lost workday case
         ☐ Restricted work case   ☐ Time away from work case   ☐ Fatality
12. Estimated number of days on restricted work _____
13. Estimated number of days away from work _____
14. INJURY DESCRIPTION Describe nature of injury or illness _____
15. Part of body affected _____
16. Degree of disability (describe) _____
                      (Temporary total; permanent partial; permanent total)
17. ACCIDENT DESCRIPTION Place incident occurred _____
18. What part of job was being performed at time of incident? _____
19. What happened? Describe in sequence: _____
_____
20. Physical surroundings at time of incident: (weather, equipment, machinery, aisles, features, etc.) _____
_____
_____
21. How was work being done? _____
22. What happened to cause incident? _____
_____
_____
23. Other factors necessary to fully describe incident _____
_____
24. PERSONAL PROTECTIVE EQUIPMENT required (Protective glasses, safety shoes, safety hat, hearing protection, respirator, etc.)
_____
_____
25. Was injured using required safety equipment? _____
26. Date employee was last trained in proper use of required safety equipment _____
27. WAS THERE A VIOLATION of a published safety/health rule, regulation, procedure or specific instructions? (Explain)
_____
_____
28. WAS EMPLOYEE PROPERLY INSTRUCTED on how to do the job safely and properly exposed in training to those items listed in previous question? (Explain) _____
_____

(Front of form)

(Figure 1 continued)

29. WERE INSTRUCTIONS ADEQUATELY related to the specific hazards involved? (Explain) _____
_____
_____

30. WERE MECHANICAL/PHYSICAL/ENVIRONMENTAL conditions safe at the time of the incident?_____
(Explain)_____
_____

31. DETAILED NARRATIVE DESCRIPTION: (How did accident occur; why; objects, tool, equipment, tools used, etc.)
_____
_____
_____

32. WHAT CORRECTIVE ACTION should be taken to avoid a reoccurence of this type of injury (state who - what - engineering changes; written procedure development or improvement, enforcement of safety rules, regulations, instructions or procedures or specific training)
_____
_____

33. ACTIONS TAKEN ALREADY to correct and/or eliminate the hazard, injury causing agent(s)_____
_____
_____
_____

34. WITNESS TO ACCIDENT _____

Date report prepared _____

Signature of investigating Foreman/Supervisor _____

Signature of reviewing Supervisor _____

SUPERINTENDENT'S APPRAISAL AND RECOMMENDATION
MANAGEMENT COMMENTS AND ADDITIONAL CORRECTIVE/PREVENTIVE ACTION REQUIRED

_____
_____
_____
_____
_____
_____
_____

Signature of Superintendent/Plant Manager_____ Date: _____

(Back of form)

Figure 2. This cost data sheet, published by the National Safety Council, provides pertinent information about an accident.

Investigator's Cost Data Sheet

Class 1_____
(Permanent partial or temporary
total disability)

Class 2_____
(Temporary partial disability or
medical treatment case requiring
outside physician's care)

Class 3_____
(Medical treatment case requiring
local dispensary care)

Class 4_____
(No injury)

Name_____

Date of injury_____Its nature_____

Department_____Operation_____Hourly wage_____

Hourly wage of supervisor $_____

Average hourly wage of workers in department where injury occurred $_____

1. Wage cost of time lost by workers who were not injured, if paid by employer $_____

   a. Number of workers who lost time because they were talking, watching,

      helping_____.

      Average amount of time lost per worker_____hours_____minutes.

   b. Number of workers who lost time because they lacked equipment damaged in ac-

      cident or because they needed output or aid of injured worker_____.

      Average amount of time lost per worker_____hours_____minutes.

2. Nature of damage to material or equipment_____

   _____

   Net cost to repair, replace, or put in order the above material or equipment $_____

3. Wage cost of time lost by injured worker while being paid by employer $_____
   (other than workmen's compensation payments)

   a. Time lost on day of injury for which worker was paid_____hrs._____mins.

   b. Number of subsequent days' absence for which worker was paid_____days.

      (other than workmen's compensation payments)_____hours per day.

   c. Number of additional trips for medical attention on employer's time on suc-

      ceeding days after worker's return to work_____.

      Average time per trip_____hrs._____mins. Total trip time_____hrs._____mins.

   d. Additional lost time by employee, for which he was paid by company_____hrs.

      _____mins.

(Front of form)

(Figure 2 continued)

4. If lost production was made up by overtime work, how much more did the work cost than if it had been done in regular hours? (Cost items: wage rate difference, extra supervision, light, heat, cleaning for overtime.) $_____

5. Cost of supervisor's time required in connection with the accident $_____

   a. Supervisor's time shown on Dept. Supervisor's Report____hrs.____mins.

   b. Additional supervisor's time required later____hrs.____mins.

6. Wage cost due to decreased output of worker after injury if paid old rate $_____

   a. Total time on light work or at reduced output____days____hours per day.

   b. Worker's average percentage of normal output during this period_____%.

7. If injured worker was replaced by new worker, wage cost of learning period $_____

   a. Time new worker's output was below normal for his own wage____days____

      hours per day. His average percentage of normal output during time____%.

      His hourly wage $____.

   b. Time of supervisor or others for training____hrs. Cost per hour $_____.

8. Medical cost to company (not covered by workmen's compensation insurance) $_____

9. Cost of time spent by higher supervision on investigation, including local processing of workmen's compensation application forms. (No safety or prevention activities should be included.) $_____

10. Other cost not covered above (e.g., public liability claims; cost of renting replacement equipment; loss of profit on contracts cancelled or orders lost if accident causes net reduction in total sales; loss of bonuses by company; cost of hiring new employee if the additional hiring expense is significant; cost of excessive spoilage by new employee; demurrage). Explain fully. $_____

        Total uninsured cost (sum of items 1 through 10) . . . . $_____

(Back of form)

Figure 3. This accident analysis chart, published by the National Safety Council, can readily be adapted by hospitals to provide a summary for the administrator and the safety committee.

Accident Analysis Chart

Report of _____

Address _____

ACCIDENT ANALYSIS CHART

(list all injuries)

Period _____ to _____

TABULATION OF DISABILITIES

1. Temporary total disab.	_____	5. Man-hours worked	_____
2. Permanent partial disab.	_____	6. Freq. rate (line 4 x 1,000,000) (Line 5)	_____
3. Deaths and perm. total disab.	_____		
4. TOTAL DISAB. (1, 2, & 3)	_____	7. First-aid cases	_____

Acc. No.	Date of Acc.	Name of Insured	Occ. or Dept.	Injury Nature and part of body	Injury Class (1,2,3,7)	Injury Days Lost	Description of Accident (use more than one line if needed) Give exact details—employee actions, equipment and part of equipment involved, contributing conditions. Avoid terms "carelessness" and "inattention."	Corrective Action Taken

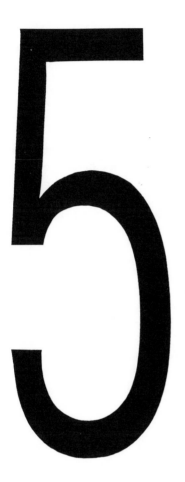

Providing the essential support services for patient care involves many people: physicians, employees, volunteers, visitors, salespeople, and service and repair personnel. To develop safety-conscious attitudes and well-defined procedures for each of these groups, all of which have different missions, responsibilities, and functions in the hospital, requires a concerted effort. Indeed a major portion of the safety drive is in the realm of human relations, because any strategy for safety must consider human behavior and the important role it plays in reducing accidents. Factors to be considered include individual personality differences, attitude, emotional makeup, and motivation.

Although some patients can follow instructions to ensure safe procedures, few can take full responsibility for their own safety. Other patients are essentially helpless and cannot care for themselves. Therefore, hospital employees are responsible for the well-being of patients. This fact cannot be overemphasized.

Orientation

Patients are entitled to the highest quality of care, which includes a safe environment and personal consideration. In addition to being in an environment where every attempt should be made to eliminate accidents, patients should have the comfort of knowing that an accident prevention policy is in force.

Patients are also entitled to know the hospital's regulations and policies that affect them. All patients except those who are critically ill, senile, or pediatric patients should be made aware of their contribution to safety and the importance of following the rules. Since many areas of the hospital present an entirely new environment for patients, they should be told or shown:

■ The importance of rails on hospital beds, which must be narrow enough to be pushed through doorways. If patients are assured that the rails are for their protection, they will cooperate in letting the rails remain up.

■ The way to request help through signaling devices and the location of light pull chains and radio and television controls. If electrically operated beds are used, patients should be given special instructions and then should be asked to demonstrate how to operate the controls.

■ The dangers of falling out of bed because of reaching, sitting up while in a weakened condition, or turning over in a comparatively narrow bed. Bedside items such as reading materials and toiletries should be so accessible to patients that overreaching is unnecessary.

■ Hospital regulations on smoking. Ambulatory patients should be permitted to smoke only in lounges or approved areas and only with the physician's approval. If a patient is bedridden, the attending physician should determine whether the patient's condition would be aggravated more by smoking or by deprivation of the habit. When permitted to smoke, a bedridden patient must have a responsible adult in attendance. Smoking in the presence of oxygen should be forbidden, and the hazards involved should be thoroughly explained.

■ The rules and procedures for fire practice drills and practice emergency evacuations that the hospital must conduct periodically to meet accreditation standards. Hospital staff should inform patients of these drills well in advance so that they are not disturbed or falsely alarmed when the practice drills and evacuations take place. To avoid panic during an actual fire, staff should use discretion in informing patients, especially those who are bedridden.

■ The need to report any excessive temperatures from appliances or from heat or radiation treatment. The nature of radiation exposure and its possible effects should be explained.

Signs describing hospital rules and regulations should be clearly worded and prominently posted. Printed instructions should be carefully prepared and presented so that they will be read. In some hospitals, multilingual instructions are necessary. Instructions that must be followed quickly and require specific, direct action, such as fire evacuation procedures, must be brief and clear.

Identification

All patients, including newborn infants, must be properly identified and must wear some type of physical identification at all times. The need for this precaution is apparent when, for example, patients are undergoing anesthesia, are incoherent, or are otherwise unable to identify themselves. In a technical advisory bulletin entitled *Identification of Hospital Patients,* the American Hospital Association states:

> Where possible, exclusive reliance on oral identification should be avoided because patients may be indifferent or inattentive, sedated, or otherwise unable to respond. In addition, patients may have language barriers, speech and hearing defects, or may be too young or too confused to comprehend.
>
> A method for affixing identifying data to the patient's body is preferred to prevent misidentification. A tamperproof, nontransferable identification band can be affixed to the patient upon admission. The band should be checked before every procedure. All persons associated with patient care, including members of the medical staff, should be trained in the use of the band. The band should never be removed unless the patient's welfare necessitates such removal. In this event, another band should be affixed immediately to the same or a different part of the patient's body.

The identification system may include not only the patient's name, hospital record number, and name of attending physician, but also information on any allergies and on the patient's religious preference, in case the patient's illness becomes grave enough to warrant notification of a member of the clergy.

The hospital may wish to establish its own policies on patients' wearing of rings, wrist or ankle bracelets, or religious medals. Such items are possible hazards during treatment with electronic equipment and should not be worn near it. However, because they may be important to the emotional state of some patients, tact should be used in persuading patients to remove them.

Metal bracelets or necklaces that indicate the wearer is allergic to certain medication or is diabetic and taking insulin should be removed and kept with the patient's other personal belongings. Just prior to discharge, the patient should be reminded by nursing staff to wear this jewelry again.

The hospital should make sure that every new-born infant is properly identified immediately at the time of birth. This should be done in the delivery room, by placing duplicate items of identification on the infant before the mother or the infant is transferred from the birth room. These identification items should be clearly visible and should be used by doctors, nurses, and the mother each time the infant is moved. Both mother and infant should be removed from the delivery room before another mother is brought in for delivery.

Every mother should be informed of the identification system used and of the mother's responsibility to check the identification on the infant each time it comes to her bedside and when she goes home. Duplicate identification devices, such as waterproof and oilproof bands, should be fastened on the wrist or ankle. The identification items should be prepared individually for each infant by the supervising nurse in the delivery room and secured to the newborn infant immediately upon delivery.

Before taking the infant to the nursery, all identification items should be checked by the supervising nurse to see that the name of the mother, her admission number, the date and time of delivery, and the sex of the infant are recorded. Simultaneously, the same identification information should be placed upon the infant's birth record.

When the infant is brought into the newborn nursery, the labor or delivery room nurse and the nursery nurse should check to see that information on all identifications and on the infant's birth record is identical. The sex of the infant should be verified, and both nurses should sign the infant's birth record. The crib card should be filled out by the nursery nurse and affixed to the infant's crib. Infant identifications and crib cards should be checked each time the infant is removed from or returned to the crib.

At the time of discharge, all identification items on the infant should be checked with the crib card and the infant's birth record in the nursery by the nurse in charge. With the assistance of the nurse, the mother should check the infant's identifications, remove one of the infant's identifications, and record her signature acknowledging her acceptance of her infant. The item of identification that has been removed should be attached to the

infant's birth record. The infant should be dressed in the presence of the mother or the person taking custody and discharged without removing the remaining item of identification.

A baby born while the mother is en route to the hospital or in the emergency room must be identified by standard hospital means until proper mother and infant documentation can be prepared by postsurgical or nursery staff.

Ambulatory Patients

Early ambulation assists the healing process, and the benefits of getting out of bed and walking around should be explained to patients in a way that will overcome feelings of insecurity without arousing any overenthusiasm. The following guidelines should prevail:

■ Before a patient walks, the patient's record should be checked for any special physician's instructions, such as deep breathing or limbering exercises in bed.

■ Patients getting on their feet for the first time should wear regular shoes or slippers, but not high-heeled shoes.

■ Areas in which patients may walk should be dry and free of obstacles and slipping hazards.

■ Corridor handrails should be provided.

■ Night lighting should be provided in patients' rooms and in all corridors.

■ Patients should not use stairs, except with permission of the physician.

■ Patients should be kept from medicine storage areas and medical records.

■ Tub baths or showers should be taken only under the supervision of a nurse.

■ Handrails and grab bars should be provided in the bathroom. Tub and shower surfaces should be of abrasive material, to provide safe footing. The bathroom should be equipped with a nurse-call button. The bathroom door lock should be operable from the outside as well as from the inside. Instructions on such details should be given to the patient.

Crutches issued to patients should be of the correct height and weight. They must have heavy suction-cup tips that are in excellent condition and are free of wax and small particles.

Proper use of wheelchairs should be explained to patients, their locking devices should be checked, and canvas seats should be examined for defects or loose stitching.

Pediatric Patients

Active children are especially subject to falls from a bed. For younger children who are able to stand upright in bed and for older children, tall side rails are necessary; the mattress and spring should be lowered to the maximum extent to prevent the youngster from climbing over the railings. Special attention must be paid to the danger that the child will choke if its head and neck are caught between bars of the railings or that the child will fall between the mattress and the side of the bed. In some cases, padded restraints may be ordered by the pediatrician.

Because smothering is always possible with small children, pillows should be firm and offer support, and plastic wrappings should never be permitted on sheets and pillows.

Children should be protected from contact with steam lines or other hot piping that may pass through their wards. Inhalators, especially the type with funnels, should be carefully adjusted. Children receiving any kind of heat treatment—pad, lamp, or water bottle—should be kept under close supervision.

Toys, where appropriate and permitted by the physician, should be contained in a common playroom area and should never be left in corridors, on the floors of children's rooms, or in the cribs of sleeping children. Children should not be given any toys made of glass or having sharp edges, flaking paint, or parts that could be detached and swallowed.

Children should never be left unsupervised while eating. Those children in high chairs should be returned to their rooms as soon as they have been fed.

Major Hazards

Despite great advances in medical technology, patients continue to be victims of three major types of accidents: *falls* from the bed or elsewhere in the room; *electrical shock,* occurring particularly during surgery or in special treatment areas but also in patient rooms; and *explosions,* primarily due to gases used during anesthesia. In the case of electrical shock and gas explosions, the primary

causes are the operator's unfamiliarity with newly developed devices and improper testing or grounding of the mechanisms before they are put into operation. Thus, new devices designed to increase patient comfort and recovery and employee effectiveness do not always achieve these goals.

A case in point involves the most basic of all hospital equipment: the patient's bed. In the history of health care, the patient's bed has progressed from a simple pallet, to a collapsible cot, to the familiar wheeled unit complete with side rails and adjustable springs controlled by hand cranks and operated usually by members of the nursing staff. Today, more and more hospitals are using electrically controlled beds. Patients usually operate the hand controls of such equipment, automatically adjusting the springs and flexible mattress into a variety of positions and elevating or lowering the bed height. These beds have permitted patients to attain the optimum in bed comfort and have effectively reduced the need to call nurses or aides to adjust beds.

But electrically operated beds also have caused many types of accidents. Staff members and visitors have tripped over the beds' electrical cords. Electrical shocks and fires, caused by damaged plugs, pinched wires, and ungrounded motors, have brought serious injuries. Fatal accidents have befallen patients in electrical beds during examination with an electronic device or after insertion of an electrode or catheter into the heart. In such tragedies, it has been determined that the fault lay in the bed motor's broken ground wire or ground connection. When the patient touches the bed frame or the nurse touches both the patient and the bed, a capacitive ground current can flow into the patient and pass through the electrode or catheter directly into the heart, producing ventricular fibrillation and death.

Hospital personnel use many mechanical devices: suction machines, nebulizers, oxygen apparatus, lighting equipment, traction devices, oxygen systems, and motorized beds. Personnel should not only know how to operate the equipment, but should also be aware of the danger to patients and themselves if it is operated unsafely or if it is returned to storage in defective condition without being tagged for repair. Equipment that is not in satisfactory working order should be tagged as defective and taken out of service immediately, and it should not be used again until it is properly repaired.

There are no simple solutions to the problems associated with the application of advanced technology. Because of both the constant turnover in personnel and the constant development of new equipment, an ongoing instructional program by qualified members of the safety surveillance team is required.

Falls

Falls are the most frequent single incident involving patients. Patients of 55 years or older are as much as 6½ times more likely to fall than younger patients. Young people, on the other hand, may be overanxious and unwilling to wait for help in whatever they require. Studies in a 491-bed convalescent and chronic care hospital showed that almost 80 percent of the 776 incidents reported over a one-year period entailed falls.

About 65 percent of all patient falls occur within 10 feet of the patient's bed. Among the causes are overreaching; attempts by irrational, incapacitated, or postsurgical patients to get into or out of bed without assistance; and faulty bed rails or casters.

Although patients may feel fine when flat on their back in bed, they may become dizzy or disoriented when they begin to get up. Beds should be lowered before the patient attempts to stand. If a footstool is used, it should have a slip-proof top surface, and its legs should be provided with rubber feet. To spare the patient from having to bend over to locate it, the stool should be kept within reach and not under the bed. Bed cranks should be retracted after use, so that they will not be a tripping hazard.

Once out of bed, a patient may trip over unfamiliar objects or slip on a spill. If the patient has not been shown how to use equipment such as a walker or crutches, or if these items are of incorrect height or are broken, he or she can readily fall. An unbraked wheelchair can roll away as a patient attempts to sit in it.

Rails should be required for all beds and should be used for sedated, unconscious, disoriented, or restless patients of all ages. Patients should be told the purpose of bed rails. Rails should be raised whenever drainage tubes, intravenous solutions, or catheters are being used, unless the physician directs otherwise. Gentle restraints also may be prescribed by the physician to keep the patient from trying to cast aside such chemicals and instruments or to lower the bed rails. Each problem of this type must be decided individually.

Bedside tables should be placed close enough to the patient's bed so that the watch, water pitcher, drinking cup, telephone, spectacles, toiletries, reading matter, bedpan, urinal, and other articles are within easy reach. Intravenous and other equipment attached to the patient should be arranged and maintained so that it is as much out of the way as possible. The nurse-call button and the radio and television controls should be readily accessible to the patient. Night-light cords and similar devices can be pinned to the patient's pillow if necessary.

The problem of patients' falls is complex in that it involves both education of patients, who may be unable to understand safety instructions, and a continuing education program for staff members. Many patient falls can be traced either to ignorance or to a sense of insecurity and disorientation. Patients who have no rapport with the attending nurse are more likely to try taking care of themselves when they should not do so. If the staff makes an effort to see that patients have the items they need and want, that they can reach them without danger of falling, and that service is prompt, patients have no need to risk a fall by leaving the bed.

Equipment not in use should be removed from the room. The sight of an unoccupied wheelchair may invite an unescorted trip. If bedside toilet facilities are left in the room, the patient may try to use them unassisted. Any piece of unnecessary equipment can cause tripping or injury. Falls brought on by equipment that breaks or malfunctions can generally be kept at a minimum through a thorough preventive maintenance program and a mandatory check before each use.

Escorting, Lifting, and Transporting Patients

Escorting

As a general rule, patients must be escorted when moved within the hospital, from the time they are admitted until the door on the vehicle taking them home is closed. Employees and volunteers are trained and authorized to escort patients. Guidelines for escorting patients are shown in figure 4 at the end of this chapter.

When a patient is unconscious, a nurse and at least one other person should be in attendance during the entire move. An anesthesiologist always escorts the patient from the operating room to the recovery room. A member of the nursing staff usually escorts pediatric patients and, with special care and attention, tries to make them less fearful.

Lifting

Hospital staff members should be made aware of their responsibilities in preventing injury to bedridden patients and of their duties and obligations to assist other staff members in transferring patients. Such cooperation among staff members is constantly needed; the employee providing assistance today may be needing it tomorrow. The rules concerning lifting should be taught to all employees to ensure that patients are lifted safely at all times. In general, staff members should follow these guidelines when moving patients:

1. Always check first with the supervising nurse as to what the patient may safely do.
2. Loosen the bed clothes for easier movement, taking care that the patient's body is properly covered.
3. Have the patient flex his or her knees, if conditions permit.
4. Get close to the patient being lifted instead of reaching for him or her. Move in and hold the patient close.
5. Place one arm under the patient's knees, the other across the patient's back under the far shoulder.
6. Stand with feet slightly apart to provide a broad base of support for proper balance. Take as much of the strain as possible with the leg muscles, not with the back. Keep the back straight; and bend only at the knees and hips.
7. Take a deep breath when about to lift a patient.
8. Straighten the legs to lift, and push with the thigh muscles, not with the spine.
9. Shift the position of the feet to turn rather than twisting with the body.

Staff members should keep the following points in mind:

■ Avoid false motions, sudden jerks, and pulls. Never pull on the patient's muscles or skin.
■ Work in unison, with the patient contributing effort, but not permitting the patient to overexert.
■ Be sure to give support to the heavy parts of the patient's body. Do not let the patient "hang" unsupported.

When lifting or moving helpless patients, staff members should decide whether they will need help in the task and should not hesitate to ask for assistance from co-workers. It is important that a helpless patient *knows* he or she is going to be lifted and knows *how* and *to which place* staff members are going to lift him or her. Two employees, lifting the patient from opposite sides of a sheet folded double under the patient, can handle the patient with relative ease, although it is safer and easier to push or pull the patient whenever possible.

When moving a patient from lying to sitting, the staff member should roll the patient to a side-lying position and move the patient's legs over the edge of the bed facing the staff person. In this way, the patient's buttocks will serve as a fulcrum or pivot point to raise the patient to a sitting position.

When moving a patient from the bed to a chair, the staff member should place the chair parallel to the bed. If a wheelchair is to be used, it should be of the nontipping type, have a security belt, and have its brakes locked. Standing directly in front of the patient, the staff member should press against the patient's ribs at the axilla or on the patient's hips. The staff member should help the patient bend forward, and then should thrust the patient further forward and upward to a standing position. The staff member should make a quarter turn by pivoting the feet, not twisting from the hips, so that the patient's back is to the chair. Then, bending at the knees, the staff member should lower the patient into the chair.

When a patient who is unable to stand is lifted from the bed to a chair, the staff member should raise the patient's trunk to a sitting position without bending the patient's knees. Standing at the patient's back, between the bed and the chair, the staff member should reach under the patient's arms to grasp the patient's forearms near the elbow. As the staff member lifts to bring the patient to the chair, the patient should press his or her elbows against his or her ribs. A co-worker's assistance should always be used to lift the patient's legs.

When lifting a patient from a cart to the bed or from the bed to a cart, one or two persons should assist the staff member and help lift the patient from one side. Caster brakes should be applied to the bed and the cart. The patient should be kept flat throughout the transfer. Using draw sheets in this instance is hazardous, because staff members can easily overextend their reach.

When a patient is transferred from the bed to a wheeled stretcher, caster brakes should be applied to the bed and the stretcher to prevent the two from separating. The bed should be raised to the same level as the stretcher before the patient is transferred. The patient should be helped from the bed to the stretcher and, if sedated or unconscious, should be moved by two employees.

Transporting

Patients being transported from their rooms to other departments within the hospital are especially prone to distractions, dizziness, and nausea. They may faint in a wheelchair or on a stretcher or examining table, and the likelihood of falling increases. When the means of transportation is specified by the attending physician, it cannot be changed. When the physician does not specify, the nurse makes this decision.

The most frequent mode of transportation in the hospital is the wheelchair. Guidelines for transporting patients in wheelchairs are listed in figure 5.

Every patient should be secured with a restraining belt while on a stretcher. The patient should be covered with a sheet, and with a blanket if needed. The escort should caution the patient to keep his or her hands, arms, and feet under the blanket and on the cart. The patient's head should be at the conveyance end nearest the escort. On a stretcher, the patient should be moved feet forward.

When irrigation stands or supports for blood or plasma containers are used on stretcher carts, they should be anchored securely to prevent their tipping and falling. Carts so equipped must be moved cautiously, particularly at intersections and in and out of elevators.

When two persons are handling a stretcher, both should face forward, and the one in front should act as a guide at corridor corners. If one

person is handling a stretcher, he or she should move to the front to brace it from there before going down a ramp.

When transporting patients in beds, including those in traction, the general procedures for stretchers outlined in figure 6 should be followed. Two persons are always required for such procedures. The side rails of the bed must be up, and the electrical cord should be wrapped around the rack provided at the head of the bed.

Certain circumstances necessitate specific equipment. Portalifts can be used to transfer helpless or disabled patients from beds to stretchers or wheelchairs. Guidelines for their use are listed in figure 7.

Burns, Cuts, and Punctures

Burns

Thermal and electrical burns and burnlike wounds are responsible for a small percentage of incidents. Generally, burns result from carelessness on the part of either the patient or the staff person. Figure 8 lists precautions for eliminating injurious burns to patients. Burns should be treated promptly, the incident described in the chart, and an incident report filed.

Employees should be aware of the potential for serious, possibly fatal, burns that can result from oxygen fires and explosions.

The delicate skin condition of many ill persons increases the effect of a burn. Adhesive tape can produce burnlike wounds, so where this probability exists, special tape or tape substitutes should be used.

Smoking in bed is a major cause of preventable burns. Bed fires that result from smoking occur frequently despite much publicity on hospital smoking rules. Staff members are responsible for pointing out to patients the hospital's smoking policy. They should also be aware of the danger to themselves and others of violating that policy.

Cuts and punctures

Although the major incidence of cuts stems from falls, there are other sources of cuts in hospitals. To avoid infection, all cuts, including paper cuts that a patient may incur in opening envelopes and handling magazines, should be treated immediately.

Cuts from broken glass can be minimized by requiring that personal items such as mouthwash and shampoo be brought to the hospital in non-breakable containers. Floral arrangements in glass containers should be placed where they are secure. Serving dishes and glassware should be selected with safety as one criterion.

Skin punctures, a source of cuts among staff members, may also happen to patients in the course of treatment when a patient's unexpected move or a doctor's or nurse's unintentional move punctures the patient's skin. All procedural precautions should be taken to avoid these mishaps.

Thermometers are a potential source of serious safety problems, especially when they break during use. Patients using an oral thermometer should be cautioned not to talk or bite. If the patient has a cough or is unconscious, use of an oral thermometer is inadvisable. When a temperature is taken rectally, the patient should be attended constantly. The attendant should hold the rectal thermometer in place when taking the temperature of children, the elderly, and persons who are confused, partly conscious, or unconscious. If a thermometer breaks, glass shards and mercury should be gathered and wiped up immediately and put in a special container for harmful waste, not in an ordinary wastebasket.

Medication

Because errors in medication carry grave consequences and can originate with the order, preparation, delivery, or administration of drugs, each staff member should take precautions to ensure that what he or she does is correct. Physicians, nurses, nursing supervisors, and pharmacists should have precise and fully defined responsibilities that ensure strict control and proper identification of all medications.

Under no circumstances should the nurse change labels, refill containers, or perform other functions recognized as the prerogative of the pharmacist. The opportunity for error is reduced when medication is prepared and packaged as unit doses by the pharmacy and then sent to the nursing service in a compartment reserved and marked for the specific patient.

There are five medication "rights": (1) the right medication must go (2) to the right patient (3) in the right dosage (4) by the right route and (5) on the right schedule.

The medication given must be exactly that prescribed; only the physician can order a substitution. An ambiguous order must be clarified by the physician.

Nonmedical products such as talcum and liquid soap should be clearly identified and labeled with instructions. They should be packaged in suitable containers, not in medicine containers.

Medication brought along to the hospital with a patient should be sent to the pharmacy for analysis and confirmation before the patient may use it. Medication brought by a patient may be confiscated and then either discarded or maintained at the nurses' station, depending on hospital policy and physician preference.

To make certain the right person receives the right medication, the nurse should always positively identify the patient by asking the patient's name and checking his or her wristband. Positive patient identification is necessary because new patients or new staff members may be unfamiliar with a hospital service, patients may exchange beds in confusion, or patients may be moved from one bed or ward to another. Patients themselves can help to minimize medication errors provided they are told what they are to be given, and why and when they are to receive it. Each medication must be charted on patients' records by the individual who administered it.

The amount of medication, as specified, must be given as ordered. When a dose is given in juice or another vehicle, this, too, must be prepared as specified. When several drugs are given in combination, the medication cup should be labeled with the name and content of each drug and the name of the patient. Some medicines must be shaken to ensure proper dosage. If the patient drops or otherwise loses a medication, or spills the liquid containing it, it should be replaced and given immediately. In such instances, the pharmacist needs all the pertinent information regarding the mishap.

Medications are taken orally, intravenously, intradermally, intramuscularly, and rectally. The route must always be clearly stated, and when the patients are allowed to take their own medications, they must be told exactly how to do it. Medication for dermal application and for other external uses should always be administered by a staff member and should be stored separately from internal medicines. When injecting a medication, the nurse must make sure the entire dosage is given in the appropriate site.

Drugs must be given at the intervals prescribed, as dosage is calculated on this basis. Realistically, staff cannot give the 6:00 p.m. medication to each patient in a given area at precisely 6:00 p.m., but the schedule should be adhered to within a few minutes.

If a medication error does occur, it should be reported to the physician and the nursing supervisor immediately upon discovery. If an antidote or procedure is specified in the standing instructions, the antidote should be given or the specified procedure initiated at once.

Intravenous Solutions

Intravenous solutions should be administered carefully and with sterile technique. Accepted injection sites should be used. IV treatment can cause tissue damage and other problems, so the site should be checked frequently for hematoma and other complications. The level of solution in the container should be checked periodically. Before a new container is used, the nurse should be certain that all solution has been drained into the IV tube. When administering an intravenous solution, the nurse must make sure the solution is infusing correctly.

The supporting stand should be placed on the side of the bed away from employees and visitors. A solution stand used on a stretcher cart should be anchored securely to prevent its tipping and falling. Stands that protrude into traffic areas (while on wheeled stretchers, for example) should be wrapped with highly visible tape to prevent injury to others.

Smoking

The use of cigarettes, cigars, and pipes by patients should be controlled. Some patients, such as those under alcoholism treatment, psychiatric care, or drug rehabilitation or those who are on antidepressant or sleep-inducing medication, should not be permitted to smoke at all. Patients who want to smoke should have their physician's written permission on their charts.

Patients have the prerogative of objecting to smoking by a roommate or a visitor. Visitors who wish to smoke should do so only with the permission of all patients in the room.

Areas where smoking is permitted should be designated as clearly as those where smoking is prohibited. Increasingly, institutions of all types are attempting to provide separate areas for smokers and nonsmokers. In the hospital, designating sections of patient wings and of the cafeteria as smoking or nonsmoking areas is an arrangement more acceptable to nonsmokers and, from a safety viewpoint, one that limits hazard.

Accredited hospitals are required to have a smoking policy, but developing an adequate, enforceable policy is difficult. Although most persons recognize that cigarettes are a fire hazard as well as a health hazard, smokers find it difficult to give them up, even temporarily. Therefore, attempts to outlaw smoking altogether may be unrealistic, inasmuch as enforcement is nearly impossible. Examples of smoking rules and policy are shown in figures 9 and 10.

Figure 4. Trained escorts are essential to patient and hospital safety.

Escorting Patients

Patients are escorted by medical staff, hospital and nursing staff, paramedical personnel, and volunteers. The escort should:
■ Take only one patient at a time.
■ Consider the patient's safety the primary responsibility.
■ Never leave the patient alone.
■ Give the patient support and undivided attention.
■ Refrain from smoking.
■ Introduce himself or herself to the patient, being polite and friendly.
■ Inform the patient, if conscious, as to destination and route to be taken.

Patients should be escorted in the following situations:
■ **Before admission.** A prospective patient may need to be escorted for preadmission testing, such as blood work, X rays, and so forth.
■ **On admission.** The patient should be escorted from the admitting office to the room. If the patient's condition warrants, a wheelchair should be used. When the patient arrives by ambulance, the driver should call for a nurse or an escort to take responsibility for escorting the patient.
■ **When moved inside the hospital.** Whenever the patient goes from one area of the hospital to another, he or she should be escorted. In rare instances, a patient may obtain permission to go unescorted to another area of the hospital. Such permission must be written on the chart, and the patient should be wearing street clothes or a robe.
■ **When discharged.** The escort is responsible until the patient is in the car with the door safely closed.

Figure 5. Transportation of patients in wheelchairs requires careful and constant attention to many details.

Transporting Patients in Wheelchairs

If the patient can lift his or her own weight, one assistant is required. If the patient is unable to support his or her own weight, a minimum of two assistants is required.

Before helping the patient into the wheelchair, the escort should:
1. Have the patient don a robe and slippers or shoes.
2. Check the wheelchair to make sure it is in safe operating condition. Faulty equipment should never be used.
3. Place the wheelchair parallel to the bed or chair, lock the wheels, and make sure footrests and leg supports are lifted for clearance.

To transfer the patient to the wheelchair, the escort should:
1. Explain the procedure to the patient.
2. Face the patient and support him or her under the arms.
3. Have the patient place his or her feet on the floor, rise, and pivot to sit down in the wheelchair.
4. Adjust footrests and leg supports.

Before starting off, the escort should:
1. Cover the patient from waist to ankles with a blanket.
2. Have the patient place arms in lap.
3. Make sure clothing, tubing, drainage bags, and other equipment are clear of wheels.
4. Make sure the patient chart is out of the patient's reach. Escorts should either carry the chart or place it in a pouch on the backrest of the wheelchair.

During the trip, the escort should:
1. Release the wheelchair lock, and move slowly.
2. Stay in the center of the corridor, and approach corners and closed doors with caution to avoid collisions.
3. Push the wheelchair. It should not be pulled except to go through doors.
4. Pull the wheelchair backward through all doors except those such as elevator doors, which are controlled by an electronic device. In such cases, wait until the door is fully open, then push through, tipping the chair so that the small front wheels pass above the gap.
5. Check the chair frequently to make sure that wheels are free and that the patient's feet are secure on the footrests.

To remove the patient from the wheelchair, the escort should:
1. Place the wheelchair parallel to the bed or chair, lock the wheels, and release leg supports and footrests.
2. Face the patient and support him or her under the arms.
3. Have the patient place feet on floor, rise, and pivot to the bed or a chair.

To transfer a patient to a car, the escort should not attempt patient removal on an incline. The escort should:
1. Lock the wheelchair wheels.
2. Open the car door.
3. Face the wheelchair toward the open door, preferably the door to the front right seat.
4. Lock the wheels, and release leg supports and footrests.
5. Face the patient, support the patient under the arms, and help the patient pivot to the carseat.

As a special precaution, the escort should check the patient's position and wheelchair function from time to time while en route. Also, when intravenous equipment is in use, the IV pole should be attached to the wheelchair with an adapter, or a member of the nursing service should push the stand and remain in attendance at all times.

Figure 6. Moving a patient onto and off a wheeled stretcher safely and steering this large piece of equipment require the skill that comes from proper training.

Transporting Patients on Wheeled Stretchers

When the patient is conscious or when the patient and the stretcher are unencumbered by attachments other than intravenous equipment, one person can handle the stretcher. Under all other circumstances, two persons are necessary.

Before transferring the patient to a wheeled stretcher, the attendant should make sure that:

- The equipment is in good condition and that all equipment necessary to ensure the patient's safety and comfort, such as side pads, is at hand.
- The stretcher is positioned directly beside the bed and *level* with it.
- The stretcher and the bed wheels are locked.

To transfer a patient to the stretcher, the attendant should either lift the patient onto the stretcher with the assistance of one or more persons or have the mobile, unencumbered patient lift himself or herself onto the stretcher with help and supervision.

Necessary equipment for the stretcher is:

- Side rails, which must be raised.
- Pads for side rails when small children, sedated patients, combative patients, or patients with convulsive disorders are transported.
- Safety straps, if only one escort attends.

Before beginning the trip, the escort should:

- Make sure the patient is covered.
- Advise the patient what is to happen, and request the patient to keep arms inside the rails and close to his or her body.
- Lock the wheels nearest the patient's feet in straight or forward position for maximum control, making sure the wheels are parallel.
- Make sure the patient's chart is placed in a pouch under the stretcher or, if there is no pouch, under the mattress-like pad of the stretcher.

During the trip, the escort should:

- Stand at the patient's head.
- Push the stretcher, not pull it.
- Push the stretcher through doorways foot first except when entering a patient's room that has insufficient turn-around space.
- Push the stretcher onto the elevator foot first.
- Ask visitors to leave the car if the elevator is also used for visitor traffic.

Oxygen administration cannisters must be held by a bracket. A nurse and at least one other person should be in attendance. Clearly visible "No Smoking" signs should be affixed to the stretcher.

If the patient is receiving fluids intravenously, a nurse must set up the intravenous fluid equipment but need not attend the patient during the trip. The IV pole must be at the head of the stretcher and must be sufficiently long to ensure proper flow. Tubing must hang free of side rails.

If restraints are necessary, they should be fastened so that the patient's circulation is not impaired. Restraints must be attached to the stretcher, never to the side rails. At least two persons are required to attend a restrained patient.

Figure 7. Portalifts are used to transfer helpless patients.

Moving Patients by Portalift

The following procedure should be followed when using a portalift:

1. Open the portalift base to its widest position and place it under the bed, taking care not to hit the patient with the overhead bar.

2. Turn the patient on his or her side, and position the canvas hammock under the patient's buttocks and the upper canvas under the patient's armpits. Turn the patient on his or her back.

3. Release the hydraulic lift valve, lower the chains, and attach them to the hammock. Make sure that the attached hooks are equidistant on each side of the hammock. For example, attach one hook to the third link on the right side and the other to the third link on the left side.

4. Fasten the chains to the overhead swinging bar.

5. Set the valve of the hydraulic lift in the position for pumping. With pumping action, raise the patient to the desired height.

6. With the patient in a sitting position, bring the patient's legs over the side of the bed.

7. Adjust the base of the portalift as necessary.

8. Position the portalift so that the patient is directly over the chair or wheelchair.

9. Slowly release the hydraulic valve and guide the patient into the chair or wheelchair by placing one hand at the patient's back or elbow.

10. Release the chains from the overhead bar, taking care that they do not strike the patient.

11. Leave the hammock in place until the patient is ready to be returned to bed.

12. To return the patient to bed, repeat steps 3 through 10, removing the canvas after the patient is in bed.

Figure 8. Use of heat requires care. The following reminders for posting at nurses' stations reinforce training.

Preventing Burns

Heating pads and hot water bottles:
- Never place a heating pad or hot water bottle directly against an unconscious person, a person in shock, an infant, or a dressing.
- Check the temperature of pads and bottles. Temperatures should never exceed 130 °F. (54.4 °C.) for adults and 120 °F. (48.8 °C.) for children.
- Check skin temperature shortly after applying a pad or bottle. Do not accept the patient's opinion on his or her comfort.
- Check soundness of each item before use. Heating pads are electrical appliances and subject to all regulations set for electrical equipment.
- Use tape, binders, or straps to keep units in place. Do not use pins or clamps.
- Use heating pad only on low setting.

Infrared lamps and light candles:
- Use infrared lamps and light cradles only on the physician's orders.
- If the site to be treated is near the head, protect the patient's eyes with a towel or washcloth.
- Place the equipment at least 18 inches from the patient's body. In a light cradle only a 25-watt bulb is used.
- Ensure that equipment has guards.
- Attend the patient the entire time the equipment is in use. The attendant must be a staff member, not a visitor.
- Inspect wiring and connections daily.

Steam inhalators:
- Inspect the steam inhalator equipment before using it to be sure it is filled with water.
- Prevent hot vapor from concentrating on the patient's body.
- Make sure the equipment does not overheat.

All burns require immediate attention and notification to the patient's physician.

Figure 9. The rules put forth in this example should be given to each employee, patient, and visitor, and should be prominently posted throughout the hospital. This example is also suitable for inclusion with preadmission forms mailed to patients and orientation packets for new employees.

Smoking on Hospital Premises

The hospital restricts and discourages the smoking of cigarettes, pipes, and cigars by employees, volunteers, visitors, and patients. Smoking is forbidden in the following locations and under the following circumstances:

■ In all areas of the hospital where flammable gases such as oxygen are in use or are stored

■ In all areas where combustible supplies or materials are stored

■ In elevators

■ In surgical and obstetrical suites, with the exception of specific dressing rooms and lounges

■ In any area where employees are in direct contact with patients

■ To any patient on antidepressant or sleep-inducing medication

■ To any patient under psychiatric care, alcoholism treatment, or treatment for drug overdose or ingestion unless a responsible adult is in attendance

Signs posted throughout the premises mark areas where smoking is forbidden or permitted. Smoking by patients is to be supervised by appropriate patient care personnel. The sale of smoking materials on hospital premises is discouraged.

Figure 10. It is incumbent that every employee know hospital smoking policy and observe it at all times. Employees should also make the policy known to visitors. This example of smoking policy can be used for posters and handouts.

Smoking Policy

In accordance with the local fire department's recommendations and for the safety and comfort of patients, employees, volunteers, and visitors, the hospital's policy on smoking is as follows:

■ In assignment of rooms, every effort is made to separate patients who smoke from patients who do not.

■ Ambulatory patients are forbidden to smoke in bed.

■ Patients confined to bed must have the physician's written permission on the chart to smoke, and when smoking, a responsible adult must be in attendance.

■ Unsupervised smoking by patients classified as not mentally or physically responsible is forbidden; this prohibition includes patients so rendered by medication.

■ Employees and volunteers are forbidden to smoke in any patient area, including rooms and corridors, and at nurses' stations. Except where signs to the contrary are posted, employees and volunteers may smoke in locker rooms, lounges, private offices or offices generally closed to the public, dining rooms, and toilets.

■ Visitors are forbidden to smoke in all areas specifically designated as nonsmoking areas.

■ Visitors are forbidden to smoke in any patient room designated as a nonsmoking room or without the permission of all patients in the room.

■ Smoking is forbidden in any area where flammable liquids or oxygen or other gases are in use or are stored. These areas include the emergency department, coronary care unit, intensive care unit, and central service.

■ Smoking is forbidden in the laundry and storeroom, except in the office area, and in linen rooms or any other storage areas where combustible materials are stored.

■ Smoking by personnel using the surgical and obstetrical suites is limited to dressing rooms and lounges. Doors leading to the suites must be kept closed.

■ Smoking is forbidden in any food preparation or service area.

■ Sale of cigarettes, cigars, and other smoking materials or related supplies on hospital premises is discouraged.

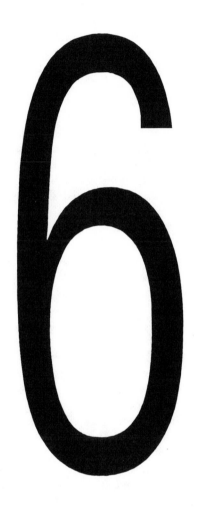

All hospital employees, in addition to safeguarding patients and visitors, who are dependent upon them, must assume the responsibility for their own on-the-job safety by using safe procedures and techniques. The expense and planning of safety programs are wasted if employees do not cooperate in preventing accidents. Good safety programs train employees in procedures that require them to maintain a safe environment by performing each job safely. Pride emanates from well-trained staff members who can act with confidence in a hazard-free workplace.

All members of the work force should follow the ten fundamental rules of safety:

1. Use approved procedures for all job functions.
2. Report all accidents/incidents to the supervisor immediately.
3. Know and comply with the safety rules, and use the safety equipment provided.
4. Report all unsafe or hazardous conditions.
5. Obey safety signs and notices.
6. Smoke only in designated areas.
7. Know personal responsibilities in the event of a fire or other disaster.
8. Keep personal work area neat and clean.
9. Refrain from horseplay.
10. When in doubt, ask the person in charge.

Hiring

Employee safety begins when the applicant is interviewed. A skilled interviewer explores and verifies information on the applicant's application and watches for personality traits and attitudes such as reliability and carefulness.

Before an applicant is hired, he or she must pass a physical examination to ensure that the applicant is healthy and physically capable of doing the work the position entails. Such an examination also exposes diseases and weaknesses that could put either the employee or others at risk. To assist the examining physician to determine the capabilities and potential problems of new employees, all prospective employees should be asked to complete a health questionnaire. From the physical examination, the prospective employee can be classified as:

Class A: Physically able to handle any work in the hospital; no physical problems.

Class B: Physically able to handle the position sought; applicant's minor physical problems unlikely to generate disability.

Class Bx: Acceptable only with the approval of the chief executive officer. Applicant has no specific physical problems but, by reason of personal hygiene, evidence of personality aberration, or unsatisfactory medical history, is potentially unsuitable. The need for hiring such persons should be carefully scrutinized by the department director.

Class C: Having problems that can be corrected, enabling applicant to be reclassified as A or B. It is specified whether or not this applicant can begin work on a temporary basis pending correction.

Class E: Physically disqualified.

Once applicants are classified, whether or not they are hired rests with the employer, except for Class E applicants.

Health

Hospital employees must demonstrate good health when they begin employment, and it is important that they continue to be healthy. In particular, hospital employees subject to unusual risks should be examined periodically to ascertain whether they may have contracted an occupational disease and whether their health may have been impaired.

In the hospital work environment, pregnant women are exposed to many hazards, such as anesthetic agents, radiation, toxic chemicals, and diseases such as rubella. All women employees of childbearing age must be informed of these dangers, with emphasis on the early onset of their effects. Mutagenesis (induction of genetic change), teratology (abnormal development of a fetus), and congenital malformations also must be carefully explained to these female employees.

Orientation and Training

Government and other regulatory agencies require that certain kinds of safety information be presented in employee orientation sessions. Safety orientation includes information about worker's compensation and the Occupational Safety and Health Act of 1970, which assures every worker the right to a safe workplace. Safety orientation also includes the hospital's procedures for coping with fire and other disasters (chapters 11 and 12) and its incident reporting system. Each new employee should be instructed in the use of fire extinguishers.

The manner in which training in these subjects is scheduled and presented demonstrates to the newcomer the importance that the hospital attaches to safety. Presentations should be carefully prepared, and adequate time allowed. On completion of training, employees should sign a form stating the type of orientation received and the date. These forms should be kept on file in the safety office and in the employee's personnel file to document the employee's training.

Work Environment

Orderliness of personal housekeeping, whereby each employee keeps his or her work station neat and clutter-free, is important in maintaining an environment free of hazards. If every unnecessary personal item, unused piece of equipment, out-of-date medicine, item needing repair, and long-range replacement were stored away from the work area or discarded, the potential for a safe environment would be greatly increased, the causes of possible accidents removed, and response to incidents and disasters expedited.

Housekeeping is the responsibility and obligation of every employee, not just the staff of the housekeeping department. Overall safety is improved when every employee takes a personal role in hospital upkeep and maintenance. Light bulbs are replaced sooner when the first person to spot a burned-out bulb reports it. Equipment is in better operating order when serviced at the first sign of disorder. Slips are fewer if everyone picks up debris and polices public areas for obstacles.

The pharmacy is obligated to inventory its stock and dispose of deteriorated, contaminated, and unlabeled drugs. The laboratory should dispose of old reagents periodically. Pathogenic wastes should be handled in accordance with approved procedures. Radioactive wastes should be stored properly until they can be safely discarded. In all cases, whether ordinary or extraordinary, specific procedures must be developed and followed in order to maintain safety; these are outlined with respect to clinical services in chapter 8.

Orderliness and attention to housekeeping generally result from training and publicity. Employee participation can be developed through publicity campaigns, newsletters, and recognition in the form of prizes and awards. To encourage persons in such activities, appreciation must be expressed. For example, when an employee calls to report a burned-out exit light, the respondent should thank him or her and express appreciation rather than tell the employee that he or she is the tenth person who has called about it.

A supply of maintenance work order forms such as those shown in chapter 10 should be readily and conveniently available in all work areas, including nurses' stations.

Communication

Many accidents result from misunderstanding or lack of communication between employees, between managers and their employees, between employees and patients, and between employees and visitors. Clear, concise directions and information must be given, and the recipient should question points he or she does not understand or does not agree with. Communicators should:

■ Know what they want to say, and be sure they actually say it.

■ Be precise and specific. For example, the nurse should say, "Swallow these tablets" rather than "Take these."

■ Be sure the persons to whom they speak understand the instructions when the language in use is not the recipient's primary language, when the person addressed is hard of hearing or has other disabilities that impede hearing or comprehension, or when the person is in an unusual or stressful situation.

■ Watch until the instructions have been carried out satisfactorily.

■ Write instructions when necessary.

Uniforms and Special-Purpose Clothing

Hospital employees wear uniforms designed to accommodate job procedures. Each employee is responsible for keeping his or her uniform clean and in good repair. Each employee also must be sure it is the proper size and kind.

Employees should not wear tight clothing that restricts movement. Overlong or flared pants can cause tripping. Shoes not only should fit properly but should be suitable for many hours of activity on the feet. Some shoe styles, such as high heels or platform shoes, are intrinsically dangerous. Jewelry, particularly rings and bracelets that can catch or be caught on equipment and supplies, presents a safety problem.

The hospital should have a written policy on clothing-related safety problems so that management can take action to prevent such hazards. Dress can present personal problems in that many persons consider clothing an extension of their personality and culture. Many do not appreciate the danger of certain clothing. Inasmuch as it is difficult to enforce dress codes, the hospital must document the safety hazards of certain apparel before the hospital can forbid its use and determine an enforceable policy.

Personal grooming habits also play a safety role. Fingernails so long that they harm patients, catch in equipment, or harbor bacteria should be forbidden. Likewise, long hair should be tied up or back so that it does not obstruct vision, fall on a patient's face, or tangle in equipment. All personal items should be secured in the employee's locker, not brought to the work station.

Certain procedures and services require special protective clothing. A partial list is shown in figure 11 at the end of this chapter. Such clothing and instructions for its use are provided to employees, who must use it as instructed.

Eating, Drinking, and Smoking

Employees should not eat, drink, or smoke at their work stations, but in lounges and lunchrooms during breaks. Alcoholic beverages should not be consumed by employees before reporting for work or while on duty. Although these regulations are sensible and reasonable, they are difficult to enforce, especially on night shifts. The social activities usually reserved for the evening hours for 9 a.m.-5 p.m. employees become afternoon activities for 11 p.m.-7 a.m. employees. A major reason for this difficulty is inconsistent enforcement of policy. Office workers generally drink coffee and smoke at their desks, and committees sometimes work over lunch trays. Employees do not appreciate the differences between environments and the problems that may result. The hospital must therefore stipulate policy on eating and smoking areas and enforce it at all levels.

Lifting and Carrying Materials

Lifting is so much a part of everyday routine that most persons give it little advance thought. This sometimes results in a pulled muscle, a hernia, or a disc lesion. Many back injuries can be prevented by proper utilization of body mechanics to avert strain when lifting and carrying heavy or bulky materials. Because of its importance as a major cause of injury, proper lifting should be taught repeatedly and persistently. (The information contained in this section pertains only to the lifting of materials. Proper techniques for the lifting of patients in daily routines or in emergency evacuations are discussed in chapters 5 and 12.)

The principles of lifting and handling are simple. However, before teaching proper lifting to any group, the instructor should issue a list of precautions that the person who is doing the lifting should follow:

1. Be sure flooring is safe from slippage.
2. Check to see that the object to be lifted is not slippery, has no protruding nails or slivers, and has no jagged edges.
3. Check the path along which an object is to be moved, to ensure a clear field of vision.
4. Where applicable, wear proper gloves to secure a better grip.
5. Squat rather than stoop to lift a heavy or bulky object. The heavy muscles of the legs and thighs, not the flat muscles of the back, should take the strain.
6. Grasp the load firmly; be sure any handles are securely fastened. Avoid jerking at the load, but keep it close to the body.
7. Avoid twisting the body when it is under a weight strain; instead, shift the footing.
8. Never lift too much; make heavy lifting a teamwork job. Request service personnel to move furniture and heavy appliances.

The following procedure is designed to make safe use of the body as a perfect and safe lifting device. This technique can be used in any lifting situation involving a carton, a drum, or a bulky sack:

1. Part the feet, with one foot alongside the object being lifted and one behind. Feet comfortably spread provide greater stability, and the rear foot is in position for the upward thrust of the lift.
2. Use the sit-down position and keep the back straight, remembering that straight does not always mean vertical. A straight back keeps the spine, back muscles, and body organs in correct alignment. It minimizes the intestinal compression that can cause hernia.
3. Tuck in the chin so that the neck and head continue the straight back line. Tucking the chin helps keep the spine straight and firm.
4. Use the palmar grip, in which the fingers and the hand are extended around the object to be lifted with the full palm. Fingers alone have very little power.
5. Draw the load close, and tuck the arms and elbows into the side of the body; when held away from the body, the arms lose much of their strength. Also, keeping the arms tucked in helps keep the body weight centered.
6. Position the body so that its weight is centered over the feet. This posture provides a more powerful line of thrust and ensures better balance. Start the lift with a thrust of the rear foot.

Twisting during a lift is one of the most common causes of back injury. By simply turning the forward foot out and pointing it in the direction of the eventual movement, the greatest danger of injury is avoided.

Employees should never attempt to lift a heavy object or load alone. When two or more persons are lifting, they should lift the load at the same time, counting "one, two, three, lift" if necessary.

Handling Materials

Improper handling of materials of all types accounts for about 22 percent of all occupational injuries, such as strains, sprains, fractures, cuts, and bruises. Improper handling includes not only improper lifting, gripping, and carrying, but also the failure to observe proper foot and hand clearances, grabbing at falling objects, unsafe actions around sharp objects, and failure to wear proper protective equipment.

All hospital personnel who handle any type of materials should:

■ Wipe off greasy, wet, slippery, or dirty objects before trying to handle them.

■ Keep hands free of oil and grease. Wear protective gloves and use extra caution around running machinery. Rope slings or holders can be attached to bulky equipment to facilitate lifting; smaller items should be placed in appropriate containers.

■ Use the appropriate equipment. Remember that hand trucks, dollies, and wheelbarrows are designed to handle heavy, bulky, or loose materials, whereas medical carts and utility carts are designed for medicines and office supplies.

■ Get a firm grip on the object.

■ Keep fingers away from pinch points, especially when setting down materials, passing through doorways, and closing drawers and doors.

■ Be alert to the hazard of burns while handling hot applications of any kind, both for the safety of the employee and of the patient.

Avoiding Cuts and Punctures

Employees who practice the following simple measures spare themselves cuts and punctures:

■ Put away sharp tools when not in use. Do not cover with cloth or papers any spindles, kitchen knives, or sharp tools that are on a desk, table, or workbench.

■ Avoid trying to catch a sharp object or a glass object if it starts to fall. Let it go; then pick it up (if it is a knife or tool) or sweep it up (if it is broken glass).

■ Dispose of broken glass and crockery immediately.

■ Wrap ampuls, glass tubing, flask stoppers, and similar items in a towel before twisting, pulling, or pushing them. If breakage occurs, shake the glass particles out into the appropriate trash receptacle and carefully rinse the towel to dispose of remaining slivers before putting the towel into the soiled-linen basket.

■ Use grinders, breakers, or safety cans, which should be available at nursing units and treatment centers, for destruction or disposal of disposable needles, lances, and the like.

■ Use the inside of special containers for breaking fluorescent light tubes and other types of tubes and bulbs, to prevent their subsequent explosion or implosion. Wear appropriate personal protective equipment while this is being done.

■ Discard aerosol spray cans and other pressure-operated containers in specially marked receptacles; they should never be incinerated. Carefully follow all directions on aerosol cans. Avoid mixing the contents of two cans, as this may result in spontaneous combustion or toxic fumes.

■ Avoid "digging into" a wastebasket; hold it by the sides and empty it onto a sheet of paper.

■ Use forceps to remove sharp objects from pans and jars or empty the container onto a flat surface.

A major hazard to employees is hypodermic needles. Accidental needle punctures can cause infection and transmit disease. The persons most frequently involved in such incidents are nurses and other medically trained staff members who use such equipment and housekeeping personnel who dispose of it. All needle cuts and punctures must be treated immediately. Those who administer injections can reduce the incidence of needle punctures by:

■ Performing the procedure carefully.

■ Breaking the needle point and returning both parts of the needle to its plastic container before discarding it.

■ Discarding the container in a receptacle reserved for this use.

Preventing Falls

Falls to employees can be prevented if employees:

■ Never, under any circumstances, leave articles on stairs or in a passageway.

■ Wet-mop only half of a corridor or stairway, leaving the other half for safe passage of traffic; use "Wet Floor" signs; and block off slippery areas.

■ Keep halls and stairs free of water, sand, flower petals, paper, and other materials that can cause slipping and serious injury.

■ Avoid climbing on storage-room shelving, and never use crates, boxes, kegs, or other substitutes for ladders.

■ Keep handholds and stair rails in good condition.

■ Appraise the hospital's need for stepladders, straight ladders, extension ladders, and stepping stools, and see that these items are provided and maintained.

Safety for Volunteers

Although volunteers are not employees, the hospital must guarantee its volunteers a safe work environment and assume responsibility for their orientation and training.

Volunteers are generally required to observe all rules that govern staff, and they should be trained and supervised on the job and encouraged or corrected in the same manner as staff members. In particular, volunteers should be instructed in any procedure they are permitted to perform, such as lifting patients, directing visitors, and handling persons who create a disturbance. Volunteers should participate in safety training and in fire and other disaster drills and, where appropriate, should be included in safety motivation campaigns.

On duty, volunteers should wear an identification badge at all times and the clothing prescribed for them. Also, they should comply with the apparel regulations pertinent to employees, such as wearing protective, low-heeled shoes and avoiding jewelry that impedes activity or catches on equipment.

Hospital policy or the volunteer's work assignment may require a health examination. Incidents involving volunteers should receive the same attention as those involving staff; incidents should be logged and reported and, if further instruction or medical attention are in order, they should be given.

The safety of volunteers must be ensured, for the services they give can take them into practically any part of the hospital and out into the community it serves. Depending on hospital policy and need, and on volunteers' abilities, they work with patients personally; interpret for foreign-language-speaking persons; assist the hearing-impaired and the blind; staff the gift shop; and take part in outpatient clinics, home care programs for the homebound and elderly, health education programs, and various other activities. Professionally qualified persons, such as technicians, for example, who may serve as volunteers, must have any license their vocation requires.

Figure 11. Employees should be taught the value of certain clothing in protecting them and should be required to wear it. This list should be given to persons employed in the departments listed below and should be posted on the site. Except where specified otherwise, appropriate footwear in the hospital consists of low-heeled nonskid shoes that completely cover the foot.

Protective Clothing for Employees

Central Service
- Impervious gloves to eliminate skin contact with irritating chemicals
- Respirator
- Chemical apron and full-face shield, when required

Food Service
- Low-heeled shoes with slip-resistant soles and boots for wet areas
- Impervious gloves for washing pots and pans and for consistently wet hands
- Metal mesh gloves for meatcutters and others who use knives frequently
- Rubber gloves and goggles or a face shield for handlers of concentrated liquid ammonia, drain cleaners, strong caustic solutions for cleaning reusable filters, and oven cleaners
- Disposable masks for persons sensitive to powdered soap or detergent dust
- Hair nets in food preparation and serving areas to minimize contamination of food

Housekeeping
- Heavy rubber aprons and impervious gloves for persons engaged primarily in removal of trash
- Protective gloves for users of soaps, detergents, or solvents
- Rubber gloves, plastic or rubber aprons, masks, and eye protection for persons using disinfectants that contain ammonia, phenols, and iodophors
- Protective clothing such as gowns, masks, and gloves when performing isolation cleaning procedures
- Non-skid shoes or boots for persons who sluice, strip, rinse, and wax floors

Laboratories
- Chemical goggles or face shields for protection from splashes
- Chemical-cartridge respirators for persons using acid gases and organic vapors to clean up spills
- Coats or aprons, which are removed when wearers leave the laboratory

Laundry
- Protective clothing and masks for sorting contaminated linen
- Gloves, aprons, and safety glasses for persons using bleaches and soaps
- Hair nets to minimize contamination of clean linen

(Figure 11 continued)

Maintenance
- Gloves for handling hot, wet, or sharp objects and for chemicals
- Safety goggles and glasses for protection from chips, sparks, glare, and splashes
- Equipment to protect ears from extraordinary noise (The current safe standard is 85 decibels.)
- Masks for persons who cut or handle insulating material
- Rubber gloves and goggles or a face shield for persons handling ammonia and drain cleaners
- Gloves and other personal protective clothing to prevent skin irritation from paints and adhesives
- Air-supplied respirators for persons who work with paint or adhesives where proper ventilation is not possible
- Masks and rubber gloves for persons applying pesticides
- Protective clothing and goggles or face shields for welders
- Slip-resistant footwear with heavy soles and heels, as well as protective toes
- Hard hats for heavy maintenance where falling objects present a hazard
- Bump caps for persons working in areas where low-hanging pipes or other obstacles may cause injury

Nursing Service
- Low-heeled shoes with slip-resistant soles
- Gloves, gowns, masks, and booties for isolation procedures

Printing Shop
- Goggles and gloves for handling solvent-based materials

Radiology
- Lead aprons and gloves for persons working in the direct field or where scatter radiation levels are high
- Radiation exposure badges for persons exposed to ionizing radiation (When a protective apron is worn, a dosimeter should be worn on the outside of all clothes.)
- Gloves, goggles, and apron for handling film-developing chemicals

Receiving
- Shoes fitted with metal toes to protect feet from falling objects and other hazards

Surgery
- Conductive clothing when required
- Conductive footwear, tested daily for conductivity, or conductive slip-on booties

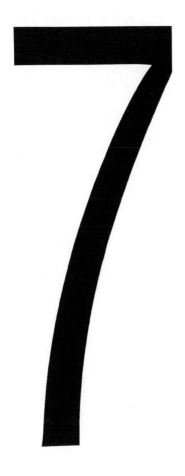

Every day many persons who have no official connection with the hospital are on its premises. They include visitors to patients and persons on business. Special events such as tours, seminars, and symposiums bring various groups to the hospital. Representatives of regulatory agencies and accrediting bodies inspect the premises periodically. When facilities undergo modifications or expansion, construction crews are on site.

From a public relations and legal viewpoint, the benefits of a concise safety program aimed at the transient public are as important as an extensive program devoted to hospital personnel. Professional staffs' direct contact with patients and the general public has given hospitals a reputation for trustworthiness, confidence, and security. When this image is abruptly shattered through an act of negligence, a hospital is at a far greater disadvantage than any other business or industry in legally defending itself and in reestablishing its former position within the community.

Virtually all hospital areas used by visitors are used also by nursing staff, maintenance personnel, or medical personnel. Consequently, the visitor is the beneficiary of the accident and fire prevention work that is done as a part of the total hospital safety program. The principles of accident prevention practiced for other persons on the premises apply to visitors. Prevention of injury to them is therefore a question of degree, not of method.

A visitor safety program provides a broad base for the overall safety surveillance program and assures that the possibility of injuries to staff is minimized. It calls for (1) internal safety while visitors are within the confines of the building and (2) external safety and security while visitors are anywhere on the plant grounds, including the parking lot, service walks, courtyards and gardens, and such ancillary buildings as the laundry and nurses' or staff residences.

Education

Most visitors are willing to comply with all hospital rules, including safety rules, but often are unaware of their safety responsibilities and of the elements of the hospital's safety program.

An effective communication tool is a flyer that is handed out along with the visitor's identification card when the visitor enters the hospital. Such material should be brief and to the point. Figure 12, at the end of this chapter, shows a sample visitor handout, detailing safety information important for all visitors.

Visitors also can be informed of hospital safety rules by a letter to prospective patients before they are admitted to the hospital. This letter, which can include information about visiting hours, reaches a small percentage of those who visit a hospital, usually patients' immediate families.

Restrictions

Visitors should be restricted to defined areas and the restriction enforced. Visitors should be permitted only in waiting rooms, patient rooms, and lounge areas. Employees are responsible for ensuring that visitors are deterred from entering restricted areas and, when off limits, are directed to their desired destination.

Persons on business that requires them to go beyond public areas should obtain authorization from the department or service they wish to visit. For example, vendors should be authorized by and should obtain an identification card from the purchasing department. Likewise, repair personnel should be authorized and identified by the engineering department. For reasons of security, areas such as central service, nursery, pharmacy, and receiving should require escorts for nonhospital personnel such as repair persons and vendors.

Unwanted Visitors

Public places such as hospitals attract persons who have no legitimate reason for being on the premises and who may pose safety problems for patients, employees, volunteers, and legitimate visitors. These unwanted persons should be reported to the security office as soon as their presence is discovered. The safety or security office should alert employees to their responsibility in requesting all unidentified persons in their working area to identify themselves, showing proof of identification, and to notify security if such a person is unauthorized to be in the hospital or refuses to show proof of identity.

Incidents

Visitors become involved in incidents despite staff efforts to prevent such occurrences. The emotional and physical condition of visitors as well as the unfamiliar surroundings are often the root causes of such problems, many of which are beyond the hospital's control.

In personal injury situations, hospitals are becoming increasingly liable to the same kind of legal action that theaters and other places of public congregation face. The best legal defense against such action is prevention: searching out and removing those acts or conditions that might later be interpreted as contributory negligence.

Visitors' legal status differs from state to state, but generally the hospital must accept responsibility for visitors when on the hospital premises. Most public liability cases against hospitals involve stairway falls, elevators, broken glass, hazardous floors, and inadequately lighted and poorly maintained premises both inside and outside the building.

Investigation

The hospital has certain obligations that it must meet if a visitor is injured on its premises. When a visitor is injured, first aid should be administered immediately. As soon as possible after the accident, an administrative officer should investigate the circumstances and, on the basis of the acquired information, decide what medical care the hospital should give, if any, beyond immediate and obvious first aid. The report of injury should be made by the department director in whose area the incident occurred. All records of visitor accidents should be reviewed by the safety committee, and the hazardous condition should be eliminated as soon as possible.

Most visitor traffic occurs during the evening hours, when the safety director is not in the hospital. Often, the nursing supervisor must handle the situation and notify the administrative representative on call.

Recommended procedures for the accident investigator to follow are:

■ Investigate all injury-producing accidents as soon after their occurrence as circumstances permit.

■ Delay any interview with the injured person until he or she has received initial medical treatment, no matter how minor the injury may appear. The investigator should always be more concerned with the victim's welfare than with determining facts and should insist that the injured person, even if quite willing to talk, receive medical attention first.

■ Postpone questioning if the victim is in pain or upset after treatment. The injured person is usually the main source of information on the accident, and the accuracy and completeness of the information obtained depend to a great extent on the way the interview is conducted.

■ Refrain from using sarcasm, appearing aggressive, or attempting to blame anyone.

■ Talk with witnesses, the nurse, or the physician in charge if the extent of the injury does not permit an interview. Avoid making them feel that they are informers; emphasize that the purpose of the investigation is to gather facts to prevent recurrence of the accident.

■ Avoid admitting any liability on the part of the hospital or any mention of insurance. An admission of liability could invalidate insurance coverage to the detriment of the injured party, the hospital, or both.

The investigator should be empathetic with the victim, show concern, be friendly and attentive, and solicit the victim's suggestions. Whether he or she is the safety director, the department director, the administrator, or the chairperson of the safety committee, the investigator should (1) compile the facts, (2) review these facts, (3) make an official report, and (4) prepare the records and reports required by the insurance carrier.

Other important procedures that must be thought out in advance, both for injuries and fatalities, include: (1) notification of the police, in the event of a fatality, (2) notification of the victim's family, (3) disposition of the injured person, (4) notification of the hospital's attorney and insurance carrier and discussion of the situation's legal aspects with them, and (5) making information available to news media.

Fatalities call for the highest level of investigation, frequently by a hospital committee and a legal group. Insurance carriers and governmental bodies also may conduct accident investigations in such cases. Thus, the need for specific detailed information, obtained as early as possible at the scene of the accident and including testimony from witnesses, is vitally important.

Policy

The following principles should be incorporated into a policy statement, which may be useful to hospitals as a basis for action in cases of injury to visitors:

■ Any hospital visitor who has an accident on the premises is entitled to immediate first aid, including control of hemorrhage, temporary splinting, emergency treatment for shock, and whatever is necessary to preserve life.

■ If deemed necessary, X rays of all possible fractures and head or spinal injuries should be taken.

■ An injured visitor requiring hospitalization should be assigned to an attending staff physician. If the visitor prefers to be hospitalized elsewhere, arrangements should be made for transfer.

■ The administrative office should investigate the accident, get the details of its circumstances, the names of witnesses, and all other pertinent information, and have the information recorded on an accident report form.

■ Regardless of provocation, the attending physician and other hospital staff members should not comment to the visitor on the injury or its causes other than to provide the usual medical report or diagnosis.

■ If an accident appears to be of a serious nature, the hospital's attorney or insurance carrier should be notified at once.

If the hospital bases its visitor injury policy on these principles and uses tact and good judgment in handling individual cases, it will meet its ethical obligations to injured persons and will not place itself under more liability than it justly should bear. Each hospital should decide for itself what charges, if any, it should set for first aid and medical services rendered to visitors injured on its premises.

Figure 12. Safety instructions should be distributed to every visitor at the reception desk, along with a visitor's badge or card.

Instructions for Visitors

Welcome to Community Hospital. Visiting hours are from 11:00 a.m. to 8:00 p.m. For your safety and the safety and well-being of the patient you are visiting, please observe these precautions while you are on the hospital premises:
- Use the main entrance when entering or exiting from the hospital.
- Walk. Do not run.
- Smoke only in specifically designated smoking areas.
- If confused, ask for assistance.
- Observe parking lot instructions.

Please remember that you are visiting a sick person.
- Do not give the patient food, candy, or beverages unless you have checked with the nurse.
- Do not smoke where oxygen is in use.
- Smoking in patient rooms is discouraged without the consent of all patients in the room.
- Check with the nursing staff before attempting to move the patient or assisting the patient in walking.
- Talk quietly.
- Observe visiting hours.

Special precautions for ICU, CCU, maternity, pediatrics, and outpatient surgery: When visiting patients in any of these areas, please check with the nursing unit in that area for special precautions and instructions.

Emergency procedures:
- In the event of a fire or other emergency, remember that the first concern of the staff must be for patients who are unable to help themselves.
- Take a moment to familiarize yourself with emergency exits and firesafe stairways. Suggested evacuation routes are marked on the attached map of the hospital.
- If a fire alarm or drill is in progress, do not use an elevator. Use the nearest stairway marked "Exit."
- If you are in a patient's room when an alarm sounds, remain in the room, keeping the door(s) closed. Wait for a staff member to evacuate the patient. When the staff member comes, you will be escorted or directed to a safe area.

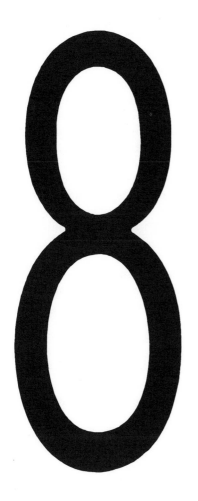

In both the delivery of patient care and in providing diagnostic data, hospital staff members in clinical services work with a wide range of equipment. Because of the complexity and technical sophistication of much of the equipment, it is essential that staff members follow instructions with care, making no assumptions about the operation of a piece of equipment. No step of an operating procedure, no matter how unimportant it may seem, should be changed unless a thorough assessment of the procedure has been undertaken. Equipment should not be modified or circumvented, and apparatus or parts should not be exchanged unless staff has first checked the manufacturer's instructions or consulted with a biomedical engineer. Questions about equipment should be referred to manufacturers' representatives or to the hospital's biomedical engineers. Whoever operates equipment must demonstrate knowledge of its proper and safe use before using it to deliver patient care.

Nursing

Of all the hospital staff members who provide services to patients, nurses have the most continuous and direct impact on patients' well-being. The nursing service delivers round-the-clock care to patients and is responsible for them over the greatest percentage of their stay in the hospital.

The first obligation of the nursing staff is to patients, and the nursing staff plays the major role in ensuring that the criteria for patient safety described in chapter 5 are met. Because patient care is administered by a nursing team, in which each member contributes to and is responsible for the entire team effort, the nursing staff should follow procedures that maintain safety for themselves and their co-workers and that guarantee the delivery of high-quality patient care.

The largest number and most serious kinds of injuries to nurses result from handling and lifting patients. Although handling and moving patients are routine, the safety measures are sometimes overlooked. Improper procedures can also cause injury to patients. The procedures described in chapter 5 enable safety handling and moving of all kinds of patients without injury to the staff or the patients.

Cuts and punctures from glassware, laboratory equipment, and hypodermic needles are frequently hazards for the nursing staff. An employee should not attempt to catch a sharp or fragile falling object, but should let it fall and then sweep it up. Glass tubing should never be forced. It is important to select the right size, use a lubricant as instructed, hold the tubing with a towel, and work it away from the palm of the hand. Only water or water-soluble jelly should be used as lubrication. Gloves should be worn. The raw cut ends of all glass tubing to be used should be fire-polished. A frozen syringe should never be "fought." If it does not come apart easily, it should be tagged as unusable and put in a surgical exchange box.

The best way to clean needles is to soak them in detergent and/or inorganic solvent preparation, and then rinse them with water. Personnel should never reach into pans and jars for hypodermic needles they are cleaning; they should either empty the container onto a flat surface or use grasping forceps to transfer the needles. After use, hypodermic needles should be returned to carrying tubes instead of being dropped onto a tray. Disposable needles and syringes should be bent or otherwise made useless immediately after they have served their purpose.

Instruments should be kept in a specific place on the dressing cart. They should never be laid on the patient's bed or chair or dropped into a pocket. Safety pins can be safely stuck into a bar of soap on the cart or tray, and should then be properly disposed of.

Surgery

The level of activity in surgical suites is high, and there can be no margin of risk. The operating room staff is responsible for keeping the area orderly, and removing any item or debris that could cause an accident. However, the responsibility for between-case and terminal cleaning of surgical suites should be clearly defined to maintain proper coordination between housekeeping and operating room staff and to ensure asepsis throughout the surgery schedule.

Patients should be transported to surgery using the precautions outlined in chapter 5. The patient should be strapped to the operating table, which should be locked before the patient is transferred to it.

Unauthorized persons should never be in the suite during surgical procedures. For safety and infection control reasons, anyone who is permitted to enter the surgical suite must wear surgery garments, masks, and hairnets and, in flammable anesthetic locations, conductive footwear.

The engineering department is responsible for preventive maintenance and for ensuring that equipment works and that there will be no failures. An increasingly wide range of equipment is operated under the direction of various health care professionals in the surgery suite and is used in the course of surgery. Information regarding the use of such equipment and any problems associated with it is necessary. Whether stationary or mobile, equipment must be positioned so that it supports activity rather than interferes with it and must be installed or stabilized so that it does not fall or move.

An effective preventive maintenance schedule requires that electrical equipment cords, plugs, and receptacles in the surgical suite be inspected at specified intervals to ensure good working order. All electrical wiring and equipment, both portable and fixed, should comply with the specifications of the NFPA *National Electrical Code* and local codes. The outlets themselves should be inspected annually for polarity, and the cords and plugs connecting equipment to its power source should be frequently inspected for defects. According to NFPA standard no. 56A, any receptacle below 5 feet must be explosionproof. Light bulbs should be changed promptly as needed, and the emergency lighting and generator system checked at regularly scheduled intervals. Before new electrical equipment or a surgeon's personal electrical equipment is to be used for the first time in the surgical area, it should be thoroughly tested and inspected by the hospital safety officer or a designated representative.

All personnel who regularly use the suite should know the location of the fire extinguishers and how to operate them.

Procedures for counting instruments, needles, and sponges must be strictly observed, both before and after a surgical procedure. Care should be taken to protect personnel who remove specimens, equipment, and used materials from the suite between surgical procedures and to protect those who handle these items after they have been removed from the suite. Contaminated linens and disposables should be double-bagged separately and labeled. Sharp items, such as needles, broken glass, and blades, should be placed in puncture-proof containers labeled with contents and destination. Equipment suspended from a ceiling or attached to a wall should be retracted following each use.

Anesthesiology

Standard III of the 1982 JCAH *Accreditation Manual for Hospitals* section on anesthesia services states: "Precautions shall be taken to assure the safe administration of anesthetic agents."

The interpretation reads: "Controls shall be established to minimize electrical hazards in all anesthetizing areas, as well as hazards of fire and explosion in areas in which flammable anesthetic agents are used. Anesthetic safety regulations should be developed by, or under the supervision of, the director of anesthesia services in conjunction with the hospital safety committee. Such regulations shall be approved by appropriate representatives of the medical staff and administration, reviewed annually to assure compatibility with current practice, and enforced....

"Written regulations for the control of electrical and anesthetic explosion hazards shall include, but should not necessarily be limited to, the following requirements:

■ Anesthetic apparatus must be inspected and tested by the anesthetist before use. If a leak or any defect is observed, the equipment must not be used until the fault is repaired.

■ When electrical equipment employing an open spark (for example, cautery or coagulation equipment) is to be used during an operation, only nonflammable agents shall be used for anesthesia or for the preoperative preparation of the surgical field.

■ Flammable anesthetic agents shall be employed only in areas in which a conductive pathway can be maintained between the patient and a conductive floor.

■ Each anesthetizing location shall be identified by a prominently posted permanent sign that clear-

ly states whether the anesthetizing location is designed for flammable or nonflammable anesthetic agents.

■ Rooms in which a flammable agent is employed for anesthesia preparation of the surgical field shall be identified by appropriate signs while the anesthetic agent is in use.

■ The administration of a flammable anesthetic to a patient being moved from one area to another shall be prohibited.

■ When required, all personnel shall wear conductive footwear, which should be tested for conductivity before entering the area.

■ When required, all equipment in the surgical suite shall be fitted with grounding devices to maintain a constant conductive pathway to the floor.

■ Fabrics permissible for use as outer garments or blankets in anesthetizing areas shall be specified in writing.

■ With the exception of certain radiologic equipment and fixed lighting more than five feet above the floor, all electrical equipment in anesthetizing areas shall be on an audiovisual line isolation monitor. When this device indicates a hazard, the administration of flammable anesthetic agents should be discontinued as soon as possible; the use of any electrical gear should be avoided, particularly the last electrical item put into use as well as any item not required for patient monitoring or support; and the hospital engineer or maintenance chief shall be notified immediately. Following completion of the procedure, the operating room from which the signal emanated should not be used until the defect is remedied. All personnel who work in such areas shall be familiar with the procedures to be followed.

■ The condition of all operating room electrical equipment shall be inspected regularly, preferably on a monthly basis, and a written record of the results and any required corrective action shall be maintained.

■ The results of any required monthly conductivity testing shall be made known to personnel who work primarily in these areas.

■ Anesthesia personnel shall familiarize themselves with the rate, volume, and mechanism of air exchange within the surgical and obstetrical suites, as well as with humidity control."

Special-Care Units

Staff members serving special-care units, which include such facilities as intensive care units, intensive cardiac care units, hyperbaric pressure chambers, and facilities for renal dialysis, require special instruction in the safe use of electrical and electronic equipment. Such instruction can be given as part of the hospital's in-service education program and also by equipment suppliers. Although videotaped instruction is often used, the best method is person-to-person instruction, which permits the staff person to question points not understood. After instruction has been completed, the supervisor should conduct a follow-up interview with each person to be certain that the procedures and precautions are understood.

Although the electrical equipment in special-care units is serviced by the engineering department, by the manufacturer, or by a contract repair service, the employees who operate it are responsible for maintaining it in readiness. Each piece should be checked every day, and the condition of the cords and plugs should receive particular attention. All equipment must be kept clean, and spills should be removed immediately. Operation of the equipment should be monitored, and any malfunction should be reported immediately.

Special-care units especially need fail-safe arrangements for keeping electrical devices and machines operating in time of electrical power failure. The emergency power generator should be in perfect working order at all times to ensure operation of the many monitors and pumps that these special units require for monitoring patients and sustaining life. Proper ventilation and humidification are vital for patients with respiratory problems, and the equipment must be constantly inspected and regulated. A special hazard in a hyperbaric pressure chamber is the high concentration of oxygen, which may cause a catastrophic fire if proper precautions are not taken.

Psychiatry

About one-third of the disabling injuries in psychiatric units result directly from combative incidents, and another substantial percentage are indirectly related to these. In any hospital that admits psychiatric patients, it is important for staff members to know that they must control their tempers and feelings if they are to bring potentially harmful situations under control. They must become instantaneous police officers, judges, and jurors under the most trying conditions without injuring patients, other staff, or themselves.

One of the most effective basic means of preventing injuries and accidents due to patient outbursts is a thorough knowledge of the patient's condition. Flagging on the patient's medical record any tendencies toward violence alerts other personnel. Personnel in a psychiatric unit have a responsibility to keep the physician informed of the patient's behavior and reactions to medication.

Psychiatric department personnel will further curb injuries and accidents if they:

■ Use good judgment and make decisions as needed. Know the individual patient well enough to determine whether a sharp command or a soft and calming approach is better.

■ Get enough help for physically handling a recalcitrant patient when he or she is taken out of seclusion, fed, given medication or nursing care, or otherwise attended.

■ Are prepared for the combative patient who may hide in the bathroom or shower room or behind some obstacle.

■ Make sure the patient for whom medication has been prescribed is actually taking it instead of spitting it out, discarding it, or saving it.

■ Keep patients' fingernails clipped and trimmed, to help prevent minor injuries.

■ Wear a ready-tied, slip-off necktie. An attendant with a standard tie can be choked by a patient.

■ Inspect all parcels brought in by visitors or patients.

Radiology

For the protection of staff and patients, the radiology department should have written policies and procedures that include safety procedures developed by the radiologist or the radiation safety committee in cooperation with the safety committee. Rules should be established for the safe use, removal, handling, and storage of radium, other radioactive elements, and their disintegration products. Radiation safety procedures should include proper safety precautions against electrical hazards, mechanical hazards, fire, and explosions.

Mechanical or electrical defects should be reported immediately. All main switches should be disconnected at night.

Before equipment is put in operation, it is essential to make sure that:

■ Only authorized personnel are present in the radiography room.

■ All persons are properly protected. The reproductive system of all patients must be shielded, and pregnant women must be shielded by a lead apron.

■ Patients on wheeled stretchers are secured with straps and side rails.

■ A minimum distance of 6 feet is maintained between staff and the source of radiation.

■ The door is closed when the radiography room is in use.

All radiologic equipment should be calibrated periodically in accordance with federal, state, and local requirements. X-ray machines should be checked regularly to ensure proper positioning of secondary radiation filters. All x-ray switches should be housed so that they cannot be activated accidentally.

When a portable x-ray unit is used, only the technician and the patient should be in the room at the time of exposure. When the unit is used in a semiprivate room, it must stand at a safe distance from the other patient and must be kept at that distance. When the equipment is to be moved, it must be packed with all parts carefully arranged so they do not protrude and cause an accident or make transporting difficult or dangerous.

Stored film constitutes a fire hazard, and should be kept in metal storage cabinets or covered metal containers, not on the floor or in passageways.

Nuclear Medicine and Radiation Therapy

The Nuclear Regulatory Commission defines the conditions under which radioactive material may be used. Only employees trained to use such material should be permitted to handle it. All rooms and areas that contain any radioactive material should be plainly identified as shown in figure 13 at the end of this chapter. Figures 14 and 15 present procedures for handling radioactive material.

Respiratory Therapy

Most safety regulations for the respiratory therapy department are directed toward prevention of oxygen fires. Signs stating that oxygen is in use and that smoking is prohibited should be posted in the department and wherever respiratory therapy is conducted.

The oxygen tent in particular, with its high concentration of oxygen, must be secure from any agent that could in any way, even under improbable circumstances, cause a fire. Any equipment that emits sparks, including all electrical equipment, must be used with caution. Motorized beds used with tents should be approved by Underwriters' Laboratories, and even approved beds should be operated manually when the patient is receiving oxygen. Electrical equipment such as heating pads, which can raise the temperature to a level at which oxygen in combination with other factors will ignite, should be prohibited.

When oxygen cylinders are used, they should be labeled, secured, and stored. If a gas cylinder must be brought to the patient's bedside, precautions should be taken to avoid obstacles and hazards en route from storage.

Special caution must be taken with children receiving respiratory therapy treatment. Toys that can generate sparks by friction must be removed from tents. Very thin disposable plastic canopies, when used, can press against a child's face and cause asphyxiation and should therefore be carefully monitored.

Physical Therapy

Special attention should be given to the physical therapy department's equipment. Wheelchairs, wheeled tables, and wheeled carts should be inspected for any mechanical defects. Equipment for hydrotherapy, ultrasonics, and the like should be inspected regularly for electrical safety. Exercise machines should be checked for frayed rope or loose pulleys. Crutches, walkers, and canes should be provided with large, nonslip tips. Tools should be issued only to patients who can properly handle them; such tools or handling devices should be free of burrs, slivers, and sharp edges. Floor surfaces should provide good footing, and any stumbling or slipping hazards should be removed.

The physical therapist or rehabilitation counselor must be aware of each patient's capabilities and each patient's limitations. Excessive exercise, by exhausting and weakening the patient, makes that patient more vulnerable to accidents.

Dialysis

Dialysis machines and ancillary equipment must be inspected according to a prescribed schedule. The lines and coils should be checked for leaks before each treatment, and electrical connections should be inspected daily. The responsible technician should be informed if malfunction is suspected or observed.

The machines should be maintained at the correct temperature range (35° to 40°C., 95° to 104°F.) and conductivity (12 to 14 millimhos). The tanks should be cleaned after each treatment, and once a week should be soaked with formaldehyde for 24 hours. The frequency and requirements for microbiological testing of the tanks are determined by the infection control committee. The equipment should be kept clean at all times; spills should be removed immediately.

Patients undergoing dialysis should be given instructions on cleaning and maintaining the cannula safely and on procedures for handling bleeding. When under treatment, patients should be monitored periodically. Reports should be prepared on incidents such as needle puncture and wound contamination that occur in the course of treatment.

Emergency

The number of persons using hospital emergency departments has doubled in the past 15 years, although only 20 percent of these persons are in life-threatening situations. Many people, particularly in large cities, do not have a doctor, and in time of need they look upon the emergency department as an outpatient department. This trend tends to overload emergency facilities and brings on problems, many with safety and security implications.

In an emergency department that sees several hundred patients during a 24-hour period, the waiting group becomes large and the wait long. Patients are in pain and may be out of temper or inebriated; for these reasons, security problems may occur. The security staff present can be expected to handle disorderly persons and to observe walk-ins.

Most persons do not understand that the way in which the emergency department functions is that the patients in greatest need are treated first and those with less acute problems thereafter. Regardless of when they check in, persons who have ordinary problems must wait until those who are in more serious condition have been attended. Assessment of the condition of all comers is called *triage,* and explaining triage can alleviate the stress generated by emergency department conditions. A card such as that shown in figure 16, which briefly and forthrightly explains the necessity for such assessment, can be handed to patients and the persons who accompany them.

Triage officers (the staff members who assess the severity of conditions) have difficult choices and are under great pressure. Heart attacks, burns, gunshot and stab wounds, and extensive injuries and bleeding from accidents are clearcut conditions for immediate care. Less clear is the condition of patients who, because of language, culture, or personal reasons, are unable to describe their symptoms or who are not sufficiently assertive to make the doctor or nurse realize their urgency. In such instances, good interviewing techniques by the triage officer are essential.

The method of treatment should be clearly explained to emergency patients. In the event that they require tests not available in the emergency department, they should be informed of procedures for utilizing the services of other departments, such as radiology or the laboratory.

Parents, relatives, or friends should be discouraged from entering the treatment rooms with patients. They should remain seated in the waiting area for their own safety and so that they do not interfere with treatment.

Housekeeping in the emergency department is important, particularly the need for fast service. Spills, tracks, and body fluids must be mopped up at once, and housekeeping equipment removed. Soiled department equipment must be cleaned. However, because most housekeeping departments do not operate on all shifts, emergency department employees should always be prepared, when necessary, to clean the surroundings with cleaning supplies provided daily by the housekeeper. Fresh uniforms should be available for those times during a shift when staff members must change clothing.

Outpatient

New medical techniques and the increased use of drugs have reduced hospitalization and shortened the period of acute illness, so more and more ambulatory patients depend on the outpatient department. The medical and health care services provided by the outpatient department are no longer concerned solely with dispensing medicine. As evidenced by an almost doubling in patient load over the past decade, the outpatient department represents a convergence of preventive, curative, and restorative medicine and health education services that strive to meet a community's total health care needs.

The outpatient department is the point of entry through which many patients are channeled to other medical services in the hospital, many for the first time. Ambulatory patients are often strangers to the hospital and come in to the outpatient department alone, so they need the staff's guidance when further medical services are necessary. Many served by the outpatient department have no personal physician. In addition to the personal attention given to patients by the outpatient staff, confusion and anxiety can be allayed by the use of posters in the waiting room, signs directing persons to clinical service departments, and pamphlets that explain the various medical services and instruct outpatients on where to find each service.

The outpatient department is unique in the location and design of its quarters. The entrance should be accessible directly from the street, but away from the main hospital entrance. It should be canopied or enclosed and free of curbs, platforms, and any impediments. The waiting area should be clearly separated from the working area and should contain suitable furnishings, a public telephone, a drinking fountain, and a restroom equipped with nurse call buttons and locks operable from the outside.

Laboratory

General guidelines

The laboratory's functions pertain to the chemistry, bacteriology, serology, and histology areas and extend to the basal metabolism, electrocardiographic, and morgue-museum rooms.

Laboratory employees routinely work with infectious matter taken from patients and also with toxic chemicals. To ensure a safe laboratory, the practices outlined in figures 17 and 18 should be followed. Laboratory employees' practices should, of course, be in compliance with all applicable state and local EPA standards.

The laboratory should be fire-resistant and large enough to prevent crowding. Rooms should be locked when unattended. A strict no-smoking rule must be maintained. Each laboratory that uses any hazardous material must post a sign on its door identifying the responsible investigator and the material; a suitable sign is shown in figure 19.

In no case should wood flooring be used. The floor should be smooth, nonporous, and free from joints. Mastic tile is less fatiguing than harder surfaces. Tile or any block form must be laid carefully to avoid cracks, which could trap mercury or other toxic materials.

Laboratory furniture should be resistant to chemicals and fire. Work surfaces and countertops should be either adjustable or of varied heights to avoid the need for technicians to stoop or to climb on stools. If stools are used, they should be broad-based and sturdy.

According to the Illuminating Engineering Society, lighting at every working surface should be at least 100 foot-candles. Natural lighting is preferred, but if fluorescent lighting is used, the tubing should be protected. Depending on the type of work, lighting fixtures can be open, vaporproof, or explosionproof.

Electrical outlets should be of the three-pole type to provide for a ground wire from all portable equipment. For new construction, it is required that the conduits carry an insulated extra wire for grounding. In existing facilities, if an extra wire is not installed, the metal conduit itself can serve as the ground conductor. However, it should be tested for continuity to ground before it is used and also on an annual basis.

The ventilating system should be designed specifically for the various laboratory functions. In most laboratory areas air changes per hour of outside air. However, in some areas containing potentially hazardous material and high-heat-producing equipment, a much higher air change rate may be needed. One approach is to use exhaust air from cleaner areas to provide supply air to areas having potential airborne hazards. Air movement in laboratory areas or rooms should always go from areas of low risk to areas of higher risks or from clean to less clean areas.

Infectious agents, fumes, and toxic materials tend to spread during laboratory procedures, making the control of airflows essential in maintaining a safe environment. If the laboratory air-handling system recirculates any portion of the general exhaust air, then it is important to have a separate exhaust duct system for fume hoods and biological safety cabinets.

Work with flammable or toxic materials should be conducted under exhaust hoods. In general, the hood exhaust system should operate independently of the laboratory exhaust system and have its own air supply. An exhaust hood or safety cabinet should be provided for chemical work and a hood or ventilated glove box for pathogenic work, for example, work with tuberculosis bacilli. Biological safety cabinets and their exhaust ductwork and purifications should be inspected and maintained in accordance with established written procedures and manufacturers' recommendations.

Sprinkler systems must meet the requirements of both local law and insurance regulations. Where a fire hazard might be made worse by the use of water, a dry chemical or carbon dioxide system should be installed permanently. Sodium and most light metals, however, will react violently to carbon dioxide.

Electrical controls on refrigerators should be located outside the storage chambers to prevent accidental ignition of vapors released inside. Circulation fans can be made safe only through the use of explosionproof motors, extension shafts with the motor outside the box, or hydraulic or air-pressure motors. When new refrigerators are ordered, laboratory-safe types should be specified.

Autoclaves and other high-pressure equipment should conform to the American Society of Mechanical Engineers standard on unfired pressure vessels. Only trained personnel should work with such equipment, which must be so insulated or isolated that contact burns are impossible. Pressure vessels should be equipped with an interlock or other device to prevent them from being opened while under pressure, and they should

not be opened until the internal pressure has been brought down to zero.

Centrifuges should have covers. Electrical heating mantles should be used instead of Bunsen burners if possible. Bunsen burners should never be used to heat flammable liquids.

Containers holding volatile liquids should have grooved stoppers or other venting devices to release built-up pressure. If such vapors are explosive or toxic, the reagent should be kept in refrigerated storage. Containers should have clear labels protected by a coating of plastic, paraffin, or transparent tape.

Reagents should be kept in as small a supply as possible; unused reagents should be returned to the storeroom. A week's supply of the common reagents and a day's supply of the hazardous ones are considered proper. Small reagent bottles should be transported in carrying racks or trays, not by hand. Larger containers should be moved in special carrying jackets, commercially available for the purpose. If possible, the reagent should be stored away from direct natural light on low, uncrowded shelves with edge rims or cleats to prevent spillage from running off them. Inert shelf material is needed for oxidizing reagents. Chemicals that react together should be stored separately.

Rubber-to-glass connections should be made with care. Lengths of glass tubing should be supported while they are being inserted. Technicians should wear gloves when making such connections or should hold the ends with towels. Glass should never be pressed toward the palm of the hand.

Glassware should be emptied and rinsed before it is set aside for cleaning. If the container has held toxic materials, it should be chemically cleaned as well as rinsed before it is sent in for washing. Strong oxidizing agents should be used with extreme care.

Disposal of laboratory wastes

Technicians should rigidly observe the requirements for disposing of dangerous chemicals. Special containers with self-closing covers should be provided for volatile liquids and chemicals that may create highly toxic fumes when in contact with other chemicals in the drain system. All containers should be clearly labeled. Oil, grease, gasoline, other solvents, mercaptans, and mercury should not be discharged into drains: grease fills traps, solvents may produce explosive mixtures, and mercury corrodes lead joints. Small amounts of corrosives, such as alkalies and acids, that are diluted by large amounts of water in accordance with state and local EPA standards can be safely emptied into drains.

Those liquid chemicals that cannot be discarded via the regular trash collection system or by flushing into drains should be disposed of by specially trained personnel. Disposal of solid chemicals such as sodium, potassium, calcium carbide, phosphoric anhydride, and phosphorus, and disposal of more-than-one-liter quantities of such liquids as thionyl chloride and phosphorus oxychloride, should be handled by qualified disposal technicians in accordance with state and local EPA standards.

In disposing of fuming or concentrated sulfuric acid, extreme care is required to prevent water from splashing into the bottle and causing a violent reaction. When more than half a liter of this acid is to be discarded, the waste liquid should first be transferred to the empty original bottle with a dipper and funnel before the bottle is removed from the building.

When an unusually toxic chemical that would require a special antidote and prompt first aid is being handled, a medical officer should be notified, who will provide pertinent advice and treatment. Examples of such chemicals are hydrogen cyanide, snake venom, nitrogen mustard, nerve gases, and hydrogen fluoride.

If hydrocyanic acid is used, a medical officer should provide a small kit of amyl nitrite pearls. The kit should be kept in a readily accessible area known to all laboratory occupants. If anyone gets cyanide poisoning, the ampul should be broken and the victim should breathe the nitrite vapors while en route to a medical station for further treatment.

When a toxic gas cylinder develops a leak, it should be placed in a fume hood, and the safety officer should be notified to remove it from the building. If the gas flow is sufficient to contaminate the laboratory area, the room door should be closed and the fire alarm sounded. Purchase of large cylinders of toxic gases is inadvisable, because they cannot be placed into an exhaust hood enclosure in the event of an uncontrollable leak and because tubing or fitting failure

or release of the safety catch during exposure to fire might dump an unmanageable excess into patient areas.

Guidelines of the Atomic Energy Commission should be followed for disposal of radioactive materials. Radioactive waste should be placed in a leakproof, noncontaminated container. Personnel should telephone the area radiation safety officer, give information about the isotope and approximate activity, and request prompt disposal. The area radiation safety officer is a person outside the hospital who is responsible for centralized radioactive waste disposal procedures within each region of the country, as designated by the Atomic Energy Commission.

To give impetus to all of these laboratory standards, it is recommended that a safety subcommittee be formed within the department. This subcommittee should meet regularly, at least monthly, and should submit reports to the general safety committee. The subcommittee should make recommendations for the purchase of safety equipment, because laboratory personnel are most knowledgeable on the requirements. Such recommendations should be reviewed by the safety committee, the safety director, and the administrator.

Coordination should be established with the housekeeping department to ensure that employees responsible for routine cleaning are not inadvertently exposed to hazardous materials.

Pharmacy

Drugs in the pharmacy and throughout the hospital must be under the supervision of the pharmacist. They must be stored under prescribed conditions with regard to sanitation, temperature, light, moisture, ventilation, segregation, and security. All substances must be adequately labeled, with accessory or cautionary statements included.

The pharmacist or a designee under the pharmacist's direct supervision must combine and dispense all drug compounds. The pharmacist should review the prescriber's original order, or a duplicate, before dispensing the initial dose of medication. The pharmacist should fill only one prescription at a time, to prevent mislabeling and other errors. In filling prescriptions for any tablet available in several sizes or similar to others in appearance, the pharmacist should exercise particular care. The patient's full name must be stated on the label. Container labels should always be checked three times: when the container is removed from the shelf, when it is actually used, and when it is returned to the shelf. Prescriptions for pharmaceutical specialties, basic drugs, and biologicals should be filled according to the product's trade name; the manufacturer's name; and the lot, control, or batch number.

In the absence of the pharmacist, only prepackaged drugs may be removed from the pharmacy, and only by a designated nurse or physician in amounts sufficient for immediate therapeutic needs. A record of such withdrawals must be kept.

Written policies and procedures are essential for patient and employee safety, for control of drugs, and for accountability. Therefore the hospital should establish policy on the use of medicines brought into the hospital by patients. This policy should be disseminated in written form and strictly followed.

The pharmacist or a designee should periodically inspect all drug storage and medication centers on nursing care units, keeping a record of such inspections, to verify that:

■ Disinfectants and drugs for external use are stored separately from oral and injectable medications.

■ Drugs requiring special storage conditions to ensure stability are stored accordingly. For example, biological and other thermolabile medications should be stored in a refrigerator in a separate compartment capable of maintaining the required temperature.

■ Stock contains no outdated drugs, which are unsuitable for use.

■ Distribution and administration of controlled drugs are documented.

■ Emergency drugs are in adequate and appropriate supply.

■ Apothecary's metric weight and liquid measure equivalent charts are posted wherever needed.

Nursing units should have locked storage areas and adequate and properly controlled drug preparation areas. These areas should be well lighted and located where nurses are free from interruption when handling drugs.

Inasmuch as the pharmacy uses explosives, flammables, caustics, corrosives, and poisons, its employees should take measures to protect themselves from these dangerous materials and to ensure safe handling of them in the pharmacy and throughout the hospital. Practices that foster safety include the following:

■ A grounded pump approved by Underwriters' Laboratories should be used to draw flammable liquids from a large grounded drum. An upright drum is preferred. However, if the drum is in a horizontal position, it should be equipped with an approved valve and vents.

■ Containers for bulk storage and handling methods for all flammable liquids used by the pharmacy should comply with National Fire Protection Association standard no. 56C, *Hospital Laboratories.*

■ Care should be taken to pour liquids below eye level and to avoid splashing. Corrosive chemicals require extreme care. A bottled liquid should be poured at such an angle that it does not spill on the label and obscure it. Technicians pouring acetic and phenolic substances should avoid standing over them, so as not to inhale toxic fumes. When materials are heated, they should be constantly attended.

■ To prevent breakage, delivery carts should be compartmented.

■ If the pharmaceutical service operates a central sterile supply department or sterilizes irrigating or parenteral solutions, employees who work there should wear wire-mesh gloves, eye protection, and headgear.

■ Discontinued and outdated drugs and containers that have illegible or worn labels or that lack a label should be returned to the pharmacy for disposition. These should be disposed of with caution.

■ Throughout the hospital, refrigerators for biologicals should be equipped with thermometers. The temperature range should be 0° to 15°C. (32° to 59°F.).

■ Supplies of flammable liquids and narcotics should be kept as small as possible. Ether, alcohol, and other flammables should be kept in safety containers and should be stored in secured areas that meet local fire and safety regulations. Narcotics and poisons should have separate and secured storage places.

■ Under no circumstances should contents of partially empty bottles of a drug be combined.

Figure 13. A notice or sign on the door of the room where radioactive materials are held warns of their presence.

Radioactive Storage Identification Means

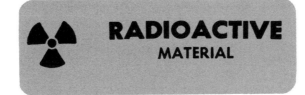

Figure 14. Only employees trained by a professional staff member versed in nuclear medicine and radiation therapy are permitted to handle radioactive material. Prudence in handling radioactive material is essential to the handler's safety.

Receiving, Handling, and Returning Radioactive Material

1. Radioactive material should be shipped directly to the hospital's receiving dock.

2. Shipping dock employees should be instructed by the radiation physicist on how to handle radioactive material.

3. Once the radioactive material is on hospital premises, it should be delivered to the radiation therapy department immediately.

4. The package should be accepted by the radiation physicist, who should examine it first visually for damage and leakage and then further with a Geiger-Muller (G-M) counter for excessive radiation levels. The radiation physicist should open the package carefully, check its contents, log it in, and place the radioactive material in a storage room specially designed for such use.

5. Measures established by the radiologist or radiation safety officer for gold therapy safety should be observed. Radioactive needles should be checked for correct strength, and radon gold seeds should be counted.

6. Employees handling radioactive material should always wear a monitoring badge.

7. Proper protective clothing and equipment should be used at all times by employees coming in contact with radioactive materials.

8. Technicians should test instruments used in handling radioactive material for activity. When radioactive, they should be removed from service and decontaminated.

9. Technicians should wear rubber gloves, face shield, and apron when handling radioactive liquids.

10. They should handle isotopes at a distance, and with instruments.

11. Spills and contamination should be reported to the radiation safety officer immediately.

12. Urine specimens from irradiated patients should be disposed of immediately.

13. Waste material should be monitored with a G-M counter, making sure the G-M reading is at background level for its disposition. "Radioactive" signs should be removed or defaced before disposing of decontaminated waste.

Figure 15. Radioactive spills must be cleaned up at once.

In the Event of a Radioactive Spill

In the event of a radioactive spill, cleanup must be initiated immediately to decontaminate the area. Until the area has been completely decontaminated and inspected, no one except the radiation safety officer or consulting physicist should be permitted access. The radiation safety officer or consulting physicist must review the following procedures thoroughly before adopting them.

The employee must:

1. Stop whatever he or she is doing.
2. Determine the contaminated area.
3. Check hands for contamination by whatever method is available. If gloves are contaminated, they should be removed, turned inside out, and put in radioactive waste receptacle.
4. Put on fresh gloves.
5. Demarcate the contaminated area with radiation-indicating tape, allowing reasonable margins.
6. Place absorbent material such as paper towels over the liquid spill, to limit and confine the spread.
7. Determine the level of radiation with a Geiger-Muller counter and record it for comparison with findings after decontamination.
8. Clean the contaminated area with a commercial decontaminant suitable for radioactivity.
9. Place all cleaning material in radioactive waste container for later disposition by approved methods.
10. After decontamination, again determine the level of radiation, using the survey meter, and compare this value with the value registered previously.

Next, the radiation physicist should make a wipe test of the decontaminated area and record the results on a special form. When the area is approved as being clean, use of the area can resume.

The employee should then check his or her body and clothing for radioactive contamination. If any part of the body is contaminated, the employee must:

■ Immediately wash the area with mild soap.

■ Examine the area for level of radiation exposure, using the appropriate instrument.

■ Continue to wash as necessary, rechecking the radiation level frequently until the area has been decontaminated.

If clothing is contaminated, the employee must:

■ Remove it.

■ Place it in a plastic bag.

■ Identify the bag with tape marked "Radioactive," on which the name of the employee, date of contamination, and contaminating material are indicated.

■ Store the bag in radioactive storage area in the radiation therapy department until disposition.

■ File an incident report providing all pertinent details.

Figure 16. This information on emergency screening can be given to patients and to the persons who accompany them. Printed on a card in easily read type and in whatever languages are prevalent in the community, it explains an unfamiliar situation in unfamiliar surroundings.

Emergency Department Screening

In the emergency department the most critically ill and injured must always be cared for first. Patients who suffer from less severe forms of illness and injury must wait: they will be treated after patients who have a critical or life-threatening emergency are treated.

The condition of all persons who come to the emergency department is assessed by a doctor or nurse. This evaluation, called *triage*, determines which patients are in urgent and which in less urgent need of emergency care. During this evaluation, a nurse hears your complaint and checks your appearance and vital signs. You can help in this evaluation by remaining calm and describing your condition as clearly and as completely as possible.

If you are waiting, please know you are waiting for the most immediate medical attention possible. Your turn for treatment is based on the nature of your emergency and on that of others in the emergency department at the same time. We request that all persons, both patients and persons who accompany them, remain as calm and quiet as possible.

Figure 17. Vigilance on the part of the technicians who staff a laboratory is essential to their safety. Rules for the particular laboratory environment, as well as those for the hospital generally, should be observed.

Safety Rules for Laboratories

- Permit only authorized personnel in the laboratory. Designate areas for other staff and for patients.

- Observe all signs denoting hazardous areas where there are infectious agents and toxic substances.

- Walk carefully. Floors in lab areas where paraffin is used are extremely slippery.

- Before and after work and if a spill occurs, wash all counter tops with a 1:500 dilution of a suitable disinfectant to destroy bacteria or with 1 percent chlorine bleach to destroy viruses.

- Wash hands often with disinfectant soap, and always wash before leaving the work area.

- Cleanse and dress a cut or puncture immediately, noting the cause of injury and the material handled.

- Treat all organisms as pathogens. Do not remove infectious materials from specified areas.

- Handle all tissue samples, bloods, and serums as though they were from infected patients. Dispose of clots in disinfectant-soaked towels. Thoroughly disinfect all tubes, needles, and syringes.

- Wear disposable gloves and mask when handling infectious materials.

- Identify highly infectious agents during use and prior to storage with a label on the container. Identify incubator trays or racks containing hazardous materials.

- Put all hazardous material in labeled plastic bags for incineration.

- Use both hands when handling large bottles and never lift them by the top alone.

- File an ampul at the demarcation prior to removing the tip, and cover the top with gauze.

- Use a mechanical pipette aid to draw material into a pipette. Do not ever use the mouth to suck any material into a pipette.

- Without splashing, used pipettes should be placed carefully, tip down, into a 1:500 dilution of a suitable disinfectant or 3 percent phenol for 24 hours before washing or disposing of them. Plug all pipettes with cotton.

- Never place pipettes or hot wire loops in culture fluid.

- Remove all broken glass from counter tops to prevent slivers from cutting hands, arms, and elbows.

- Discard all glassware, syringes, and needles into labeled special containers for this purpose. Disinfect such items if necessary.

- Place petri dishes containing infected cultures first in a closed container and then in an open bag with an airtight seal. Autoclave the bag and contents at the usual temperature and pressure for at least 45 minutes. After autoclaving, seal the bag and dispose of it.

- Wear gloves to remove materials from ovens and autoclaves.

- Observe usage rules on all laminar flow hoods.

- Chain gas cylinders in place. If empty, label them. When removing them, use a dolly.

- Use only self-adhesive labels.

- Never remove materials and equipment from one laboratory to another laboratory without permission.

Figure 18. Chemicals and unidentified substances constitute a great hazard, and they must be expertly handled.

Handling and Storing Chemicals and Unidentified Substances

■ When working with chemicals dangerous to the eyes, employees should wear goggles that have side shields. Persons wearing contact lenses should be especially cautious.

■ When working in mist and vapor atmospheres, employees should wear chemical goggles and full-face shields.

■ When working with unknown materials or carcinogens, employees should wear gloves, appropriate respirator mask, and protective apron and should work under a ventilation hood suitable for these purposes.

■ Employees should know the location and operation of the eyewash centers and safety showers.

■ Only trained laboratory personnel should operate autoclaves, and manufacturers' procedures should be followed. The fast exhaust should never be used when autoclaving liquids. The internal pressure must be zero before opening an autoclave.

■ Proper methods should be used for lifting and carrying reagents, especially corrosives, flammables, and unidentified chemicals.

■ All reagents should be labeled with the following information:
  Contents
  Storage requirements
  Date of preparation or receipt
  Initials of preparer
  Date opened for use
  Expiration date
  Specifications for special care when contents are toxic or are an irritant
  Specifications for handling and for disposition
  Antidote if it is necessary

■ Always carry large containers of acid in an acid carrier.

■ Store reactive agents, such as acetic acid, sulfuric acid, and nitric acid, in separate areas.

■ Keep ether, acetone, and other flammable liquids in the place provided for them especially, and keep only in quantities necessary for current work.

■ Dilute acid by pouring it *into water;* never pour water into acid. Pour slowly to prevent splashing.

■ Never work with radioactive materials unless properly instructed.

■ Moisten pipettes and glass tubing before inserting them into rubber tubing or corking them. Protect hands with gloves or gauze.

■ Protect hands when cleaning sharp objects or instruments.

■ Return each instrument to its prescribed space.

■ Employ proper means to dispose of the various substances used.

■ *Do not* take empty containers and bottles home from the laborotory.

Figure 19. This particular sign is required to be posted on a laboratory door wherever a biohazard exists.

Laboratory Hazard Sign

Admittance to Authorized Personnel Only

Hazard identity _____

Responsible investigator _____

In case of emergency, call: _____

    Daytime phone _____ Home phone _____

Authorization for entrance must be obtained from the responsible investigator named above.

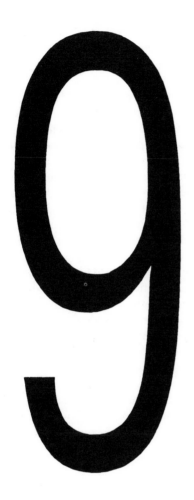

Safety is unique in that it is measured not by its level of success but more often by its failure, that is, the frequency and severity of accidents and injuries. As a consequence, safety communications to staff often become problem-oriented and not well accepted, because few people consider their work habits unsafe. Safety memos and reminders of a general nature often fall on deaf ears. However, safety communication made *personal*—on a one-to-one basis through well-trained supervisors—and *specific*—by providing enough detail on a particular incident to enable staff to identify with the unnamed victim's circumstances—will improve safety awareness and attitudes.

Support service staff, whose daily functions are essential to the efficient operation of the hospital, deserve the benefits that directly result from adequate safety training and enforcement of safety rules, procedures, and standards. Because many of the job functions require the use of mechanical power equipment, heating elements, pressure vessels, and so forth, the safety-related problems associated with support services differ from those in the clinical and nursing areas. The potential for slips and fall from wet floors or unsafe floor coverings, incidents involving mechanical equipment failures or misuse, and injuries from sharp edges, unprotected surfaces, protruding objects, or moving parts all present major challenges to department directors and safety staff to develop effective safety programs relevant to the needs of support service employees.

Administrative Offices

Administrative offices such as the business office, public relations, and purchasing should be set up for efficient, convenient, and safe operation. In general, personnel in administrative departments are best guided by the information contained in chapter 7, Safety for Visitors. Work flow patterns govern arrangement of furniture and equipment. In many instances, small structural or mechanical modifications can eliminate problems.

Floors are the most significant contributor to office accidents. They should be as maintenance-free as possible. Floor finishes should be selected for resistance to slipping. Defective tiles, boards, or carpeting should be repaired or replaced immediately. Special anti-slip protection should be used on stairways and at elevator entrances. Floor mats and runners often are relatively slip-resistant.

A recommended minimum width for aisles is 4 feet. Passages through work areas should be unobstructed. Wastebaskets, telephone and electrical cords and outlets, pencil sharpeners, typewriter carriages, and such equipment should not protrude into aisles. Step-offs from one level to another should be avoided; they should be converted into ramps with nonskid surfaces or at least be well marked and provided with a hand railing. File drawers should not open into aisles.

Adequate light should be provided, in conformity with levels recommended by the Illuminating Engineering Society. Employees should not face windows, unshielded lamps, or other sources of glare. Fluorescent lamps are particularly desirable, because they produce high levels of illumination without glare.

All mechanical ventilation and air-conditioning systems should be tested periodically to ensure an adequate flow of air at proper temperature. Fans should be placed where they cannot cause tripping or falling. They should have substantial bases and convenient means for being moved and carried.

Adequate ventilation should be supplied for duplicating machines, especially those using spirits or such toxic liquids as ammonia or methanol. If these machines are kept in a small room, mechanical ventilation is vital.

Protection against hazards from electrical equipment should be provided. Outlets should accommodate three-wire grounding plugs to protect operators from electric shock; they should not be located where they create tripping hazards or where they will be used as footrests. Wherever possible, enough receptacles should be installed to make extension cords unnecessary. If cords must cross the floor, they should be covered with special rubber channels designed for the purpose; they should not be laid under rugs or carpeting, where they are both a fire and a tripping hazard.

Materials should be stored where no heavy traffic can prevent their being reached and where they are not likely to fall on anyone. Nothing should be allowed on passageway floors. Piles of materials should be stable and secure. If materials are stored on shelves, the heavy objects should be on the lower shelves.

Chairs should be sturdily built, with a wide enough base to prevent easy tipping. Casters on swivel chairs should have a base at least 20 inches in diameter and should be securely fixed to the chair base.

Spring-loaded typing desks should be inspected to ensure that they work properly. Employees should be shown the correct way of operating the desks to release the typewriter. New desks and file cabinets should be examined for burrs and slivers. Glass tops on desks and tables may crack or shard; durable synthetic surfaces do not. Drawers on desks and file cabinets should have safety stops. Paper cutters should be placed to provide ample room for the blade to slice cleanly and should be on a stable surface.

Many hazards are peculiar to filing cabinets and warrant special mention. Employees can suffer head bumps from getting up too quickly under open drawers, mashed fingers from closing drawers improperly, and hand injuries and strains from moving the cabinets. The following precautions are necessary:

■ No part of the body except the hand should be used to close file drawers. Fingers should be placed in the drawer handles, not curled over the top of the drawer. All file drawers should be closed immediately after use.

■ Only one file drawer at a time should be opened. Otherwise the cabinet may topple over.

■ When a file drawer is open, others in the area should be warned so that they do not turn around or straighten up so quickly that they bump the drawer.

■ Climbing on file drawers should be forbidden.

■ Small stools used in filing areas should not be left in passageways, where they are tipping hazards.

■ Filing personnel should wear rubber finger guards to avoid cutting their fingers on metal fasteners or paper edges.

Corridors and Other Public Areas

For fire and life safety purposes, compliance with the National Fire Protection Association standard no. 101, *Life Safety Code,* should be followed. Floors and wall openings should comply with standards of the American National Standards Institute (ANSI). Handrails are required for both sides of stairs that are 44 inches wide or less, and center rails for stairs wider than 44 inches.

Glass doors should have some conspicuous design, such as a painted emblem or a decal, about 4½ feet above the floor at the door's center, to keep people from walking into them. Safety glass, complying with ANSI standard no. Z97.1, should be installed in preference to plate glass.

A solid door can also present a hazard, because someone may be struck when it is approached from both sides and opened. Frosted glass in such a door gives a sufficient view for accident prevention, yet preserves privacy. As an additional warning, the swing path of a door should be marked on the floor by special yellow and black striped tape, painted a bright color, or outlined by yellow plastic circles. If that area is carpeted, a quarter circle or half circle of differently colored carpet can be laid. It is a good practice for the door hinges to be on the "upstream" side of traffic, that is, on the right-hand side as one faces the door from the hallway; this keeps people from walking into the edge of an open door.

Housekeeping

Much of the responsibility for maintaining a safe and healthful environment in the hospital rests with the housekeeping department. Every day, the housekeeping department must deal with such practices as the safe storage of materials, disposal of hazardous wastes, and pest management. Without a well-trained housekeeping department, the opportunity for fire, accidental injury, or infection is greatly increased.

When a housekeeping situation arises that could cause an accident, it should be reported immediately to the housekeeping staff unless immediate corrective action is required to avoid a hazard. During hours when housekeeping personnel are off duty, either the maintenance staff or the unit staff should take responsibility for cleanup.

The hospital is responsible for providing housekeeping staff and equipment sufficient to do all work expeditiously and for training housekeeping staff in proper procedures. Housekeeping employees should be made aware of their own safety responsibilities: to safely use the equipment pro-

vided, to know and understand the safety rules and regulations applicable to the housekeeping department as well as the department(s) in which they work, and to watch for hazards and to report them. The safety rationale for each procedure should be explained in a way that each employee understands. Lists such as those in figures 20 through 22, at the end of this chapter, are useful ways of making general instructions available. Such instructions should be prepared according to the hospital's specific requirements. It may be necessary to print the instructions in more than one language.

Electrical equipment

Electrical power equipment, a frequent source of incidents involving support service staff, should be handled only with dry hands. Before cleaning, power equipment should always be disconnected. Extension cords should be pulled out by the plug, only after the equipment has been switched off.

Lighting equipment should be checked every day, and burned-out bulbs and tubes replaced. Electric lamps should be unplugged before they are wiped with a dry-damp cloth. Bulbs, fluorescent tubes, and other glass fixtures should not be changed while a patient is directly underneath. Overhead lamp fixtures should be swung away from patient-occupied areas before they are cleaned, to protect patients from falling dust and possible shattering glass. Special care must be taken to prevent breakage of fluorescent tubes.

Caution must be exercised in the use of a scrub machine where water is likely to enter electrical receptacles. Such receptacles should have moisture-resistant fittings. Operators should wear insulated boots and gloves.

Special instructions should be followed where electrical cables are strung across floors or near x-ray apparatus, electronic equipment, transformers, control panels, and the like.

New personnel must demonstrate proficient use of power equipment before being permitted to operate it in patient areas. The supervisor should be prepared to remove the plug of power equipment immediately from the electrical outlet until the employee demonstrates the ability to control the equipment. This is especially important when training new employees in the use of rotary floor-buffing machines.

Before unidentified spillages are removed, a staff professional from the laboratory should determine whether a hazard such as possible pathogenic, radioactive, or mercury contamination is involved.

Cleaning and polishing agents

Only the specific amount and type of cleaner for a particular job should be used. Excessive quantities or the wrong type may cause dermatitis, slipping, or fires, or cause the cleaned article to deteriorate. Only relatively safe organic-solvent degreasing agents and spot removers should be used. The flash point should be at least 135 °F. The toxicity TLV (threshold limit value) should be as high as that of methyl chloroform—350 parts per million. Use of gasoline, benzene, and carbon tetrachloride should be prohibited.

The least toxic and the least flammable kinds of spot cleaners should be used for removal of water-immiscible substances. High-flashpoint solvents or relatively low-toxicity liquids such as methyl chloroform are recommended. Abundant ventilation, short exposure periods, and proper containers for cloths are essential, even if the solvent has a "safety solvent" or similar label.

Cleaners should not be mixed. Some mixtures may produce hazardous gases or violent reactions. For example, chlorine bleaches mixed with such substances as vinegar, toilet bowl cleaners, or ammonia will produce chlorine dioxide, which is extremely toxic. Such "thirsty" chemicals as lye may react violently with water. Pouring of water into acids or alkalies may cause a spray. The mixing of acids and alkalies may produce a violent reaction.

Skin contact with caustics and degreasing agents, such as lye, drain cleaners, or methyl chloroform, should be avoided. Even diluted lye solutions can cause skin burns. Caustics are particularly dangerous, because the skin-burning sensation is slower than that from acids. Grease solvents can readily defat hand tissue, and ugly wounds result after repeated exposures. Clothing that has been splattered with chemicals should be promptly replaced; even relatively safe flammables can readily ignite it, because cloth reacts in much the same way as the wick in a kerosene lamp. Phenol can be lethal if allowed to remain in contact with the skin.

If foreign substances spray into the eyes or on the skin, first aid should be given by flushing with considerable quantities of water, not chemical neutralizers, for at least 10 minutes. Medical attention should be sought promptly after flushing. If possible, a physician should be asked to examine the victim while the flushing continues.

Careful attention should be given to the selection of slip-resistant waxes. For example, water waxes should contain colloidal silica. Purchases of such materials should be cleared with a staff professional from the laboratory, because there are times when buffing of floors in patient care areas might spread infections.

Special instructions should be provided for the proper cleansing of conductive floors. Floor coatings may negate the electrical conductivity. Any floor coatings used on conductive floors must be approved by the director of the department in which they are used, and a check for conductivity must be performed by the engineering staff.

Containers for cleaning agents should be labeled and should not be too heavy, too large, or made of unsafe or incompatible materials. Flammables should not be handled in glass containers or in incompatible plastic containers. Liquids should be transferred only to containers that have been purged of noncompatible substances. Sufficient void space to permit adequate expansion of the liquid should be allowed. Flammable liquids should be handled in approved safety cans.

Waste Disposal

Every day hospitals generate many kinds of waste in large amounts that require constant disposition. Each kind of waste requires particular attention.

Waste receptacles should be placed next to each patient's bed at all nurses' stations and offices and throughout the hospital in areas where visitors will have access to them.

Containers and other equipment should be readily cleaned and should be small and light enough to handle easily without strain. They should be constructed from noncombustible material, preferably steel, which is more likely to contain any outbreak of fire than aluminum, magnesium, or plastic and does not produce toxic smoke. Containers should have at least ½ inch of space between the base of the basket and the floor.

Large containers for collecting and storing waste and lids for these containers should be constructed of thermosetting material, which does not produce toxic smoke when burned. Collection-type containers should never be kept in unconfined areas, such as corridors or receiving areas. They should be kept within a confinable space, such as a utility room equipped with a door or some other type of smoke barrier.

Refuse containers should be marked with the name of the area to which they belong, so that they remain there. This arrangement prevents the problem of containers being used in infectious areas one day and in the kitchen the next day.

Where their use is permitted by law, trash chutes should be properly designed. They should be sealed off if they create jamming hazards. Loading doors should be located in soiled-equipment areas or in closets separated from corridors or clean areas; they should be tightly fitted with flexible gaskets. Trash chutes should be equipped with self-closing doors; the catches must hold securely and be electronically interlocked to prevent the opening of more than one door at a time. Chutes should discharge to a receiving room that is provided with exhaust ventilation and is separate from the incinerator charging room. The chute itself should be under negative pressure, so that air will flow into and not out of it. Combustibles and hazardous wastes, such as infectious, chemical, or radioactive waste, should not be discarded in chute systems. Requirements for sprinkling systems in trash chutes should be checked to ensure compliance with the appropriate Life Safety Code referenced by jurisdictional authorities.

Garbage grinders should be an approved type that can be cleaned easily. They should be equipped with backflow preventers, impellers, flywheels that resist corrosion and jamming, and a deflector made of elastomeric material. All should be equipped with a protective screen, which must be in place before the grinder can be actuated.

Personnel who collect waste and trash and dispose of it should:
■ Wear gloves of fabric or heavy-duty rubber.
■ Never dig into a wastebasket. Close plastic liners securely before transferring a wastebasket's contents to collecting receptacles. Grasp a wastebasket by the sides and tip to let contents fall into the receptacle.
■ Empty ashtrays into a container with a small amount of water.
■ Dispose of broken glass so that no one is harmed during any stage of the waste-handling process. A separate container labeled "Glass Only" is helpful. Fluorescent tubes should be broken into covered containers.
■ Know the hazards of each area, for it cannot be assumed that safety precautions have been taken. For example, staff of a nurses' station could improperly dispose of hypodermic needles, and laboratory staff could put chemicals in unidentified cans.
■ Not collect waste in areas where food is being prepared or served, in patients' rooms during mealtimes, or at any time that would disturb the delivery of patient care.

Chemical, pathogenic, and radioactive spills require immediate attention, as follows:
■ **Chemical spills** should be absorbed with suitable material, such as sand. The material should be placed in a suitable closed container and the container marked and removed directly to the proper disposal site. The floor, equipment, and furniture should be cleaned with a neutralizing agent by employees wearing suitable protective equipment. Suitable absorbent materials and neutralizing agents should be designated by the safety director or another qualified staff member.
■ **Pathogenic spills** should be cleaned up immediately by employees wearing protective masks, gowns, and gloves. Suitable disinfectants should be applied immediately, the area restricted, and the packaged waste removed directly to the disposal site.
■ **Radioactive spills** should be handled immediately by the radiation safety officer. See figure 15, chapter 8.

Waste should be removed from the hospital frequently and before trash receptacles overflow. Large bags should be carried or wheeled away; they should *not* be put into trash chutes, where they could jam and ignite. Bulky waste should be removed from buildings at least once by the end of each work shift or as often as the availability of work force permits. Bulk refuse containers should be shut tightly. Isolation trash containers should be located where the public cannot come in contact with them.

Many hospitals use incinerators to dispose of waste material. The incinerator room, which usually is located outside the main hospital building, should be locked when no one is present, and access to the room should be limited to incinerator attendants.

Waste should be separated before it is sent to the incinerator station. Glass items and pressurized cans should be separated out, and the cans punctured. Chemicals should be put in special containers, never in containers used for conventional waste. Nonroutine waste should be delivered by hand to the incinerator station, and its nature described to the incinerator operator. This practice eliminates the need for the station attendants to sort the waste to ensure that it contains no freshly etherized waste, ether cans, chemicals, pressurized cans, and glass.

For safety's sake, a face shield, impervious gloves, and long-sleeved clothing buttoned to the neck should be worn during loading of the incinerator. Operators should change coveralls daily. Special care should be taken against the possibilities of infectious contamination and of backfire caused by etherized materials or aerosol cans.

Incinerators should be of the high-temperature type and be equipped with auxiliary fuel burners. They should be fitted with appropriate air pollution controls and ensure complete destruction of pathological materials.

Laundry

The laundry department is responsible for the safe and proper collection, cleaning, and distribution of linens within the hospital.

The soiled-linen sorting and washing area in the laundry should be separated from the clean-linen processing area, from patient rooms, from areas of food preparation and storage, and from areas in which clean material and equipment are stored. Commercial linen processing companies contracted by the hospital must ensure that clean linen is completely packaged and is protected from contamination when delivered to the hospital. Whether the health care facility handles its own laundry or contracts with an outside firm, soiled linen should be placed into bags or containers at the site of collection and separate containers should be used for transporting clean linen and soiled linen.

The laundry area should be arranged and operated so that so that work flow and pathways for transporting clean linen and soiled linen are separate to minimize the possibility of contaminating clean linen.

Although isolation rooms use disposable linens to an extent, contaminated linens must be handled so that no one has to touch the linen itself after it leaves the isolation ward. Isolation linens should be sorted in the isolation ward and soiled linens put in water-soluble plastic or mesh bags. These are then placed in a second bag made of canvas or plastic, which is marked to indicate that its contents are contaminated and are from an infectious area.

All such specially marked bags should be segregated from the rest of the linen and handled in one operation. The laundry attendant should use tongs to remove the contaminated bag from its canvas or plastic shell and should deposit the water-soluble or mesh bag inside the washer without touching anything en route. The tongs should be sterilized before they are used again.

There is always the possibility that the outer bags containing contaminated linen will be damaged and allow contact with their contents. For this reason, some hospitals require that bags containing contaminated laundry be taken directly to the laundry room from the infectious area, instead of permitting these bags to be put down laundry chutes or through the routine linen collection process.

Employees should be instructed to use only the equipment that they are trained and authorized to operate, to check safety devices at the start of each work cycle, to use scoops and containers to handle cleaning compounds, to make sure lids are closed, to balance loads in extractors, to open valves on steam lines with great care, to shut off equipment before making any adjustments or repairs, and to avoid touching hot surfaces and standing beneath suspended loads.

Before clothing is removed from the dryers, cooling air should be turned on to prevent burns and to keep the clothing from igniting after it has been folded. Wool blankets may ignite and should be cooled before folding.

Lint is flammable and should not be left to accumulate on overhead duct work, pipes, wiring, lighting fixtures, or the floor. Lint and wax accumulation at the mangle-operating temperature of about 340°F. can be a fire hazard, particularly if the operator fails to turn off the steam supply at the end of the shift.

In order to prevent injuries to laundry employees, equipment should be maintained and inspected regularly. Twice a year, condensate tanks should be pumped up until they overflow, to show that vents are clear. Flatwork rolls should be inspected at regular intervals for hairline cracks. Electrical lines should be checked regularly for corrosion. Hot-water tanks should be checked for corrosion. To extend the life of such tanks, they should be opened once a year and the inner surfaces coated with rust-preventive paint. Any corrosion spots uncovered should be filled by deposits of weld metal, not stoppered with plugs.

Moving parts lower than 7 feet above floor level should be enclosed. Steam or hot water lines should be insulated if they are lower than 7 feet from the floor or if they are in an area higher than 7 feet where maintenance personnel may come in contact with them.

Insect and Pest Control

The control of insects, rodents, and other vermin is a problem in every hospital, although such pests are rarely incriminated in disease outbreaks. They enter the hospital by way of packing cartons, food deliveries, or crevices in the building. Although control programs will inevitably entail the use of pesticides, it is important that their use is minimized by eliminating the opportunity for pests to enter the building, sources of harborage, and food sources.

Control programs can be contracted to professional pest control operators, or the hospital can develop its own program. If the hospital contracts for control service, it should ascertain that the operator selected is licensed by appropriate authorities and should inquire into the operator's reputation in the community. His operation should be checked constantly by the hospital engineer. Such monitoring includes examining the types of materials used and the manner in which the program is carried out. Particular attention should be given to toxicity of pesticides used in sensitive areas, such as those for food service and patient care. The pesticide operator should be well versed regarding safety and should follow directions on labels closely.

If the hospital chooses to operate its own pest control program, it must make certain that the staff is properly trained. Those involved should attend training courses provided by health agencies or universities and, if possible, become registered with local authorities as pest control operators. University extension services often provide useful pesticide control programs and necessary training for pest control operators.

The following guidelines are suggested for a safe and effective pest control program:

■ Whether the institution uses the services of a pest control company or establishes its own program, specific guidelines for the use of the pesticides must be formulated. Only EPA-regulated pesticides should be used in the hospital.

■ Personnel must document the ongoing program.

■ Pesticides should be used according to manufacturers' precautions and directions.

■ Personnel must follow state, county, and local health codes.

Food Service

Hospital food service employees suffer about 20 percent of the total disabling injuries received by all hospital employees. The most frequent injuries are burns, cuts, and falls. The hazards of the food service department are many and include considerable handling of glass and crockery, sharp instruments, power machinery, pressure vessels, and heating elements.

Training of all new employees and review training for all regular employees are important functions of the food service department managers. Special attention must be given to personnel who are unable to read job instruction rules and operation manuals.

Although cautious, trained workers are the primary source of safety in the food service department, factors such as cleanliness, proper clothing, good housekeeping, proper quality and arrangement of equipment, and preventive maintenance contribute in large measure.

Receiving and storage

Adequate storage space should be provided for foodstuffs in process and in storage. Safe and sanitary working conditions cannot be maintained in a crowded area.

Pest control is one of the most important duties of the food service department. Insecticides and poisons, along with cleaning powders, should be stored in rooms separate from the storage room for foodstuffs. If sodium fluoride is used for insect control, it should be tinted blue and segregated, so that it is not mistaken for sugar, salt, or other seasoning.

Shelving should be ample and strong. Heavy and bulky materials should be kept on lower shelves. Employees should be provided with steps, stands, or ladders to reach upper shelves safely. Climbing on shelves should be forbidden.

Personnel should be instructed in safe lifting procedures; back injuries are frequent among handlers of bulk produce. Dollies and hand trucks should be provided for handling of materials bulked in burlap bags, crates, boxes, or barrels.

Stairs, rails, loading docks, and similar facilities in the receiving room should be kept in good repair. These busy areas are subject to frequent damage and should not be allowed to deteriorate.

Walk-in refrigerators and freezers should have buzzers or alarms on the inside. When an employee enters a cold-storage room, a sign indicating "Person Inside" should be posted on the outside door, to prevent fellow employees from locking it. An illuminated sign can be interlocked with the light switch as an additional safety precaution.

Food preparation and cooking

Cutlery should be kept in good condition. Proper kinds of knives, skewers, cleaners, and other cutlery should be provided so that no one uses hazardous substitutes. Knives should be used with extreme caution. Personnel should cut away from the torso and should not hack. Cutting edges should be turned away from the body when cleaning or drying a knife. Cutlery should be kept sharp and should be cleaned and checked for burrs after sharpening. Knives should be returned to storage after use and should be stored separately in magnetic racks.

All cooking should be done under a range canopy. Grease filters in the canopy should be washed at regular intervals, but not during cooking operations. Removing the filter allows unfiltered oil vapor to coat the ducts and raises the threat of food pollution from duct drippings. Special care should be taken when frying food in grease. Guidelines to prevent grease fires are listed in figure 23.

Pop-off safety valves and gauges on pressure equipment and coffee urns should be kept in working order. All pressure vessels should be vented before the lid is removed.

Utensil handles should be kept away from burners and pilot lights and from extending over the front edge of the range, where they may be burned. Oven doors should never be left open, as they are a tripping and bumping hazard. To prevent burns, employees should assume that all pots, pans, stoves, steam kettles, coffee urns, and pipes are hot and should use dry, fire-resistant mitts or potholders.

Exhaust fans should be run whenever food is being cooked, to prevent the buildup of highly flammable oil vapors. The exhaust system should be designed so that the exhaust fan control will shut off automatically upon sensing a fire in the duct and so that the dampers will close at a fixed temperature. Requirements for automatic fire-extinguishing systems on exhaust hoods should be checked to ensure compliance with applicable codes. Although the fan is wired to enable it to shut off automatically, it should also be wired to allow for manual control. The fan switch and its instructions should be well marked.

Containers of food to be served should be arranged in steam tables so that servers do not have to reach across them. Containers should be tilted away from the person and then inserted into the well of the steam table. Before cleaning steam tables, dishwashers, dishwarmers, and such equipment, the steam should be shut off and the equipment permitted to cool enough to be handled. Steam tables should be shut off when they are not in use.

Serving

Food service employees who serve meals to patients should:

■ Observe feeding schedules, so that food carts can be cleared quickly.

■ Make space for a tray before taking it into the patient's room.

■ Serve no foods that have been subject to unsanitary handling or into which broken glass may have fallen.

■ Not overload trays or liquid containers. Place the heaviest objects and liquid containers in the center to keep them from falling or spilling.

■ Keep food covered when in transit.

■ Clean up spilled food promptly.

■ Remove the tray as soon as possible after the patient has finished the meal.

■ Be cautious when wheeling food carts. Keep to the center in corridors; use extra care at intersecting corridors and at swinging doors. In passing through doorways, always pull the cart, not push it through the door.

■ Not let the cart block corridors or doorways. Keep large swivel wheels in line with the cart, so that they do not trip anyone.

■ Operate electric carts in a safe manner. Check their cords and plugs. Be sure that grounding fittings are provided.

China and glassware

Broken china or glass should never be picked up with bare hands; it should be brushed into a pan or collected under dampened paper or cloth. If the broken glass is in a sink, the sink should be drained before the glass is removed. Glass or china should not be put in the pot sink; it may be broken by metal pots.

Chipped ware of any kind is both unsafe and unsanitary and should be discarded. Broken glass should be deposited in receptacles other than those used for paper or routinely emptied by hand.

China should be stacked with like sizes together. It should not be stacked near the floor or where it is subject to contamination from floor splashes.

Machines

All power equipment should be used cautiously and only by authorized personnel. Slicing, chopping, and mixing machines and other equipment should have guards, which should be used each time the machine is operated. Attachments should be firmly secured. After a machine has been turned off, food should not be removed until all moving parts have stopped.

A mixing machine should be stopped before testing, stirring, or moving its contents. A nonmetallic spatula should be used, and all beaters and bowls should be securely fastened.

When cleaning a meat slicer, the cleaning motion should be from the center of the blade to the rim, using a mesh glove. The blade can be kept stationary by holding one side of it with a protective cloth.

Employees should never place their hands inside a garbage disposal unit. If retrieval of silverware or other items becomes necessary, the operator must turn off the machine's power and keep the switch under his or her supervision.

All electrical equipment should be grounded with either a three-way plug or a separate ground wire. Electrical equipment, especially cords and plugs, should not be handled by employees with wet hands. Employees should not attempt to pry out burned toast from a toaster until the device has been unplugged and cooled.

Dishwashing

Sinks should be provided with drain plugs that allow the drain of a sink to be opened without having to reach to the bottom of the sink.

When washing glassware, utensils, and china, employees should:

■ Keep glassware separate from metal utensils. See that knives on mesh trays point in the same direction.

■ Not use steel wool to clean food-handling ware. Use scouring pads designed for such work, or a stiff brush.

■ Inspect pots and pans for loose handles.

■ Alert the pot washer to pans that have just been removed from the oven.

■ Before cleaning the dishwasher, turn off the steam and cool the interior by spraying it with cold water.

■ Report any signs of skin irritation to the supervisor, particularly if the skin has been exposed to dishwashing detergents.

Floor care

The following rules will help reduce floor hazards in the food service department:

■ Floors should be kept clean, dry, uncluttered, and free of broken tiles and defective boards. Such care reduces tripping hazards as well as the possibility of contamination.

■ Care should be taken to keep wet mops, cloths, and used tea or coffee bags and strainers from dripping across the floor.

■ Leaking or sweating pipes should be reported to the supervisor.

■ Spillage should be mopped up immediately with a clean mop. If spillage occurs during rush periods, powdered feldspar or a commercial compound can be sprinkled on the floor.

■ A "Wet Floor" placard should be posted to alert all personnel. Steps taken on wet floors should be short and unhurried.

■ Floor drains should not be permitted where contamination by sewage backflow is a possibility. All floor drains should be periodically filled with fresh water to prevent fumes and odors from seeping into the kitchen area.

Central Service

The central service department furnishes most of the nondrug supplies for the nursing, surgery, emergency, laboratory, x-ray, and outpatient departments. Sterilization is generally considered to be the main function of the central service department.

Instruments, operating packs, trays, and so forth are normally sterilized by autoclaving, which consists of heating with pressurized steam exceeding 121°C. (250°F.) in a stainless steel pressure tank. Particular attention must be given to the maintenance of autoclaves to provide continuous, troublefree operation. Cleaning and maintenance of the chamber drain screen and the exhaust system are crucial to ensure that air will not be trapped in the chamber. Frequent inspection of gauges, thermostatic devices, thermometers, and other appurtenances must be made to further ensure reliability. Gauges and pressure release valves need to be checked against standard test gauges. These items are essential to the hospital's preventive maintenance program. Equal attention must be given to plumbing connections. Proper installation of vents, drains, and air gaps or siphon breakers prevents contamination of the interior of the autoclave chamber.

Many articles, particularly plastics and lensed instruments, are damaged by 121°C. (250°F.) temperature. If sterilization of such materials is required, it is necessary to provide an autoclave equipped for the injection of ethylene oxide (EO). EO sterilization procedures vary, depending on the materials to be processed. For example, EO concentrations range from 450 to 1,000 milligrams per liter. Other factors that vary are relative humidity, from 30 to 50 percent; temperature, from 21.1 to 60°C. (70 to 140°F.); and exposure time, from one to several hours. Because of the potential hazards of EO identified by the National Institutes of Occupational Safety and Health, stringent controls should be placed on procedures and ventilation.

Because EO has both toxic and mutagenic properties, it should be used only when another sterilization process would be less effective or more toxic. The following control measures will minimize employees' exposure and the contaminant risk.

■ The EO sterilization process must be done in an approved (commercial) sterilizer.

■ All personnel operating EO sterilizers must be completely oriented to the EO process: the gas injection and ejection mechanisms, chamber residual, product residual, handling of materials, safety factors, and hazards associated with EO.

■ All EO sterilizers and aerators, or materials to be aerated at ambient conditions, should be located in a restricted area so that access by unauthorized personnel is prevented. This restricted area, which includes the recess room, if appropriate, should have a mechanical air-ventilation system. If the gas sterilizer is a built-in model (extended through the wall), the recess room must have an exhaust ventilation system and be under negative pressure (airflow into room). The air exhaust should be directed to the outside atmosphere. If the gas sterilizer is a portable model, it must be used in a room that has negative pressure (exhaust ventilation system), and the exhaust air should be directed to the outside atmosphere.

■ All EO cylinders must be stored in a special area that meets appropriate building codes and the gas manufacturer's temperature specification. The tank must be secured (chained) at all times.

■ There must be a manual shut-off gas valve between the gas cylinders and the line that feeds gas to the sterilizer. This valve should be located on the end of the feed line that attaches to the cylinder. (This is not necessary if the gas sterilizer uses a single-copy gas canister.)

■ When the sterilizer cycle is completed, the door should be cracked open about 3 to 6 inches. Then, a 15-minute waiting period should be imposed before the items are removed from the chamber.

■ Protective gloves (cloth) should be used when removing items from the sterilizer.

■ Persons responsible for operating the gas sterilizer, changing the cylinder, and providing maintenance should attend an in-service program of instruction relating to the EO process.

■ A preventive maintenance program for the sterilizer should be established.

Accidental excessive exposure to EO by either inhalation or skin contact should be recorded and reported to the medical department.

Figure 20. Attention to equipment and care in handling it contribute to the safety of everyone in the hospital. The reminders listed here are suitable for posting in work areas.

Equipment Safety

■ Read the instructions that accompany a new piece of equipment before using it.

■ Carry portable equipment such as a mop or broom close to the body to avoid injuring anyone.

■ Station equipment out of the way. Never permit it to block exits, fire doors, fire extinguisher or fire hose cabinets, stairwells, or elevators.

■ Clean equipment after use. Turn buckets upside down to dry thoroughly. Mops and cleaning cloths should be changed with each shift.

■ Keep equipment in good repair: nuts and bolts tight, broken parts repaired or replaced.

■ Report broken equipment immediately, remove it from service, and label the equipment as defective until reparied. Do not put broken equipment in a storage area containing operable equipment.

■ Make sure electrical equipment is in working order and is grounded when in use. Do not use adapters. When using electrical rotary cleaning machines on wet floors, make sure all wiring and connections are sound.

■ Wear rubber-soled shoes or rubber slipovers to prevent slipping.

■ Do not clean ramps with power equipment.

■ Make sure an adequate number of various sizes of ladders are available and in good repair. Set the ladder firmly in position, and never stand on the top two rungs or steps. Do not use chairs, tables, or other furniture as stools or ladders.

Figure 21. Regular and careful attention to floors throughout the hospital promotes safety. This list of reminders is suitable for training-period handouts and for posting.

Floor Care

- Make sure corridors, aisles, and passageways are clear at all times.

- Mop up fluids, including rain and snow near doorways, immediately.

- Determine the nature of spills, and clean them accordingly. Display ''Wet Floor'' signs prominently when floors are washed, waxed, sealed, or stripped.

- Mop areas so that there is a dry passageway. Half of a corridor should always be free for traffic. All equipment should stand in the section being cleaned.

- Make sure wet areas are marked. ''Wet Floor'' signs should be placed at the beginning, middle, and end of the section being mopped. Such signs should be displayed whenever floors are washed, waxed, sealed, or stripped.

- Before leaving a work area temporarily, remove water pails from floors or stairs, secure equipment, and pull out all plugs.

- Schedule floor care in heavy-traffic areas to correlate with periods of least traffic, and clean only a small section at a time.

- Maintain floors on a schedule to prevent wax buildup and resulting slippery conditions.

- After floors have been cleaned, all furniture should be returned to its original position and all bed casters should be locked. Wrongly placed beds may lead to wrong identification of patients; mislocation of other furniture may cause tripping hazards.

- Wear rubber footwear when stripping and refinishing hard-surface floors.

- During wet weather, put rubber mats or runners near entrances. Do not use carpet runners on top of carpeting.

- Put down absorbent walk-off runners at the point where carpeting that has just been shampooed joins a hard-surface floor, so that slippery shampoo residue can be removed from people's shoes before they walk on hard-surface floors.

- Provide absorbent mats for patient rooms adjacent to the corridor being cleaned, and warn patients of wet floors.

Figure 22. Carts are designed to expedite work, so they should be kept ready for use, with every item in its prescribed place.

Equipment Cart

■ Load equipment and supplies on the cart in prescribed order.

■ Move the cart carefully in corridors, keeping to the center and looking ahead.

■ Move carefully when approaching corridor intersections, stairways, elevators, and standing groups of people. Move carefully on ramps.

■ Pull the cart through swinging doors. Do not push the cart through.

■ Keep hands away from the cart's sides when pushing it.

■ Never leave the cart, equipment, or supplies where anyone could bump into or trip over them.

■ Report repair requirements immediately.

■ Never ride on the cart or permit others to ride on it.

Figure 23. The following guidelines will help to prevent grease fires in the food service department.

Preventing Grease Fires

- Keep appliances such as deep-fat containers, broilers, ovens, chicken fryers, ranges, and grills from accumulating a film of grease, which, in turn, collects dust and lint. Such a buildup can be ignited by the pilot flame.

- Remove grease drippings from broiler trays immediately after each use; overheated grease can ignite. Do not reuse deep-fat oil too often; excessive use of an oil results in a chemical change that can make a relatively safe liquid highly flammable.

- Keep the oil level of deep fryers at least 3 inches below the top. Sudden immersion of frozen or wet produce releases water into the oil and may cause foaming, overflow, or ignition of the oil vapors.

- Remove spilled fats, oil, sugar, sauces, and other flammable substances from grills or ranges. They may overheat, vaporize, and ignite.

- Know how to operate the fire extinguishers, canopy, fans, and the sprinkler system. To smother a grease fire in a pan or container, use a snug-fitting lid. To extinguish it, use bicarbonate of soda, salt, or special grease absorbents. Water or flour makes a grease fire spread and should never be used.

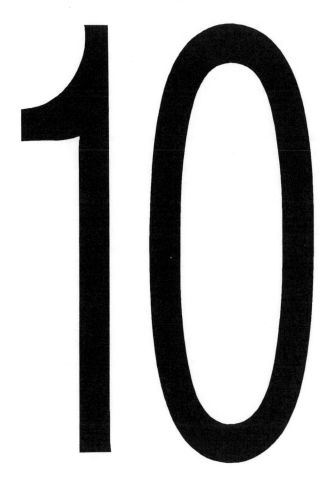

The goal of hospital engineering—the effective operation and maintenance of plant and equipment—is essential to safety. Lives rely directly on the safe operating conditions of the structure, systems, and equipment of the hospital.

To ensure the correct, precise functioning of the entire hospital complex, hospital engineers and maintenance personnel must be thoroughly familiar with a myriad of devices, machines, and work procedures. All sorts of equipment, from beds to CT scanners, are potential causes of injury to patients and employees.

Another possible source of injury to employees is the level of noise that may emanate from certain areas of the physical plant. Figure 24 at the end of this chapter outlines the steps a hospital should take to prevent hearing loss or damage to employees whose work exposes them to high levels of noise for prolonged periods.

Organization and Responsibility

The engineering department is responsible for plant operations and maintenance, which include equipment, the physical plant, utilities, electronic communication, and medical instrumentation. Organizing these related engineering and maintenance functions has become increasingly challenging as hospitals continue to grow.

Operation and maintenance are, for the most part, technical procedures performed by trained persons. Staff outside the engineering and maintenance department, patients, or visitors should never fix or otherwise tamper with anything, but should refer problems and adjustments to the department. For this purpose, maintenance requisition forms (see figures 25 through 27) should be readily available throughout the hospital.

Because of their complementary responsibilities, close cooperation between the engineering and the housekeeping departments is essential to the continuous safe operation of the hospital.

Hand Tools and Equipment

Tools used by engineering and maintenance personnel are the source of many types of injuries. Neglected minor hand wounds from improper use of tools compound the dangers from such injury.

The shop superintendent can build job instruction in hand tools around four basic principles: (1) have the right tool for the job; (2) use it correctly; (3) keep it in good condition; (4) put it away properly.

Having the right tool for the right job means that the employee should know which tool is appropriate for the job to be done and that the tool must be available. Tools should be purchased by a staff member who knows what engineers and maintenance personnel require. Also, they should be purchased in sufficient quantity so that employees are not tempted or required to use improper substitutes.

Tools should not be abused by being used for tasks other than those for which they were designed. For example, wrenches should not be used as hammers; files and screwdrivers should not be used as tools for prying. Misuse of tools leads to their rapid deterioration and, more important, is an unsafe practice that can cause injury.

Supervisors should not assume that all employees know the *proper* procedure for using common hand tools. Individual or departmental review sessions may be required. There is a proper procedure for the use of hammers and screwdrivers, just as there is for syringes and hemostats.

The good condition of a tool is as important to the safety of the user as it is to the effectiveness of the job done with it. Tools require care to prevent loss and deterioration. They should be kept free of rust and damage. Knives and other tools must be kept sharpened, and the handles and striking faces of hammers, chisels, and other impact tools must be kept tightly secure. The mushroomed head of a hammer or chisel is a serious menace to the eyes. The toolbox is the safest way to carry tools and to keep them together on the job. Edged tools should not be thrown with others into a common workbox or onto a bench; instead, they should be encased in protective leather pockets. The availability and serviceability of tools can be vital in an emergency.

The hospital should work out a policy on the ownership of hand tools and equipment. If any of these items are to be personal property, agreement should be reached on standards of maintenance. Substandard equipment is a safety hazard.

Ladder Safety

Wood ladders should be straight-grained, thoroughly seasoned, and free of shakers, decay, or injurious knots. They should never be painted; a periodical coating of linseed oil is recommended because it prevents drying of the wood, yet permits a visual check on the ladder. After coating with linseed oil, the ladder should not be used until the oil has been fully absorbed and the ladder is no longer slippery.

Metal ladders should not be used around electrical circuits or in places where they might come in contact with electricity.

Ladders should be kept clean; dirt might conceal defects. It is a good policy to scrape mud and debris from shoes before the ladder is climbed.

Care should be taken not to place ladders in front of a door that opens toward the ladder unless the door is locked, blocked, or guarded. Ladders should never lean against glass or plastic. Public areas where ladders are being used should have warning signs or be roped off.

Users should face the ladder both as they climb and as they work. Users should not lean too far to the side of the ladder and should never stand on the top two rungs. If materials must be handled, they should be hauled up by rope and bucket. Paint buckets should be held to the ladder rung by S hooks rather than by one hand.

For more information consult the standards of the American National Standards Institute.

Power Tools

Power tools should be used and maintained in strict accord with the manufacturer's instructions. All instruction sheets received with new equipment should be retained and filed.

Power tools should be operated only by authorized personnel, who should inspect such tools before using them. Any defects, such as frayed cords or broken plugs, as well as any minor shocks that occur while using power tools, should be reported to the supervisor.

All personnel should wear safety glasses when using portable power equipment or when using shop equipment. Guards should be kept in place on portable grinders and saws. Plugs should be disconnected from receptacles when changing the guards or accessories on a tool in use.

Machine Guards

Guards on machinery are necessary at the point of operation and on power transmission parts.

Specifically, machine guarding can also protect against or prevent injury from these sources:

■ Direct contact with the moving parts of a machine

■ Work in process such as kickbacks on a circular ripsaw, metal chips from a machine tool, or splashing of hot metal or chemicals

■ Mechanical failure

■ Electrical failure

■ Human error, prompted by such things as curiosity, distraction, fatigue, anger, or illness

Prior to ordering any machine, medical equipment, or device, guarding requirements should be reviewed. Manufacturers should be requested to supply guarding as a requirement of the purchasing agreement. However, whether a guard has been delivered with new equipment or has been designed by the chief engineer in the engineering department, it must conform to the standards of the American National Standards Institute or the state inspection department that has jurisdiction.

A guard should be considered a permanent part of the machine or equipment, should afford maximum protection, should prevent access to the dangerous area during operation, and should not weaken the structure of the machine. A guard should also be designed for the specific job and specific machine, with provision for oiling, inspection, adjustment, and repair of the machine parts. It should not interfere with efficient operation of the machine or cause any discomfort to the operator. It should be constructed strongly enough to resist normal wear and shock and withstand long use with a minimum of maintenance. It should be durable, resistant to fire and corrosion, and easily repaired. The guard itself should not present hazards, such as splinters, pinch points, shear points, sharp corners, and rough edges.

If a fixed guard cannot be used, an interlocking guard fitted onto the machine should be the first alternative. This guard can be of the mechanical, electrical, or pneumatic type, or it can be a combination of these types. The interlocking guard keeps the control that sets the machine in motion from operating until the guard is moved into position; thus, the operator cannot reach the point of operation or the point of danger. When the guard is open, permitting access to dangerous parts, the starting mechanism is locked. When the machine is in motion, the guard cannot be opened; it can be opened only when the machine has come to rest or has reached a fixed position in its travel.

Comprehensive details on specific guards are to be found in the *Accident Prevention Manual for Industrial Operations,* published by the National Safety Council.

Flame-Cutting, Welding, and Soldering

Flame-cutting and welding preferably should be done only in the maintenance shop. If it is done elsewhere in the hospital, the adjacent areas and related equipment such as pipelines, combustible structural materials, and so forth must be properly inspected beforehand.

Personnel should wear proper protective equipment, including gloves, hood, goggles, appropriate respirator mask, and apron. They should wear ankle-high shoes with trousers secured outside them to prevent molten material from falling into the shoes. Adequate screening and warning devices should be set up to prevent eye injuries to workers nearby. Authorization to perform hot work should be obtained from the chief engineer before any welding or cutting is done. If flame-cutting, welding, or soldering is being done in a high-traffic or a high-risk area, an employee should be stationed there to act as a fire-watcher.

Acetylene gas tanks should be capped at all times when not in use. They should be stored upright and secured with a chain or other form of holding device. They should be kept from heat and flame. Smoking and open flame should be prohibited in areas where acetylene gas tanks or flammable liquids are located.

Containers of flammable liquids or empty containers that previously contained flammable liquids should be thoroughly decontaminated before they are welded. Such procedures are described in *Safe Practices for Welding and Cutting Containers That Have Held Combustibles,* published by the American Welding Society.

While soldering, personnel should wear gloves and either goggles or a face shield. Sleeves should be kept rolled down, shirt collars buttoned, and trouser legs over the shoe tops.

Solder should be melted in a thoroughly dry pot or a ladle secured against upsets. Chilled solder or moist objects should never be put in a hot solder pot or ladle.

Before beginning to work on any container, the employee should check to be sure that all explosive vapors have been removed. The temperature of a soldering iron should never be tested by holding it near the hands or face. Hot solder should never be removed from an iron by snapping the iron or throwing the solder.

Hot soldering irons should be placed on racks or holders away from all combustible materials. The current of the iron should be turned off before leaving the work area. The iron's cord and connection should be kept in good condition.

Painting and Spraying

It is important that a no-smoking rule be enforced in paint and wood shops and other locations where paints, thinner, and turpentine are used or stored. Proper and adequate fire extinguishers must be available in the paint shop. All lacquers and thinners should be kept only in safety cans approved by Underwriters' Laboratories. They should be stored in approved fire-resistant metal cabinets in accordance with state and local fire codes.

When spray painting, adequate protective equipment—air respirator mask, goggles, gloves, and so forth—should be worn by maintenance personnel. Spray-painting tools should be nonferrous and nonsparking. Paint spraying must be done away from areas having open-flame appliances, such as gas water heaters and ranges. Spraying in kitchen and laboratory areas also raises the possibility of contamination.

Gasoline-powered air compressors with paint spraying equipment should not be used indoors because of the potential fire hazard from the exhaust.

Paint-spray booths should be used in the spraying of paint, enamel, or lacquer. The booths must be in conformance with the state codes established to control occupational disease exposures and with local codes pertaining to fire hazards. They also should conform with National Fire Protection Association standard no. 33, *Spray Finishing Using Flammable and Combustible Materials;* the NFPA *National Electrical Code* requirements on electrical equipment in spraying areas; and American National Standards Institute standard no. Z9.3-1964, *Design, Construction, and Ventilation of Spray Finishing Operations.*

Electrical Safety

Safe electrical equipment must be provided. Outlets should be installed wherever permanent operations are to be performed. Extension cords used in operating rooms must comply with National Fire Protection Association standard no. 56A, Section 2484. Cord taps (plugs) should be purchased with hand pulls, to eliminate strain on the wiring connections. Electrically operated vending machines should be provided with a grounding cord and cap. Wiring and all other electrical equipment should bear the Underwriters' Laboratories label. Panel-board circuit identification directories should be kept current. Equipment should not be modified or circumvented, and apparatus or parts should not be exchanged unless staff has first checked the manufacturer's instructions or consulted with a biomedical engineer.

In all nonfixed electrical equipment furnished with power cords, any exposed metal parts not carrying current should be grounded through a special cord or plug. Equipment should not be used until all outlets can be converted to the grounding type. Equipment that is especially critical is:

■ Equipment used around moisture, such as water baths, physiotherapy equipment, drinking fountains, stirrers, and water pickup machines

■ Readily movable equipment used with or around moisture, such as centrifuges, ovens, and hot plates

■ An electrical supply of more than 150 volts

■ Hand-held motor-operated equipment

The wattage rating for lamps should be limited to the design value. Bulbs extending past the rim of the reflector present hazards to fire, burns, and shattering glass.

Electricians should not repair, service, or perform any operations on energized electrical lines or equipment except for testing of line voltage and current, cutting of power lines when they present an immediate hazard to life, and replacement of fuses in circuits of 150 volts or less. Only journeymen electricians should replace higher-rated fuses.

After a determination that power cannot be interrupted, work on circuits of more than 440 volts should be performed by a public utility contractor; work on circuits of 440 volts or less may be performed by a qualified installation electrician. If the voltage adjacent to equipment being worked on exceeds 250 volts, two or more electricians should be present. If it is necessary to switch off high-voltage circuit breakers or disconnect switches or other equipment to clear a supply feeder or apparatus, two qualified electricians should be present while switching is in progress.

Before machinery is worked on, the electrical controls should be shut off, tagged, and locked. Tags and one-key locks should be removed only by the person who originated their use.

All electrical workers should be trained in artificial respiration techniques.

Television installations should be approved by the building maintenance chief, who will determine the need for grounding and for lighting of protective devices.

Emergency electrical power should be provided for the public address system, telephone bells, fire pump, elevator lights, suction in the operating suite, resuscitation equipment, and so forth. A battery-operated wall-mounted emergency light in corridors will be sufficient to allow personnel to adjust to a power failure; its batteries should be tested at least monthly.

Further guidelines on electrical safety can be found in Article 700 of the *National Electrical Code,* in Section 52 of the *Life Safety Code* (NFPA no. 101), in NFPA no. 76A, and in pertinent ANSI standards.

Boiler and Heater Rooms

The greatest single safety need in the boiler room is a qualified person in charge, with a competent staff. Boilers can be operated efficiently and safely for many years, but only if the accepted rules of safety are followed and only if the boiler and piping system are kept in first-class operating condition through regularly scheduled operational inspections, proper maintenance, and repair.

A boiler should not be placed in service until an operating certificate has been obtained from the governing authority. After a new or used boiler installation has passed inspection by a qualified engineer, the custom in states having boiler laws is to stamp a state number on the boiler and to send a report to the state department having jurisdiction. A hospital should consult its attorney for guidance in complying with state requirements.

An adequately installed boiler should include the following:

■ Ample room for proper maintenance and for any expansion required by additions to the health care facility.

■ Ample lighting for reading of the water column, pressure gauges, valves, and so forth.

■ Two or more exits with doors opening outwards, one at either end of the boiler.

■ Stairs, ladders, and runways around boilers that extend 10 feet above floor level, kept free of grease and with walking surfaces of expanded metal.

■ Brick, concrete, or steel stacks equipped with grounded lightning arresters. Steel stacks should not be mounted directly on the boiler.

■ Safety glass or glass with guards on water gauges.

■ Signs prohibiting any but authorized persons from entering the boiler-room area.

Boiler safety valves should be set in accordance with the code specifications of the American Society of Mechanical Engineers. Only a qualified boiler inspector or a person specially trained should change the setting of a safety valve. Valves should be hand-tested at least once a day.

Steam safety valves of hot-water-heating boilers should be set at 15 pounds above the water working pressure of boilers in which such pressure is not greater than 50 p.s.i. Hand testing of these safety valves is unsuitable, because it may cause them to leak. They should be removed from the boiler for testing and then be reinstalled.

Blowing down of boilers in service should be done at frequent and regular intervals to remove dirt, sludge, and precipitated chemical solids and should be carefully regulated, especially in large boilers. On small installations, the blowdowns should be done at least once during each shift or each 8-hour period.

Oil or grease introduced into a boiler during repair should be removed. A thin film of oil on the shell or tubes of a boiler insulates the metal from the water and can cause the metal to fail. An extremely important responsibility is to locate and prevent any oil entering the boiler from sources other than repair work. Personnel may have to boil out the contaminated auxiliary equipment to clean it of oil deposits. A safety check on boiler flue gases should be conducted regularly to ensure that they have no perceptible level of carbon monoxide, which could cause a boiler explosion.

In many hospitals, one engineer has charge of the heating and hot-water systems. So that the boiler is not left unattended in the event of this engineer's illness or absence, the hospital administrator should be certain that someone else in the plant is trained to take over in an emergency.

A substitute operator should be taught the operations of the safety valve, water column, water-feeding apparatus, and fuel supply and firing apparatus. He should know how to check the water level in the boiler and how to start or stop the water-feeding apparatus. In coal-using hand-fired plants, he should know the location of the dampers in the boiler. In plants with mechanically fired boilers, he should know how to locate the control apparatus and how to shut off the equipment in case of emergency.

Manufacturers should be consulted concerning emergency procedures to be followed in the boiler room.

Standards of the American National Standards Institute that pertain to boilers include no. Z21.13-1977, *Gas-Fired Steam and Hot Water Boilers*, including addenda Z21.13a-1979; and no. Z21.52-1967, *Gas-Fired Single Firebox Boilers*, including addenda Z21.52a-1968. State codes also should be reviewed.

Inspection and Maintenance Schedules

A well-kept schedule of periodic inspection and testing should be set up and adhered to strictly. Appropriate criteria and a record-keeping system based on the following standards should be enforced.

Boilers. Every steam boiler should be inspected annually in accordance with applicable sections of the American Society of Mechanical Engineers *Boiler Construction Codes* and possibly more stringent local codes. The inspections should include any steam boiler used for hot-water supply if (1) its pressure exceeds 15 p.s.i. or (2) its pressure is below 15 p.s.i. but its gravity return is unassisted. Inspections should be made by qualified personnel commissioned by the National Board of Boiler and Pressure Vessel Inspectors (NBBPVI) of the ASME. They should be performed by an outside firm rather than by hospital staff engineers. A certificate of approval should be posted at the boiler.

Unfired pressure vessels. Every unfired pressure vessel operating at a pressure above 60 p.s.i. and having a capacity of 15 gallons should be inspected annually by a person qualified by NBBPVI and in accordance with the ASME *Boiler Construction Codes*. The inspectors should make an external observation of safety devices and other appurtenances. If the vessel has a manhole, the inspectors should also make an internal inspection. A certificate should be posted at the vessel.

Hot-water tanks and heaters. Temperature and pressure-relief devices on hot-water tanks and heaters should be inspected monthly.

Steam-heated equipment. Urns, kettles, vegetable steamers, autoclaves, and the like should be inspected semiannually for operation of thermostats, steam traps, safety valves, control or pressure-reducing valves, and vacuum breakers.

Lightning protection. Lightning protection equipment should be inspected annually for condition of air terminals, conductors, bonding grounding connections, and system resistance to ground, in accordance with NFPA standard no. 78, *Lightning Protection Code*.

Elevators and dumbwaiters. Elevators and dumbwaiters should be inspected according to ANSI standard no. A17.1-1981, *Safety Code for Elevators, Dumbwaiters, and Moving Walks*, and no. A17.2-1979, *Practice for the Inspection of Elevators* (Inspectors' Manual), including supplements. The inspections should be conducted by an authorized inspector and at intervals not exceeding 3 months for power passenger elevators, 6 months for escalators and power freight elevators, and 12 months for hand elevators and power and hand dumbwaiters.

Incinerators. Semiannual inspections should be made to check the posting of light-off procedures and existence of operating instructions, condition of guards around charging ports if located in the floor, presence and condition of flues or stacks, presence and condition of stack spark-arrester screens, condition of sprinkler heads and hopper doors in trash chutes, general condition and functioning of fire doors, methods of handling waste, and handling and cleaning of trash cans, in accordance with NFPA standard no. 82, *Incinerators*.

Surgical suite. Tests should be performed as described in NFPA standard no. 56A for conductivity of floors, equipment, and materials; continuity of grounding; effectiveness of the ground indicator system; and so forth.

Safety showers. A monthly inspection should be made to determine that the water supply is on, that actuation by the chain and lever is proper, and that silt accumulation does not interfere with effective operation. Unless silt has accumulated or unless it is impossible to determine whether the water is shut off, flow tests need not be made. However, each installation should bear an inspection tag certifying that the actuating device is in operating order (that the chain is not tangled or otherwise not functioning properly and that the water supply valves are open).

Autoclaves. Autoclaves should be inspected semiannually to ascertain any faults, such as inaccurate recording by pressure and temperature gauges. A sterility indicator should be used as a cross-check. Safety valves should be blown off at least monthly to ascertain that they are in working order.

Figure 24. The Hearing Conservation Amendment to the Occupational Noise Exposure Standard requires employers to establish a hearing conservation program wherever employees are exposed to noise of 85 decibels or above for an 8-hour day. The following mandatory components of such a program can be posted as a reminder to employees and their supervisors.

Hearing Preservation

■ Hearing tests (audiometric testing) must be made available to all employees who are exposed to noise of 85 decibels or above for an 8-hour day. Annual audiograms are required for all employees so exposed who wear hearing protection and who show significant hearing loss as determined by a physician, otolaryngologist, or audiologist.

■ A choice of hearing protection must be made available to all employees exposed to noise of 85 decibels or more. Employees exposed to 85 decibels who show significant hearing loss and those exposed to 90 decibels without such loss *must* wear hearing protection provided by the employer.

■ An annual training program must be given to all employees exposed to 85 decibels or more for 8 hours. Training must address the effects of noise on hearing, types of hearing protection available, and audiometric testing.

■ Employees or their representatives must be allowed to observe the noise monitoring process that measures noise exposure in a particular area.

■ Employees or their representatives must be provided with copies of the hearing conservation program and must, on request, be provided with records of exposure and of audiometric testing.

For more detailed information concerning OSHA requirements, the hospital is encouraged to consult the Hearing Conservation Amendment (46 FR 4078) to the Occupational Noise Exposure Standard (29 CFR 1910.95).

Figure 25. This four-part color-coded work request form is for work that is done for a specific department and charged to that department. Such a form should be readily available in every department. One copy is for the maintenance department, another for maintenance deparment office control, another for the building and grounds manager, and another for the department in which the request originates. Reprinted with permission of Elmhurst Memorial Hospital, Elmhurst, IL.

Work Request Form

	CONTROL NO.	PRIORITY

TOTAL LABOR HRS._____DOLLAR AMT._____
TOTAL MATERIAL COST_____
THIS EXPENSE WILL BE CHARGED TO YOUR DEPARTMENT.

FROM		DATE	TIME
DEPARTMENT	WORK TO BE CHARGED TO:	LOCATION	
PERSON MAKING REQUEST	TELEPHONE EXT.	VERBAL REQUEST PLACED ____ YES ____ NO	

ITEM

BRIEF DESCRIPTION OF WORK TO BE PERFORMED:

ENGINEERING DEPT.:-WORK PERFORMED   MATERIAL USED:

(Front of form)

(Figure 25 continued)

MAINTENANCE SERVICE
PRIORITY

JOB DESCRIPTION	EQUIPMENT DESCRIPTION
1: Critical Safety Work	1: Plant Utilities
2: Preventive Maintenance	2: Key Operating Equipment
3: Corrective Maintenance	3: Multiple Operating Equipment
4: Shutdown Work	4: Mobile In-Plant Equipment
5: Routine Maintenance	5: Service Facilities
6: Sanitation	6: Office Facilities
7: Housekeeping	7: Material Handling Equipment
8: Quality Improvement	8: Building (Functional)
9: Cost Reduction	9: Grounds

PRIORITY KEY: 1-1 Critical Safety Work-Plant UTILITIES = TOP PRIORITY

9-9 Cost Reduction-Grounds = LOWEST PRIORITY

PRIORITY SEQUENCE: 1-1 thru 1-9, -2-1 thru 2-9, -3-1 thru 3-9, etc.

(Back of form)

Figure 26. This two-part maintenance service order is used for work done throughout the hospital in repairing the building and its related equipment. The originator sends the original to the maintenance department and retains the copy. Reprinted with permission of Elmhurst Memorial Hospital, Elmhurst, IL.

Maintenance Service Order

	CONTROL NO.	PRIORITY

NAME	DATE	HRS.	O.T.	DEPT.	DATE REQUESTED
				REQUESTER	

MATERIAL USED

WORK PERFORMED

EMPLOYEE SIGNATURE_____

(Front of form)

(Figure 26 continued)

MAINTENANCE SERVICE
PRIORITY

JOB DESCRIPTION

1:   Critical Safety Work

2:   Preventive Maintenance

3:   Corrective Maintenance

4:   Shutdown Work

5:   Routine Maintenance

6:   Sanitation

7:   Housekeeping

8:   Quality Improvement

9:   Cost Reduction

EQUIPMENT DESCRIPTION

1:   Plant Utilities

2:   Key Operating Equipment

3:   Multiple Operating Equipment

4:   Mobile In-Plant Equipment

5:   Service Facilities

6:   Office Facilities

7:   Material Handling Equipment

8:   Building (Functional)

9:   Grounds

PRIORITY KEY: 1-1 Critical Safety Work-Plant UTILITIES = TOP PRIORITY

9-9 Cost Reduction-Grounds = LOWEST PRIORITY

PRIORITY SEQUENCE: 1-1 thru 1-9, -2-1 thru 2-9, -3-1 thru 3-9, etc.

(Back of form)

Figure 27. Preventive maintenance forms usually specify the equipment to be checked and how often. All forms show a number that corresponds to a master sheet kept by the maintenance department. This enables the department to evaluate the preventive maintenance program from time to time. When completed and filed, these records demonstrate to inspecting agencies how well the hospital complies with applicable codes and standards. The seven categories of preventive maintenance forms that the maintenance department uses to initiate work can be color-coded. These categories are: general maintenance; electrical work; plumbing; heating, ventilating, and air conditioning; fire equipment; food service; and laundry. Reprinted with permission of Elmhurst Memorial Hospital, Elmhurst, IL.

Preventive Maintenance Form

Date _____   Week & Shift _____

SMOKE & FIRE DOORS: CHECK ALL SMOKE & FIRE DOORS
TO BE SURE THAT THEY WORK PROPERLY.   M.S. No. _____

Job Description	B	1	2	3	4	5	—	East Building									
Handles																	
Locks																	
Hinges																	
Latches																	
Magnetic Holders																	

Time

Work Performed_____

Additional Work Needed _____

Material Used _____

Period _____ Weekly _____Signature _____

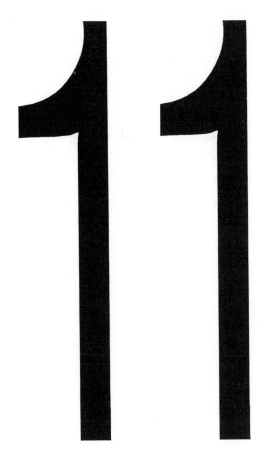

A medical disaster occurs when an incident produces casualties of such number that the routine methods for patient care are not adequate. There is no event affecting commercial or industrial organizations that is comparable to the demands placed upon hospital and community resources during a disaster. The disaster's impact on the community's medical resources is immediate and dramatic, whether or not the hospital is prepared to care for a mass influx of casualties. A disaster requires the hospital to maintain essential care and services for its current patient load while simultaneously serving as the focal point for post-disaster medical care.

The primary objective of disaster planning is to ensure efficient utilization of local health resources so that they will not be overwhelmed during the initial disaster relief period when emergency medical care and first aid are needed. In a disaster, hospitals may be called upon not only to care for the injured but also to provide for the needs of persons who are temporarily without food or shelter. Responding effectively to these demands requires comprehensive planning between the hospital and those community organizations and agencies that have emergency response capabilities.

This chapter offers a broad view of the factors to be considered in planning for disasters. It provides an outline of general principles to guide plan development, a series of checklists for use in evaluating a hospital's existing disaster plan, and a list of references for more detailed information. The responsibility for preparing a detailed disaster plan, designating the internal capability to implement the plan, and then integrating the plan with other community resources rests with the hospital disaster committee.

Historical Perspective

General disaster planning was stimulated by World War II and experienced a renewed interest in the early 1950s, when nuclear devastation became a frightening reality. The urban riots of the 1960s again raised concern for the treatment of mass casualties, but the focus centered on facility-specific planning rather than a communitywide, coordinated response. Studies conducted in the late 1960s and early 1970s pointed to deficiencies in facility and community preparedness for handling natural and other disasters. Federal legislation adopted during this period established requirements for ambulance personnel training, the use of radio frequencies for communication between emergency vehicles and the hospital, and areawide coordination and medical resource planning.

The Emergency Medical Service Systems (EMSS) Act of 1973 (Public Law 93-154) provided grant funds for the development of emergency medical service (EMS) systems to demonstrate the effectiveness of regionalized resource management in responding to medical disasters. The EMSS Act stressed the importance of communication links among the EMS system components and encouraged the use of a universal emergency telephone number (911) to solve the problem of citizen access to emergency services.

The Disaster Relief Act of 1974 gave the President authority to provide financial assistance and federal-agency support to state and local governments for Presidentially-declared or state-declared disasters.

The Federal Emergency Management Agency (FEMA) monitors disaster occurrences, surveys disaster relief requirements, evaluates the damage, and recommends appropriate federal assistance.

At the state level, more than half of the states have legislation creating statutory authority for provision of prehospital care to victims of medical emergencies by nonphysicians (paramedics).

Although the majority of mass injuries are the result of transportation accidents, explosions, building collapses, fires, and weather incidents, events such as the nuclear reactor incident at Three Mile Island (PA), the eruption of Mount St. Helens (WA), and derailments of tank cars containing toxic chemicals have surfaced the need for flexibility in disaster plans to handle hospital and community evacuation, as well as treatment of a large number of radiation-exposure victims and victims experiencing respiratory problems. The possibility of having to treat these types of victims is not restricted to a particular geographical area, because many industries use radioactive isotopes

in their manufacturing processes and transport nuclear wastes and dangerous chemicals on highways and railways. The many excellent publications on disaster preparedness include *Emergency Handling of Radiation Accident Cases.*

For many years, disaster planning has been both a standard for accreditation by the Joint Commission on Accreditation of Hospitals and a requirement by most states for licensure. The specific components and the required frequency of plan rehearsals differ for external disaster planning and internal disaster planning. More details on external and internal disaster planning, as well as procedures for disasters involving radioactive contamination, can be found in the *Accreditation Manual for Hospitals,* published annually by the JCAH. The hospital should also consult state licensure requirements, which may be more stringent.

Preparing a Disaster Plan

A detailed disaster plan prepared specifically for the hospital, then rehearsed after in-depth staff training, provides a firm foundation for disaster preparedness. The disaster planning process is neither short nor inexpensive, but it is a necessary effort. Figure 28 is a disaster preparedness plan checklist that can be used to critique the hospital's plan. The plan of another hospital in the community also can serve as a useful model.

Developing a plan should be the responsibility of a committee established by hospital administration. The committee should secure the input of hospital departments and local authorities and agencies. The hospital disaster committee, which may be a subcommittee of the safety committee, should include members of the hospital administration and medical staff; volunteers; members from each shift of the nursing, engineering, security, housekeeping, and food service departments; and the safety director. Representatives from local fire and police departments and from other emergency services in the community should also be included.

In determining the type of information and procedures to be included in the hospital's disaster plan, the committee should assess the probability and potential severity of natural and other disasters that may occur in the community environment. When a hospital's catchment area includes an airport, for example, the hospital must be prepared for aircraft disasters. Similarly, a hospital located in a heavily industrialized area must assess the potential for major industrial accidents occurring in the manufacturing and chemical processing plants in its community. Hospitals should be informed of all toxicologic and treatment data for hazardous chemicals, pollutants, and wastes handled in such plants.

Although the plan should address specifically those types of disasters with the highest probability of occurring, the plan should not be so detailed that it is inflexible for adaptation to a wide variety of disaster conditions. There must be one plan that works on all three shifts, on weekends, and on holidays. A plan that can effectively mobilize resources and staff and that can guide management decision-making during the initial post-disaster reaction period requires ongoing training, evaluation, and revision. Maintenance functions include instruction of employees in disaster procedures and in scheduling, coordination, and documentation of drills.

After the plan has been prepared and given a trial, hospital administration should designate someone such as the safety director to maintain it. This person should also be the hospital's liaison with community authorities and local emergency services. Plans require constant updating, especially when the hospital undergoes major structural changes in medical services. The plan should be comprehensively reviewed annually.

External Disasters

The hospital's written plan for the timely care of emergency casualties from an external disaster should be based on its own capabilities and should be developed in conjunction with local civil authorities and other medical agencies.

With respect to preparations within the facility, the hospital should have adequate medical and supportive materials and a system of notifying and assigning additional personnel as needed to expand the facility's emergency care activities. These preparations should include a plan for converting suitable space (separate from emergency services areas) to provide triage, observation, and treatment. There should be restricted use of elevators, well-identified access and entrance routes to the hospital, a public information center, and sufficient security to minimize the presence of unauthorized individuals and vehicles.

The preparations should also include a method for identifying patients who can be discharged immediately. A special medical record or tag should be used for disaster victims, and there should be a mechanism for physician identification. This information should be included in the patient's permanent record.

External coordination and support responsibilities include a preestablished radio communication system for use when telephone communications are out or overtaxed; disaster-site logistical and medical triage support as needed, coordinated through a unified medical command; a system, including transportation, for the prompt transfer of patients to the facility most appropriate for rendering definitive care; and a means of keeping local police, rescue squads, and ambulance teams informed of the hospital's capabilities and resources.

Realistic disaster drills should be conducted twice a year and should involve medical staff and other hospital personnel, as well as other community emergency service agencies. A written report and evaluation of each drill, including recommended corrective actions, should be maintained.

Components of external disaster medical care

The four components of disaster medical care are (1) scene response, (2) transportation, (3) hospital facilities, and (4) communication and command. The following brief description of each component is intended to guide the hospital in identifying the subcomponents that need to be addressed in preparing a workable and coordinated disaster response plan.

Scene response refers to the efforts conducted at the disaster scene in supplying treatment to people who have suddenly become patients as a result of a disaster. This treatment may be in one or all of four forms: triage, supportive and stabilizing treatment, definitive treatment, or no attention required. During the initial confusion that invariably occurs in the first minutes after a disaster, rapid response of a well-coordinated medical team that has received mass-casualty triage training can provide effective triage and the stabilizing and supportive care necessary prior to the patient's arrival at the hospital.

While there is no question that physicians are needed at the disaster site, it is important to enumerate how many and what kind are needed. The major emphasis should be directed toward the rapid transport of casualties to hospitals. With that objective in mind, the function of the field physician becomes triage, with actual care kept to a minimum. A senior physician must be designated who can decide on the amount of care that will be rendered at the scene and who can supervise the triage function. It is impossible to gauge a physician-patient ratio because the degree and the type of casualty determine the amount of effort required by the physician. For example, whereas a single physician could easily perform triage for 25 to 50 uncomplicated injuries, one physician could not attend a similar number of burn patients. Each planning area should have a number of these disaster teams ready to supply extra physicians if needed or to cover multiple disaster sites that may arise simultaneously.

The role and responsibilities of the disaster-team coordinator should be outlined. The coordinator should be a permanent employee, either administrative or medical, who is completely familiar with what is expected at the scene. The coordinator should be responsible for in-hospital operations to ensure that ancillary measures are taken for the support of overall patient care.

The plan should specify the type and amount of supplies and medications that will be sent to the scene. Provision must also be made for patient recordkeeping at the scene, and transportation for both personnel and supplies should be spelled out. Local authorities generally are responsible for coordination of nonmedical activities at the disaster site.

The prime concern with respect to **transportation** is the transporting of patients by ambulance. Conveying the injured to hospitals is of paramount importance, but provision must also be made for the movement of the team and supplies to the disaster site. Vehicles for moving the team must be available at all times, whether they be specific standby vehicles or part of an existing fire, police, or ambulance service. Ideally, a van or bus should be on standby in which equipment and supplies are checked according to a schedule and arranged so as to be identified and used quickly.

As much as possible, ambulances should be utilized before other improvised vehicles that depend on personnel unfamiliar with patient transport procedures. Because it is not always advisable to depend strictly on ambulances, thought should be given to alternative means of transportation that can be easily employed for ambulatory injured persons. Planning for the quick notification and response of these additional vehicles is important. Effective two-way communication between the disaster site coordinator, the ambulance and other vehicle drivers, and hospital staff must be maintained. Transportation to and from the disaster scene must be coordinated with the local police department.

The equipment for emergency vehicles will depend on an assessment of the need for general life-support services as opposed to mobile intensive-care services. Designing and supplying emergency vehicles should be accomplished in close cooperation with the hospitals to which patients will be transported. Because the useful life of the typical ambulance vehicle is less than four years, it is important to maintain liaison with community emergency services regarding current needs and to revise the hospital plan accordingly.

The third component of external disaster medical care is **facilities**. Depending upon the resources available, each hospital and, subsequently, each community must examine its medical capability to determine at what point its normal resources will be exhausted and at what point even extraordinary measures will be insufficient.

The hospital in immediate proximity of the disaster should evaluate whether or not it should send a medical team to the disaster site, because it will receive the most victims.

While the number of beds available for disaster victims may be adequate, the way in which they are used is important. A small hospital may be totally occupied when called upon to care for six or eight seriously injured persons, but may be able to handle three to four times this number of less seriously or ambulatory injured victims.

In the planning process, therefore, hospitals should be categorized into three groups. The first group would include those hospitals prepared and able to take care of the most seriously injured, and it is to these that the majority of such patients should be sent. The second group would be sent the less serious cases, including many of the ambulatory injured. The third group would receive only ambulatory patients requiring basic emergency care. Even though hospitals in the third group would be small hospitals, in some cases their bed availability might permit receipt of patients from the larger medical centers following secondary triage. Although this plan may seem oversimplified, it must be remembered that, at least initially, patients will arrive at hospitals randomly. Planning should prevent the difficulties involved when the small hospital is sent many seriously injured patients while a large center is inundated with minor injuries that could be treated as well elsewhere.

Among the useful criteria for categorizing hospital capabilities are factors such as the size of the emergency department, operating suites, and staff; overall bed capacity; and ancillary services. Changes in facility services or capabilities should be reflected in the disaster plan. Additional information regarding categorization can be found in the American Medical Association publication entitled *Categorization of Hospital Emergency Capabilities* and the *Accreditation Manual for Hospitals*, published by the JCAH.

In areawide disaster responses, it is important that one entity, whether a sponsoring hospital or a governmental agency, take overall responsibility for the control of disaster response activities. Additional information concerning the disaster control responsibilities is contained in the following section on communications and command.

Communications and command is the fourth component of external disaster medical care. While disaster-scene response, transportation, and hospitals comprise the resources needed to get the disaster victim from the site of injury, an efficient communication and command system ties these resources together.

In order to minimize the confusion that inevitably results in the initial few minutes of a disaster response, the operational control of the system by means of radio communication should be clearly defined in the disaster plan. The govern-

mental agency or hospital facility that forms the training, continuing education, supply, and policy base must retain control over direction of remote field personnel. To be effective, the communication system must encompass much more than the ability to converse. It must also be a command system with a central coordinating point where information can be received, evaluated, and used in making decisions and taking action.

The disaster plan must designate such a location and must further designate a person and alternates who will have overall charge of disaster operations. The location for a command communication center should be in a place that is normally in 24-hour operation and can be adapted readily to the disaster coordinating role. In the majority of cities, this center will be part of the fire or police communication system, because these are in continuous operation and are staffed by personnel trained to work in stressful circumstances. Although police or fire communication systems have obvious advantages, it should also be recognized that they are not primarily health and hospital oriented. It is essential that someone completely familiar with area hospital and transportation resources and with some medical knowledge direct the activities of the communication center, preferably from it, but, if necessary, by communication from the actual scene.

Ideally, a medical disaster control center should be incorporated as part of an ambulance dispatch office, because an ambulance service, run as an entity apart from police or fire services, will be accustomed to health and hospital activities. Furthermore, an ambulance dispatch center will have the necessary communication links, which ideally are direct telephone communication with each hospital, radio communication with each hospital and with vehicles, and direct radio and telephone communication with other emergency and municipal agencies. The ideal ambulance dispatch center will also have up-to-date information on the bed and emergency room status of all hospitals, thereby precluding the need for obtaining census information during the early stages of disaster response.

Whatever the center selected, the person normally in charge must have guidelines to follow, such as criteria for putting the areawide plan into effect and for immediate escalation of disaster efforts.

The disaster-team coordinator at the scene, in addition to seeing to it that the primary team function of triage and treatment is carried out, must also provide information on the need for additional help; on the degree to which the disaster effort must expand; and on the number, type, and tentative hospital assignment of patients. In return, the disaster-team coordinator must receive information about the status of the requests made, as well as the location to which hospital patients should be sent.

Hospitals must be kept informed about the disaster so that they can react accordingly and also can receive specific information as to the number and type of patients being sent to them. Hospitals must be able, in turn, to provide information as to their ability to treat and admit patients.

The transportation element must be coordinated by a communication system that is able to contact vehicles and to direct them to the appropriate hospital or treatment center.

Legal and insurance considerations

Because all the safety measures used in the hospital are generally not available at the disaster site, the legal ramifications of a disaster should be thoroughly evaluated in advance. Any disaster plan, therefore, should be reviewed by the hospital's legal counsel before it is accepted as final. As additional security for the hospital and its staff, a comprehensive review of the hospital's insurance coverage is advisable. Efforts to educate key personnel on liability problems will prove worthwhile. Potential legal and malpractice problems can be avoided in the design and implementation of the plan if all its features guarantee safety for the patient and guarantee that medical judgments will remain in the hands of those who are licensed to make them.

Staff alert

A hospital's ability to respond rapidly to a disaster depends on the time of day and the day of the week. Although the methods of alerting hospital staff vary from hospital to hospital, the basic alert system procedures are the same. Coded messages communicated over the public address system, coded light signals, and verbal messages

transmitted through personal paging receivers can be used to alert the general staff and key individuals within the facility.

When additional staff must be recalled from their homes, the use of existing portable receiver systems that have group alert activators through the switchboard operator avoids time delays in contacting key disaster personnel. Because staff notification and recall require a considerable amount of time if conducted by telephone, it is important that some type of pyramid or fan-out alert system be developed. One method is to alert department directors, who, in turn, are responsible for informing other members of the department. A more complicated system that has the advantage of releasing department heads for other disaster duties is the pyramid system, in which individuals who have no direct role in disaster activities take responsibility for alerting key staff on a predetermined priority basis, taking into consideration the role of the individual as well as traveling time. Some of the staff members contacted would be responsible for contacting other staff prior to departing for the hospital.

Using a hospital computer to maintain up-to-date employee addresses and telephone numbers will simplify the recall process. Since failure of the staff alert and recall system will significantly alter disaster response operations, it is important that the system be tested frequently and be maintained as part of the hospital's disaster plan.

Internal Disasters

An internal disaster plan should take effect when the safety and welfare of patients and staff is threatened as a result of fire, explosion, or any other incident that renders all or a portion of the hospital incapable of functioning. The plan should be developed with the assistance of local police and fire officials. It should include procedures for notifying appropriate authorities in the event of any disaster that disrupts normal hospital activities. Such events may include bomb threats, fire, natural phenomena, facility evacuation, and utility failure, including telephone service. The plan should specify evacuation routes and procedures and should provide for the management of casualties. All personnel should receive instructions on their assigned responsibilities and the use of alarm systems and signals. The internal disaster plan should receive maximum exposure throughout the hospital to ensure that all staff have the essential information readily available at their work stations.

Internal disaster plans should include provisions for dealing with the following various types of internal disasters that reduce the hospital capability to provide care for patients.

Fire

Effective staff training should allow each staff member to use firefighting equipment and to practice procedures for containing the spread of fire and smoke (see chapter 12). Fire drills should be held at least quarterly for each work shift in each separate patient-occupied building. A written record documenting an evaluation of each drill, including recommended corrective actions, should be maintained.

Fires can occur in hospitals despite extensive efforts to prevent them. Fire disaster planning should be a part of the hospital's fire safety program, which includes minimizing the chance of fire through inspections and surveillance; establishing and communicating the procedures to follow when discovering and reporting a fire; restricting the spread of fire; training on the use of fire extinguishers; evacuating patients; and maintaining codes and standards related to fire safety. Fire disaster planning and fire safety programs are covered in detail in chapter 12.

Power Loss

Health care institutions are dependent upon electrical power, so an outage of any proportion can be disastrous. As required by regulatory and accrediting agencies, hospitals have emergency generators that can be expected to function during public power outages, and they should continue to run smoothly.

But emergency generators are not always failsafe. During the massive electrical failure in the metropolitan New York City area in July 1977, hospitals experienced problems with their emergency generators such as overheating, automatic starting delays, and difficulty with transfer switches. A special task force investigation pointed to the need for formal, written, and supervised preventive maintenance of emergency generators and associated equipment; testing procedures that simulate actual power failure; a method to ensure that electrical loads connected to the generator do not exceed nameplate rating; adjustable timers with a bypass to delay transfer from the generator back to normal supply; and written institutional plans and training programs to cope with power failures. These considerations should be received within the context of code requirements of the hospital's jurisdiction and standards on emergency power by the Joint Commission on Accreditation of Hospitals.

Bomb Threats

Because of the hazards placed on patients in possible evacuation situations, bomb threats are particularly vicious and cruel. The hospital's first line of defense is the switchboard operator who receives the call. A trained person can often keep the caller on the line until the call can be traced and, in some instances, can coax information from the caller so that evacuation will not be necessary.

Anyone receiving a bomb threat phone call should:
1. Remain calm.
2. Devote one's entire attention to what the caller says, not even diverting attention to alert others.
3. Note the time the call is received.
4. Ask the caller for information not volunteered, such as when the bomb is timed to explode, where it is, what it looks like, what kind of explosive is used, and why the caller wants to harm the hospital.
5. Make notes of details, recording as much as possible the exact words of the caller.
6. Add to the notes any personal impressions of the call, such as the caller's familiarity with the hospital, voice and speech characteristics, background noise, and other particulars.
7. Promptly alert the responsible person in the hospital.
8. Turn the notes over to authorities.

Strikes

As the number of strikes and sit-ins among health care institutions has increased, primarily in urban facilities, disaster preparedness committees have considered the problem and have developed strike contingency plans. Unlike such natural disasters as floods and tornadoes, strikes usually are preceded by a negotiation period, which the hospital can use for crisis planning.

Long-range preparation for coping with a strike should include policies and procedures that anticipate a sudden large-scale reduction of the labor force. When the extent of the strike and the groups likely to participate become somewhat apparent, plans can be made for temporary reassignment of personnel and responsibilities and for subcontracting services that can be provided from outside the hospital. Laundry, laboratory, and many food services, for example, can be provided by outside firms, and a supply of easy-to-prepare frozen meals can be stocked.

Strikes present the possibility of violence and sabotage. Security and safety personnel should be given special training in handling these possibilities. Altercations such as picket-line confrontations should be treated as incidents, and an immediate and thorough report prepared. The injured, including strikers and pickets, should be treated.

Water and Fuel Shortages

The hospital's usual source of water could be interrupted or contaminated as a result of both natural and other disasters. The extent of the disruption should be investigated by contacting the local water department, which may serve as a source of emergency water supply. Recognizing that water and fuel are essential to most hospital functions, the JCAH states that a hospital's disaster plan should include preestablished mechanisms for immediate supply of certain major critical items such as water, food, and fuel. Although there are currently no specific requirements for on-site storage of water within a hospital, the JCAH states: "...there shall be a written plan for an emergency supply of water when the usual source of water is neither usable nor available. The plan shall include provision of water for sanitation purposes as well as potable water for life-support purposes. Failure to provide such water supply when needed carries the contingency of total or partial evacuation of patients from the hospital."

Few data exist on the actual quantities of water required for basic life support and for essential hospital services. At minimum, however, one quart of safe drinking water per person per day is an absolute essential. An additional quart per person will provide sufficient water for food preparation purposes. Water exposed to radioactive contamination should not be used unless it is approved by qualified radiological personnel or qualified civil defense officials as fit to drink.

The quantity of water used for clinical, dietary, and laundry services will vary from hospital to hospital. Figure 29 indicates the average amount of *hot* water used by a hospital per hour per bed.

The hospital plan should establish the priority uses of water during an emergency. Strict water conservation should be in effect. When contracting with a supplier of bottled water for disaster purposes, the hospital should coordinate with other hospitals in the community to ensure that a single supplier is not the sole source of water for all the community's hospitals or that the supplier has sufficient supply to meet all the hospitals' needs.

During this era of uncertain energy supplies, it is essential that hospitals anticipate and minimize the effect potential energy shortages will have on the hospital's ability to provide patient care services. Because all hospital functions will be directly or indirectly affected by shortages of various energy supplies, it is important that each department be represented in the planning process. The hospital engineer, as the individual most knowledgeable about energy systems and supplies, should have a major role in planning for and operating under an energy shortage situation.

In the planning process, the following steps should be taken:

1. Gather fuel-use data by each separate type of fuel, noting trends in seasonal consumption in order to gain a historical perspective on needs.

2. Determine, in order of importance, which energy-use systems are critical to patient care and which are for convenience; these priorities may change with the different seasons.

3. Assess the need for an alternative fuel capability in the event the primary fuel used by the hospital becomes unavailable.

4. Review and evaluate contracts with fuel suppliers to determine fuel allocation and priority procedures in the event of a shortage. (More than 30 states now have fuel allocation and curtailment plans in the event of a severe shortage. Information regarding these plans can be obtained from the state energy office or state public service commission.)

5. Develop an analysis of the impact on individual services of shortfalls of various fuels. Prepare

guidelines for continuing patient care services under moderate and severe shortage situations for periods of short and long duration.

6. Develop an energy-shortage action plan for the engineering staff to employ in reducing noncritical usage in a progression consistent with the severity of the shortage.

7. Develop a training program for hospital staff.

Figure 28. A checklist is useful for critiquing the hospital's disaster plan. Reprinted with permission of St. Elizabeth's Hospital, Chicago.

Disaster Preparedness Plan Checklist

Administration

1. Is there a committee that reviews the emergency operations plan?   Yes   No
   Name of committee: _____

2. Does this committee plan drills for all parts of the plan?   Yes   No

3. Date entire plan last reviewed: _____

4. Does the plan include:
   A. Mass casualty management plan   Yes   No
   B. Fire emergency plan   Yes   No
   C. Civil disorder plan   Yes   No
   D. Bomb threat plan   Yes   No
   E. Severe weather plan   Yes   No
   F. Electrical power failure plan   Yes   No
   G. Emergency water plan   Yes   No
   H. Telephone service failure plan   Yes   No
   I. Other emergency plan (specify):

   _____
   _____
   _____

5. Have these plans been reviewed and approved by:
   A. The medical staff?   Yes   No
      Date of last review by medical staff: _____
   B. The hospital's legal counsel   Yes   No
      Date of last review by legal counsel _____

6. Has a comprehensive review of the hospital's insurance coverage been conducted?   Yes   No

7. Dates of drills over the previous 12 months (specify type of drill and time):

   _____
   _____
   _____
   _____

Attach critiques of last three drills.

8. Is a complete manual available in:
   A. Administration   Yes   No
   B. Nursing service   Yes   No
   C. Emergency department   Yes   No
   D. Other (specify): _____   Yes   No

(Figure 28 continued)

Mass Casualty Management Plan

9. Can information about the disaster be received in several ways?   Yes   No
   A. List the ways information can be received: _____

   _____

       B. Can this information be verified?   Yes   No
         How? _____

10. Is specific disaster site information requested using a preplanned format?   Yes   No

11. Is the authority for implementing the hospital's disaster plan clearly defined?   Yes   No

12. Are the implementation steps for various levels of disaster response clearly specified?   Yes   No

13. Is the plan flexible enough to meet a number of possible conditions and circumstances?   Yes   No

14. Are key personnel to be notified clearly identified?   Yes   No

15. Is there a procedure for making the required notifications?   Yes   No

16. Is notification made by priority of need of service?   Yes   No

17. Is a place for assembly of recalled staff provided for?   Yes   No
   Location of assembly area: _____

18. Is the plan specific in providing facilities and staffing for:
   A. Triage   Yes   No
   B. First-aid cases   Yes   No
   C. Burns   Yes   No
   D. Definitive treatment areas   Yes   No
   E. Decontamination   Yes   No
   Other (specify): _____

   _____

   _____

19. Does the plan provide facilities and staffing for:
   A. News media   Yes   No
   B. Relatives of victims   Yes   No
   C. Auxiliary agencies   Yes   No
       Red Cross   Yes   No
       Police department   Yes   No
       Fire department   Yes   No
       Civil defense   Yes   No
       Salvation Army   Yes   No
       Social services   Yes   No

20. Are there provisions for expansion of inpatient facilities?   Yes   No

21. Are there provisions for the discharge of nonemergency outpatients?   Yes   No

22. Is there a defined location and staff for a command/control center?   Yes   No

(Figure 28 continued)

23. Is release of information to press specified and controlled?   Yes   No

24. Is release of information to community agencies controlled?   Yes   No

25. Is the function of the security staff clearly defined?   Yes   No

26. Are there provisions to augment the security staff?   Yes   No
    Attach the augmentation plan.

27. Are there provisions for limiting and controlling access to the facility?   Yes   No

28. Is there a plan for controlling and directing vehicle traffic?   Yes   No

29. Is the authority to initiate actions and/or make decisions clearly defined?   Yes   No

30. Are there provisions to control and maintain communications?   Yes   No

31. Is there a provision for augmenting telephone service?   Yes   No

32. Is two-way radio equipment available?   Yes   No

33. Is a messenger/runner service provided for in the plan?   Yes   No

34. Is there consideration of alternative means of communication in the event of primary system failure?   Yes   No
    Specify: _____
    _____
    _____

35. Is a reception area for incoming patients clearly specified?   Yes   No

36. Is there a plan for the recording of information and data?   Yes   No
    Attach copy of plan.

37. Is there a specified system for patient sorting by priority of care required?   Yes   No

38. Is there a system for identification of incoming patients?   Yes   No

39. Is this system compatible with the areawide plan?   Yes   No

40. Is there a specified medical record format for all incoming patients?   Yes   No

41. Are medical records controlled from reception to permanent filing?   Yes   No

42. Is there a plan for compiling of casualty lists and patient condition reports?   Yes   No

43. Are adequate records maintained for legal requirements, including:

    A. Payroll/accounting   Yes   No
    B. Census   Yes   No
    C. Police reports   Yes   No
    D. Coroner   Yes   No
    E. Patient accounting   Yes   No
    F. Postemergency critique   Yes   No
    G. Other (specify): _____   Yes   No

44. Is there a specified plan for collection and safeguarding of valuables and personal property of patients?   Yes   No

45. Is the admitting function controlled by specified procedures for the duration of the emergency?   Yes   No

116

(Figure 28 continued)

46. Is there a procedure for handling and control of:
   A. DOA casualties   Yes No
   B. Expirations in treatment areas   Yes No
   C. Expirations after admission   Yes No

47. Is there a specified plan for the transportation of patients to other medical facilities for specialized treatment?   Yes No

48. Are disaster supplies and equipment pre-positioned in designated locations?   Yes No

49. Is there a procedure for getting these supplies after duty hours?   Yes No

50. Are supply/equipment requirements reviewed at least annually?   Yes No
   Date of last revision: _____

51. Are supplies and equipment requirements specified in the plan?   Yes No

52. Has the medical staff, nursing staff, and other departments provided input into the supply and equipment requirements?   Yes No
   If no, explain. _____
   _____

53. Is there a master inventory of the pre-positioned supplies and equipment?   Yes No

54. Where is this master inventory kept?_____
   _____

55. Are all pre-positioned supplies and equipment accompanied by individual inventory listings?   Yes No

56. Is the control of supplies and equipment specified?   Yes No

57. Is there a control for periodic inventory and replacement of outdated items?   Yes No

58. Is there a provision in the plan for:
   A. Chemical contamination   Yes No
   B. Biological contamination   Yes No
   C. Radiological contamination   Yes No

59. Is the chemical, biological, and radiological monitoring and decontamination material prepositioned and readily available?   Yes No

60. Is the participation by civil and community agencies specified in the plan?   Yes No

61. Is information concerning the plan made available to the community?   Yes No

62. Are plans formulated to provide the services of clergy to patients?   Yes No

63. Is there a provision in the plan to assure that hospital staff can get to and from the hospital during the emergency?   Yes No

Fire Emergency Plan

64. Are all exit facilities:
   A. Correctly marked   Yes No
   B. Clearly marked   Yes No
   C. Unlocked from inside   Yes No
   D. Clear of debris and equipment   Yes No
   E. Connected to emergency lighting circuit   Yes No

(Figure 28 continued)

65. Does the plan include instructions on what employees are to do when they discover a fire? Yes No

66. Does the plan include instructions on what employees are to do when they hear the alarm? Yes No

67. Is there a clear line of authority to initiate action described? Yes No

68. Is there an evacuation plan? Yes No

69. Is the evacuation plan posted in a prominent location? Yes No

70. Does the evacuation plan include instructions on how patients are to be moved? Yes No

71. Does the relocation plan include:
     A. Horizontal evacuation Yes No
     B. Vertical evacuation Yes No

72. Does the manual include information on the fire alarm system? Yes No

73. Has someone been designated to direct firefighting personnel to the scene of the fire? Yes No

74. Have arrangements been made to relocate patients to nearby shelters until permanent arrangements are made? Yes No
     Relocation sites:_____
     _____

75. Have local authorities been familiarized with your facility? Yes No
     Date of last visit: _____

76. Have hospital personnel been trained in:
     A. Use of fire extinguishers Yes No
     B. Evacuation techniques Yes No
     C. Fire prevention Yes No
     Date of last class_____

77. Is a daily "head count" available so that all may be accounted for if a general evacuation is ordered? Yes No

78. Are fire drills conducted once per shift per quarter? Yes No
     Date of last drills:
     a.m. _____
     p.m. _____
     Nights _____

79. Are fire drills critiqued and reports maintained? Yes No
     Attach critiques of last three drills.

Civil Disorder Plan

80. Is the authority to initiate action clearly defined? Yes No

81. Are internal security procedures described? Yes No

82. Is there a procedure for obtaining information on:
     A. Extent of disorder Yes No
     B. Number of people involved Yes No
     C. Area of disorder Yes No
     D. Streets closed to traffic Yes No
     Attach copy of procedure.

(Figure 28 continued)

83. Is there a provision for getting personnel in and out of the hospital area? Yes No

84. Have assembly points been designated? Yes No
    A. Were local law enforcement agencies involved with the selection? Yes No
    B. Has a method of transportation from the assembly point to the hospital been clearly described? Yes No
    If no, explain: _____
    _____

85. Title of individual who has responsibility for assembly point locations: _____

86. Is this information made known to all employees? Yes No

Bomb Threat Plan

87. Was the plan developed in cooperation with local law enforcement and fire authorities? Yes No

88. Is there a procedure described when the threat is made by:
    A. Telephone Yes No
    B. Letter Yes No
    C. Note left on a door Yes No

89. Is the authority to initiate action clearly defined? Yes No

90. Is there a provision for search teams? Yes No
    What is the composition of the search teams? (titles only) _____
    _____

91. Is there a procedure described for removal of a suspect package? Yes No

92. Are all hospital personnel aware of the plan? Yes No
    Date of last inservice training: _____

93. Is there a provision for relocation of patients and personnel when a suspect package is found? Yes No

Severe Weather Plan

94. Are the types of severe weather described? Yes No

95. Is the authority to initiate action described? Yes No

96. Is there a provision for relocation of patients? Yes No

97. Is there a departmental notification plan? Yes No

98. Is there a plan to house personnel and visitors overnight? Yes No

99. Have all hospital personnel been made aware of the plan? Yes No
    Date of last inservice training: _____

Electrical Power Failure Plan

100. Is there a description of the location of emergency receptacles? Yes No

101. Have personnel assignments been described? Yes No

102. Is there a provision for testing of the generator? Yes No
    Date of last test: _____
    Attach test reports for past 3 months.

(Figure 28 continued)

103. Have all hospital personnel been made aware of the plan?   Yes   No
    Date of last inservice training: _____

Emergency Water Plan

104. Is there a description of alternative sources and how to obtain water?   Yes   No

105. Are water conservation measures described?   Yes   No

106. Have personnel been informed of the plan?   Yes   No
    Date of last training session: _____

107. Are there any problem areas that have not been covered in the questionnaire? Yes   No

108. Additional comments:

_____

_____

_____

_____

_____

Figure 29. This figure shows the average amount of hot water used by a hospital per hour per bed. The hospital can use this information to make an assessment of its hot-water needs for emergency purposes. For additional information on water use and temperatures, check with the local authorities having jurisdiction and with the Joint Commission on Accreditation of Hospitals.

Hot Water Use

	Clinical	Dietary	Laundry
Gallons, per hour per bed	6½	4	4½
Liters, per second per bed	.007	.004	.005

Source: *Minimum Requirements of Construction and Equipment for Hospital and Medical Facilities* (HRA 79-14500), published in 1979 by the U.S. Department of Human Services, Public Health Service, Health Resources Administration, Bureau of Health Facilities Financing, Compliance, and Conversion.

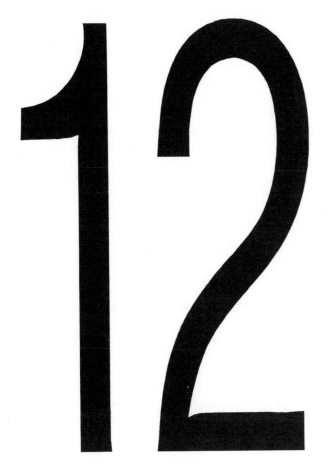

Despite staff vigilance, preventive maintenance of all equipment, and fire prevention training for all employees, fires are a constant threat in hospitals. All fires are potential disaster situations. Fires not only threaten the safety and welfare of patients, staff members, and visitors, but may reduce the hospital's ability to provide patient care services.

This chapter provides guidance in establishing a fire safety plan and program. The chapter includes a fire prevention and hazard detection checklist, recommended procedures for responding to fire disasters and restricting the spread of fire and smoke, information for staff training on fire-extinguishing equipment and patient evacuation techniques, and references from codes and standards pertaining to fire safety. When developing a fire safety plan and program, it is recommended that local fire authorities be consulted.

Organizing a Fire Safety Program

The first purpose of the fire safety program is to save life. A tailor-made program is needed for each hospital, and no plan can be adopted "as is" from another hospital or from any manual.

If a hospital does not have a fire safety program, it should develop one. With the help of safety engineers and the local fire department, the hospital should fully appraise its vulnerability to the consequences of fire. Plans should be made to fit the actual situation.

The following are the major steps in organizing a fire safety program:

■ **Establish a safety committee.** The hospital should use the existing safety committee or establish a separate fire safety subcommittee to develop and oversee the fire safety program. The subcommittee should include the chief executive officer or a designated representative, the safety officer, department directors, and selected supervisors from each work shift.

■ **Appoint a fire marshal.** The committee should appoint a committee member who is familiar with the requirements of the fire safety program to coordinate the program and act as a liaison with local fire officials.

■ **Appoint a fire brigade.** Each hospital should have its own fire brigade, at least one member of which should be on duty during each shift. The brigade should have a member directly responsible to the administrator and authorized to carry out the administrator's assignment. The local fire department may be able to help train fire brigades.

■ **Develop a fire safety manual.** The manual should stipulate emergency procedures, evacuation plans, fire safety policies and procedures, staff training, inspection frequencies, fire drill procedures, inspection and fire-drill evaluation reports, and the members of the safety committee and fire brigade.

■ **Train and orient staff.** All staff, including new personnel prior to assuming their work assignments, should receive training on fire prevention, extinguishment, and emergency procedures. All staff members should have the opportunity to operate a fire extinguisher; this can be done when extinguishers are serviced and recharged. The local fire department will assist in demonstration and training programs. The information provided in this chapter, coupled with the AHA book *Fire Safety Training in Health Care Institutions,* provides a sound basis for staff training on fire safety.

■ **Conduct fire drills.** Institutionwide fire drills should be conducted on all shifts at regularly scheduled intervals. The hospital's record of all drills should include an evaluation and recommended corrective actions.

■ **Conduct fire hazard inspections.** Inspections should be conducted throughout the hospital on a regular schedule to ensure compliance with codes, policy, and safety and fire prevention measures. Documentation of inspections and corrective actions implemented should be maintained in the fire safety manual.

■ **Investigate fire incidents.** Procedures and forms should be developed for follow-up investigations of fire incidents and for initiating corrective actions as required. Insurance company safety engineers will be helpful in establishing these procedures.

■ **Maintain a current library of applicable code requirements.**

The plan and program should be reviewed and revised as needed to ensure the safest possible environment for the hospital.

Codes and Regulations

The hospital should maintain an up-to-date library of applicable codes, regulations, and manuals pertaining to fire safety and disaster preparedness. It will be valuable during the preparation of initial detailed plans and as a ready reference for staff members and hospital officials.

The National Fire Protection Association (NFPA) annually publishes ten volumes of *National Fire Codes*, which contain codes, standards, and recommended practices. However, these codes have no regulatory impact unless adopted by the hospital's legal jurisdictions. It is important that hospitals be familiar with state and local fire codes and those required by the Conditions for Medicare Participation. The Joint Commission on Accreditation of Hospitals (JCAH) publishes its standards in the *Accreditation Manual for Hospitals.* Since JCAH and Medicare standards are reviewed and revised periodically, it is important that hospitals have the most recent applicable editions for ready reference in order to maintain the hospital's accreditation and licensure.

The JCAH standards, which provide references to specific NFPA standards, specify requirements related to fire safety and provide additional information to aid the hospital in interpreting each standard. The standards require compliance in each of the following areas related to fire protection and safety:

■ The facility is to be designed, constructed, equipped, and furnished in compliance with applicable codes, fire prevention codes, state and/or federal occupational safety and health codes and standards, and the specifically referenced edition of the NFPA *Life Safety Code.*

■ Documented evidence of structural safety in the form of a comprehensive statement of construction and fire safety is to be furnished by the hospital. Consideration is given to equivalency in meeting these requirements when an element of safety is provided as well as or better than the applicable standard, provided no other safety element or system is compromised or adversely altered.

■ Each building must have an electrically supervised and manually operated fire alarm system that automatically transmits an alarm throughout the facility and to the local fire department by the most direct means acceptable to the authority having jurisdiction. Some systems are designed to shut off designated fans in ventilation systems and activate protective doors and dampers.

■ Manual fire alarm boxes are to be distributed throughout the facility in readily accessible locations and in the normal path of exits from the building. The audible alarm must exceed the level of operations noise in the area. However, it is advisable to have a visual component of the alarm system in areas such as the boiler room, laundry, and kitchen to supplement the audible alarm signal.

■ Where provided, automatic fire extinguishing systems must be compatible with the area to be protected.

■ Automatic sprinkler systems that serve as both a heat-detection system and a fire-extinguishing system must be connected to the fire alarm system.

■ The establishment of a fire brigade in the hospital is recommended. For each work shift the brigade should be staffed with members who are well-trained and knowledgeable on the use of fire extinguishing equipment. Fire brigade members should know the specified procedures for shutting off oxygen and air-conditioning when such actions are not an automatic component of the fire-safety system.

■ Fire extinguishers must be of the type required for the class of fire normally anticipated in the area. Maximum travel distance to extinguishers must not exceed 75 feet in any area. The travel distance should be less in areas with an increased degree of hazard. A record of monthly extinguisher inspections and annual maintenance service must be maintained.

■ Automatic extinguishing systems must be installed on exhaust hoods, grease-removal devices, and ducts for cooking ranges.

■ Handling, storage, and disposing of flammable gases and liquids, nonflammable gases, and compressed-gas cylinders require special consideration as potential hazards and are addressed in detail in both the NFPA and JCAH standards.

■ Fire and safety systems that must be connected to the hospital's emergency power source to ensure adequate power within 10 seconds of failure of the normal power source include: egress

illumination (corridors, stairways, landings, and exit doors); exit signs and exit directional signs; alarms (fire, smoke, sprinkler, oxygen); hospital communications systems when used for issuing instructions during emergency conditions; and at least one elevator per bank of elevators. These requirements relate specifically to fire and safety systems. Other essential and life-support systems that must be connected to the emergency generator are listed in the JCAH's *Accreditation Manual for Hospitals* and the NFPA's code publication *Essential Electrical Systems for Health Care Facilities*.

■ A fire blanket and self-contained breathing apparatus are recommended for the clinical laboratory.

■ Written regulations governing smoking must be adopted, conspicuously posted, and made known to all personnel, patients, and the public. These regulations must include provisions that prohibit smoking in areas where flammable liquids or gases or oxygen are in use or stored; identify and clearly mark hazardous areas with "No Smoking" universally understood symbols and/or multilingual signs; prohibit ambulatory patients from smoking in bed; discourage smoking by patients confined to bed; prohibit smoking by patients classified as not mentally or physically responsible; require the use of noncombustible wastebaskets and ashtrays; prohibit smoking in areas where combustible supplies or materials are stored; and restrict smoking in surgical and obstetrical areas to dressing rooms and lounges.

■ Written electrical safety policies and procedures are required to ensure a safe environment free of the hazards associated with electrical failure and equipment malfunctions.

JCAH requirements for internal disaster planning appear in chapter 11. The JCAH *Accreditation Manual for Hospitals* and the NFPA *Life Safety Code* provide more detailed compliance requirements and equipment and construction specifications on each of the areas mentioned above.

The *Hospital Engineering Handbook* published by the American Hospital Association and NFPA codes provide useful information on specification and testing procedures for standpipes, fire pumps, and hydrants.

The hospital may also be required to comply with the various state and local codes, which may be more restrictive, and should keep copies of such code requirements available for reference. However, before the hospital expends any resources on such compliance, it should consider the many possible equivalency or waiver options it may have available.

General Guidelines

Recommendations for action against specific fire hazards in hospital departments were given in previous chapters. In addition, the following general guidelines should be observed:

■ A hospital building should be divided into sections with corridor separations, stairwell enclosures, and sealed vertical openings. In such a building, a fire may be well enough isolated for emergency action to get under way.

■ There should be exits from each floor, at floor level, that lead to an adjacent safe refuge compartment, directly to the outside, or to other means of egress. With such outlets, no one will be trapped in dead ends at any floor level.

■ Stairwells should be protected with automatic doors. Such smoke-free towers will protect their users from fire and smoke during evacuation of all or part of the building.

■ Stairways should be of sufficient width and of such a pitch that litters and stretchers can be carried down.

■ Outside contractors and suppliers should be alerted to the locations of flammable liquids, gases, and materials. They should demonstrate safe ways to handle salamanders, torches, and irons.

■ Control must be established over shop materials such as paints, thinners, scrap, shavings, upholstery materials, and fabrics and over housekeeping department materials such as solvents and caustics.

■ Explosionproof electrical equipment should be used with all refrigerators in which explosive or flammable agents are stored. Circulating fans inside the boxes can be made safe only by having explosionproof fan motors with leads in sealed circuits or external motors and extension drive shafts. Improved room ventilation around the refrigerator may lessen the fire hazard.

■ Waste rags and cloths used with solvents should be stored only in proper containers.

■ Electrical installations should be made in accordance with the NFPA standard no. 70, *National Electrical Code,* and applicable state and local codes. Heating and ventilating equipment also should meet appropriate codes and may be changed only by qualified engineers. Changes in wiring should always have a permit from the local authorities, plus a post-installation inspection, if required.

■ Standpipe hose should be kept clean and dry and be thoroughly examined periodically. Hose should be refolded periodically to avoid permanent creases. Gaskets should be inspected regularly. Racks should permit circulation of air. All interior and exterior fire department connection caps should be checked for corrosion.

■ All electrical devices should be fitted with three-prong plugs; wall outlets should make provision for such plugs.

■ High-voltage equipment should be subject to a strict schedule of inspection and maintenance, because it creates corona discharge and ozone, which eat away insulation.

■ Employees who are not qualified electricians should be prohibited from attempting electrical repairs or temporary installations of any kind.

■ If the load of appliances has been increased substantially since the hospital's electrical system was installed, the power company should check the panel load to prevent overloading and the hospital's emergency power generator should be reassessed to be sure it can handle the increased load.

■ The interior finish for all means of egress and for rooms should be in conformance with the NFPA *Life Safety Code.* Interior finish materials, floor coverings, draperies, curtains, and so forth should be in compliance with NFPA standards.

Causes of Hospital Fires

To minimize the causes of fires, it is important to know how and where fires start. In tabulating reports on 381 hospital fires and explosions, the NFPA found that the causes and frequencies were as follows:

Matches and smoking		73
Electrical		66
Fixed services	35	
Appliances	31	
Malfunction of heater		30
Mishandling of flammable liquids		23
Spontaneous ignition		20
Anesthesia accidents		18
Oxygen accidents		18
Incendiary, suspicious		12
Kitchen hazards		10
Combustibles too close to heater		8
Welding or cutting		8
Incinerator spark		7
Static other than anesthesia		5
Miscellaneous known		19
Unknown		64

The need for fire prevention in all hospital departments is underscored by the following NFPA statistics on the 381 hospital fires in terms of sites of origin within the facility:

Patients' rooms		63
Oxygen tent	30	
Bedding, including mattress	24	
Other	9	
Employees' quarters		57
Heat or power plant		42
Storeroom		28
Laboratory		27
Operating Room		25
Chute (laundry or rubbish)		19
Utility shaft		18
Lounge		15
Kitchen		14
Laundry		13
Incinerator		11
Linen closet		7
Other closet		7
Maintenance area		5
Walls, other concealed spaces		5
Miscellaneous known locations		6
No data		19

This analysis and the NFPA study show where priority fire prevention efforts can best be applied. Although the hospital's fire safety plan must be set up to accommodate the particular needs and circumstances of the individual facility, emphasis should generally be given to fire hazards created by smoking and by electrical arrangements throughout the hospital. Useful information on policies and procedures for the prevention of fire hazards from smoking and faulty electrical arrangements appears in chapters 5 and 10.

Classes of Fires

The NFPA has adopted four general classifications of fires on the basis of the types of extinguishing media they need. Of course, the components of all four types of fires are fuel, oxygen, and heat, plus the necessary chain reaction. The classifications are:

■ **Class A fires.** These occur in ordinary combustible materials, such as wood, paper, excelsior, rags, and rubbish. The quenching and cooling effects of water, or of solutions containing large percentages of water, are initially important in extinguishing these fires. Special (multipurpose) dry chemical agents rapidly knock down the flames and form a coating that tends to retard further combustion.

■ **Class B fires.** This type occurs in a vapor-air mixture over the surface of such flammable liquids as anesthetics, gasoline, oil, grease, paints, and thinners. Limiting the air (oxygen) or inhibiting the combustion is important at the outset of such fires. Solid streams of water are likely to spread the fire, but water fog (adjustable-spray) nozzles prove effective under certain circumstances. Generally, regular dry chemical, multipurpose dry chemical, carbon dioxide, foam, and halogenated hydrocarbon agents are used.

■ **Class C fires.** These occur in or near electrical equipment and require nonconducting extinguishing agents. Dry chemical, carbon dioxide, compressed gas, and vaporizing liquid extinguishing agents are suitable. Foam or a stream of water should not be used, because each is a good conductor and can expose the operator to severe shock. A very fine spray of water sometimes can be used on fires in such electrical equipment as transformers, because it is less of a conductor than a solid stream of water.

■ **Class D fires.** These are fires in combustible metals rarely used in health care facilities.

Extinguishers

Even though the health care facility may be equipped with automatic sprinklers or other stationary fire protection, portable fire extinguishers should be available for emergencies. *Portable* means manual equipment used on small fires or temporarily used on large fires until the automatic equipment functions or professional fire fighters arrive.

To be effective, portable extinguishers must be:

■ A reliable type, approved by Underwriters' Laboratories *Fire Protection Equipment List,* Factory Mutual Engineering Corporation's *Approved Equipment for Industrial Fire Protection,* or other acceptable testing laboratory.

■ The right type for each class of fire that may occur in the area (see figure 31 at the end of this chapter).

■ Provided in sufficient quantity for protection against exposure in the area (refer to NFPA standard no. 10, *Installation of Portable Fire Extinguishers* and NFPA standard no. 10A, *Maintenance and Use of Portable Fire Extinguishers*).

■ Located where they are readily accessible for immediate use. If they are enclosed, their cabinet should be marked to show that an extinguisher is inside.

■ Maintained in perfect operating condition, inspected frequently, checked against tampering, and recharged as necessary.

■ Operable by area personnel who know how to find them and use them effectively and promptly.

Portable extinguishers are classified in terms of their ability to handle specific classes and sizes of fires. The reason for such classification includes the frequency of improved or new extinguishing agents and larger portable extinguishers.

Labels on extinguishers indicate the class and size of fire that they can be expected to handle. In addition, the extinguishers and their locations should have distinctive standard markings to further indicate their suitability to extinguish specific types of fires.

Corresponding with the classes of fires are the classes of portable extinguishers as adapted from NFPA standard no. 10:

■ **Class A extinguishers.** These should be identified by a green triangle containing the letter *A.* The marking should be applied by decal, painting, or a similar method. It should be located on the front of the shell above or below the extinguisher nameplate. It should be of a size and form that

make it easily legible at a distance of 3 feet. Class A extinguishers can employ soda and acid, pressure-cartridge-operated water, air-pressurized water, a water pump tank, all-purpose dry chemical, or interior hose lines.

■ **Class B extinguishers.** The marking should be a red square containing the letter *B.* Class B extinguishers can employ foam, dry chemical, or carbon dioxide

■ **Class C extinguishers.** Aside from their electrical aspects, Class C fires are essentially the same as Class A or Class B ones, although using a Class A or Class B extinguisher on a Class C fire is extremely dangerous. Therefore, proper identification of the extinguisher is essential. The marking for Class C extinguishers should be a blue circle containing the letter *C.* They can employ carbon dioxide or dry chemical.

■ **Multipurpose (ABC) extinguishers.** This type of extinguisher is recommended for all classes of fires. It has more fire-fighting efficiency than the water-base type. When it is the only type installed throughout an institution, it reduces the confusion that operation and maintenance of varied types entail. It should be noted, however, that the smaller sizes do not carry an A rating. Because ABC extinguishers leave a sticky residue, the hospital may choose to purchase the carbon dioxide type of extinguisher for Class B and Class C fire sites, where flammable liquids or electrical fires may occur. ABC extinguishers may not be completely effective on fires in warehouses containing mattresses or in storerooms, so the safety director may choose to select water-base extinguishers, preferably the stored pressure type.

Use of the wrong type of extinguisher may not only fail to put out the fire but can actually spread it. All staff should be familiar with the instructions attached to all extinguishers; these tell the operating procedures and the classes of fires on which the equipment can be used. If markings are applied to wall panels in the vicinity of extinguishers, they should be of a size and form that provide easy legibility at a distance of 25 feet.

Figure 31, the guide to the location of fire extinguishers, provides minimum recommendations. Each health care facility must evaluate the guidelines on type and number of extinguishers, hose cabinets, and wheeled extinguishers in terms of its particular needs. More complete guidance appears in the NFPA standard no. 10, *Portable Fire Extinguishers*.

The National Safety Council suggests that, for easy lifting, extinguishers should be placed so that their tops are 5 feet above the floor if the extinguisher's gross weight is 40 pounds or less and 3½ feet above the floor if it is more than 40 pounds. Normal distribution of fire extinguishers calls for a travel distance of not more than 75 feet to an extinguisher. It is recommended that the hospital check codes for requirements regarding height of fire extinguishers and travel distance.

Fire Drills

Drills are an indispensable part of an effective emergency action program. They must be called at various and unspecified hours of the day and night and should be held at least three times a year on each work shift for each patient-occupied building. Hospitals have found that drills arouse no apprehension in patients who have been informed that these are necessary and likely to be held at any time. However, to avoid panic in the event of an actual fire, discretion should be used in informing patients, especially bedridden patients. If patients are aware of the fire, assure them they will receive assistance.

It is highly desirable to have a local fire official attend to observe and evaluate the drills. Weaknesses found in any drill detail indicate that extra instruction and drilling are needed.

Even if the alarm system is connected directly to the fire department, the fire department should be telephoned. Because the hospital's telephone service may be destroyed, employees should know the nearest outside means of contacting the fire department; this could be a street fire-alarm box, a public telephone booth, or the fire station itself.

During the drill, key personnel should be questioned on their knowledge of shutoff valves and switches, especially with regard to oxygen and to air-conditioning systems. In each drill, all areas in the building should be checked to determine whether each receives the fire alarm. If personnel within a high-noise area, such as the boiler room, laundry, or kitchen, do not hear the alarm, checks should be made on the alarm sounding device in that area to determine whether it has a malfunc-

tion and to check on the level of operational noise in that area. If the sounding device is not adequate for that particular section of the building, the problem will require immediate correction. A system of flashing red lights might be incorporated into the sounding system in high-noise areas.

During the drill, alarm-actuated and smoke-barrier fire doors and automatic smoke dampers should be checked to ensure proper functioning and complete closing.

Figures 32, 33, and 34 illustrate fire drill procedures, information for patients, and a drill report, respectively.

Discovering a Fire

When a fire is discovered, the action taken should be planned in terms of three distinct areas: (1) Area A—a room occupied by a patient; (2) Area B—a nursing unit in an area not occupied by patients; and (3) Area C—a nonpatient area.

In an Area A fire, the first step is to remove the patient from the room of fire origin; the next step is to begin the planned emergency action. In an Area B situation, the first step is to close the corridor doors; the second, to report the fire. It is important to have the corridor doors closed as soon as possible. In an Area C fire, the action will be in accord with the combustibility of the building or its contents and the degree of hazard to the more populated portions of the building.

A sequence usually applicable in a fire emergency is as follows:

1. Any patient in immediate danger is removed from the room of fire origin, and all doors to the corridor are closed.
2. The person discovering the fire sounds the alarm, or, while removing the patient, assigns a co-worker to sound the alarm.
3. The fire department is notified.
4. Personnel throughout the hospital are alerted.
5. Patients are evacuated from the threatened area if needed.
6. A hand extinguisher or even a pitcher of water or a wet blanket is used to smother the fire.
7. Utilities such as gas, oxygen, and ventilating equipment are controlled or shut off.
8. The fire brigade is brought into action.
9. Control of activities is turned over to the fire department when it arrives.

Patient Evacuation

In making arrangements for evacuation, the hospital's procedures must take into account the physical facilities of the institution, activities that may be in progress, kinds of patients and their disabilities, weather, visitors, and standby personnel.

In a fire-resistive building that has firesafe areas, patients can be moved to an adjacent area on the same floor or on another floor. In a building that is combustible and has no sprinkler system, the need for evacuation from the building is greater. In any event, the evacuation procedure should be completely understood by all staff and employees and should be part of every drill.

But a plan for removal of patients from the building is incomplete unless it provides for subsequent attention to them. It must include provisions for their protection and continuing care elsewhere. The protection, transportation, and relocation of patients present an even greater and more complex problem than their actual removal.

The plan should also provide for visitors. Visitors should be directed to remain in the patient's room, leaving the doors closed; escorted to the lobby or a safe area; or directed to leave the building.

When conditions hazardous to patients are obvious and immediate, the chief executive officer, the vice-president for patient care, the safety officer, or the local fire chief will give the order to evacuate. The following are minimum guidelines for hospital personnel to follow:

■ Begin evacuation with the patients nearest the fire area.

■ Remove ambulatory patients first, to ensure unimpeded passage for transported patients.

■ Instruct ambulatory patients to form a chain and to proceed single file, following the lead of a staff member to a safe area.

■ Remove semi-ambulatory patients next, using all available wheelchairs and wheeled carts, walking only those who are able to walk.

■ Evacuate nonambulatory patients by wheeled cart, wheelchair, hand-carried stretcher, bedding or blanket drag, or by carry. (See the next section, Patient Removal Methods.)

■ Evacuate visitors and others in the building simultaneously with patients.

■ Evacuate babies by blanket carry. Although a calm mother can assist in the evacuation, it is impractical to give each baby to its mother.

■ Keep incubator babies in the nursery as long as feasible. A nurse must stay with these babies at all times. If necessary, a small emergency oxygen tank should be taken along when the babies are evacuated.

■ Move patients to areas on the same floor but in another wing or other suitable quarters prescribed in the fire preparedness plan until the fire is extinguished and they can return to their rooms, or until other arrangements are made for them. If necessary, move patients down stairways. Do not use elevators.

■ Make a final check of all rooms and bathrooms, and look under beds. Close doors and windows when leaving the room.

■ Notify the staff member in charge of the hospital when removal of patients from the fire area has been accomplished.

■ If danger is not imminent, load charts and patient card files and remove them to a safe area.

■ Account for all patients against the patient card file to make sure they are present in the safe or holding area.

It is customary for patients in a delivery room to be moved to the surgical suite. If that suite is not accessible, the emergency treatment room may be the next best refuge. Both areas offer greater protection against fires and explosions than does the delivery room, because their special purposes and needs were recognized in the original design of the hospital.

Because of the danger of power failure, elevators generally should not be used to evacuate patients. Any elevators used for evacuation should be specifically designed for that purpose; they should be able to bypass certain floors and be adaptable to manual operation. In an emergency, they should be operated by fire department personnel and be used only for wheelchair and stretcher patients.

Orthopedic patients should be given wet towels with which to cover their faces, and they should be assured that help will come. Stretchers should be reserved for them. If these patients have to be moved bodily, their ropes and straps must be cut.

Patients in the operating room must be handled according to instructions issued in writing to the medical staff or announced at the time by the surgeon in charge.

The following distinction merits reemphasis. In fire-resistive buildings divided into fire areas, the evacuation plan can be based on removal of patients to the safe areas; the movement could be on the same floor or to a different floor. In combustible buildings lacking a sprinkler system, the need for complete evacuation becomes greater, and the plan for it should be completely understood by all employees.

Patient Removal Methods

Patient moving is comprehensively discussed in the National Safety Council-American Hospital Association publication *Emergency Removal of Patients and First-Aid Fire Fighting in Hospitals.* It describes specific carries and techniques for immediate patient rescue, as well as fire-fighting devices and methods.

Every employee should be trained to remove patients from endangered areas in time of disaster. Although certain conditions require special arrangements, the methods described here are generally useful.

Infant and child removal

The following guidelines are to be used when removing infants and children:
1. Place blanket or sheet on the floor.
2. Place two infants in each bassinet, using diapers or small blankets for padding.
3. Place the bassinet in the middle of the blanket.
4. Fold the blanket over one end, fold the corners in, then roll the sides in to form a pocket.
5. Grasp the folded corners of the blanket and pull the infants to safety. Two or, if necessary, one person can drag eight babies to the prescribed area.
6. Place as many children as possible in one crib, and pull the crib to the prescribed area.

Universal carry

The universal carry is a method of removing a patient from a bed to the floor. It is a quick and effective method for removing a patient who is in immediate danger. This carry can be used by anyone regardless of the size of the patient.
1. Spread a blanket, sheet, or bedspread on the floor alongside the bed, placing one-third of it

under the bed and leaving about 8 inches to extend beyond the patient's head.
2. Grasp the patient's ankles, and move the patient's legs until they fall at the knee over the edge of the bed.
3. Grasp each shoulder, slowly pulling the patient to a sitting position.
4. From the back, encircle the patient with your arms, place your arms under the patient's armpits, and lock your hands over the patient's chest.
5. Slide the patient slowly to the edge of the bed and lower him or her to the blanket. If the bed is high, instruct the patient to slide down one of your legs.
6. Taking care to protect the patient's head, gently lower the head and upper torso to the blanket and wrap the blanket around the patient.
7. At the patient's head, grip the blanket with both hands, one above each shoulder, holding the patient's head firmly in the 8 inches of blanket. Do not let the patient's head snap back.
8. Lift the patient to a half-sitting position, and pull the blanketed patient to safety.

Swing carry

The swing carry requires two trained persons.
1. One carrier, feet together, slides an arm under the patient's neck and grasps the patient's far shoulder. The carrier's free hand is slipped under the patient's other upper arm, grasping it, and taking one step toward the foot of the bed, the carrier brings the patient to a sitting position.
2. The second carrier now grasps the patient's ankles, bringing the patient's legs at the knee over the edge of the bed.
3. Each carrier takes one of the patient's wrists and pulls it down over the carrier's shoulder, supporting the patient's body.
4. Each carrier reaches across the patient's back, placing one carrier's free hand on the other's shoulder.
5. Each carrier reaches under the patient's knees to lock hands with the other.
6. Standing close to the patient, the carriers bring their shoulders up and remove the patient from the bed, carrying the patient to a safe area.
7. At the safe area, each carrier drops on the knee closest to the patient, leans against the patient, and rests the patient's buttocks on the floor. The patient's torso is lowered to the floor, and the

patient's head is placed on a pillow or like protection. The patient's head must always be carefully protected.

Blanket drag

If vertical or downward evacuation by an interior stairway is necessary, in many cases one person can handle a helpless patient by using the blanket drag.

1. Double a blanket lengthwise, place it on the floor parallel and next to the bed, leaving 8 inches to extend above the patient's head.

2. Using cradle drop, kneel drop, or other suitable means, remove the patient from the bed to the folded blanket on the floor alongside the bed.

3. Grasping the blanket above the patient's head with both hands, drag the patient headfirst to the stairway.

4. Position yourself one, two, or three steps lower than the patient, depending on your height and the patient's height. The patient's lower body inclines upward.

5. Place your arms under the patient's arms and clasp your hands over the patient's chest.

6. Back slowly down the stairs, constantly maintaining close contact with the patient, keeping one leg against the patient's back.

Fire Safety Inspection

Frequent routine inspections are an essential part of any fire safety surveillance program. Adequate fire hazard inspection forms should be prepared for each health care facility and for each of its departments. Different departments will present different hazards, and the report forms should be adapted accordingly.

All completed fire hazard inspection forms should be reviewed at a meeting of the administrator, the fire safety committee, and a representative of the local fire department.

Figure 30. The following inspection checklist is a guide. Items should be added or deleted, in accordance with the size and operation of the particular facility. Each feature is to be checked monthly, unless a different interval is indicated.

Fire Safety Inspection Checklist

Sprinkler and Fire Detection System

____ Tested every 30 days by local fire department, unless other arrangements have been made.

____ Sprinkler system serviced annually by qualified agency.

____ Sprinkler valves accessible (with no recently stored material forming obstructions) and sealed open.

____ Sprinkler valves operate easily. No leaks, corrosion, or other defects noted in system.

____ Sprinkler water flow alarm tested.

____ Fire-detection (alarm) system tested.

Fire-Alarm Facilities

____ Location signs in place.

____ Boxes unobstructed.

____ Date of last test: _____

____ Auxiliary boxes have sign indicating whether system is connected to fire department.

Fire Doors

____ Operative.

____ Unobstructed (no wedges to hold doors open).

Fire Hose (Standpipes)

____ Cabinet door operative.

____ Hose condition (rotted, wet, moldy, and so forth).

____ Nozzle in place; proper type.

____ Hose properly hung in rack; aired; rehung to avoid creases.

Fire Extinguishers

____ All extinguishers mounted in properly designated locations (refer to figure 31).

____ Extinguisher seals intact and inspection tags properly initiated. To be inspected monthly, and serviced at least once a year.

____ Proper decals or other markings on extinguisher and wall to indicate type of fire on which extinguisher can be used.

____ No leaks, corrosion, or other defects noted.

____ Extinguishers unobstructed, ready for instant use.

____ No carbon tetrachloride or other vaporizing liquid used in any extinguisher.

____ Personnel informed on proper use.

Exits and Exitways

____ All exits clearly marked and exit lights on.

____ All exit lights clean and of proper wattage.

____ Exitways free from obstructions.

____ Furniture placed so that occupants can quickly and safety evacuate rooms.

____ Exterior grounds kept clear of objects that might impede evacuation or fire-fighting equipment.

(Figure 30 continued)

Stairways
____ Doors at each level operate satisfactorily and are kept closed.
____ Stairways free of obstructions.
____ Landings properly lighted.

Fire Drills
____ Date of last fire drill: _____
____ All employees and staff members participate in drill.

Auxiliary Lighting
____ Auxiliary emergency generator operative: maintenance and operating condition.
____ Fire door properly maintained.
____ Lighting checked weekly; date of last test: _____

Careless Smoking Hazards
____ No smoking in bed a rule.
____ "No Smoking" signs placed where required.
____ Adequate supply of large-sized noncombustible ashtrays in every room, lounge areas, and other approved smoking areas.

Electrical Wiring and Equipment
____ All electrical equipment purchased and installed is tested for performance and safety.
____ Appliances properly grounded.
____ All motors of proper size; clean, free of lint; cords not frayed; grounded.
____ Only qualified electricians are allowed to install or extend wiring.
____ Use of extension cords discouraged. When their use is absolutely necessary, they should be checked to ensure they are not frayed or covered with grease or lint; length not over 10 feet; no multiple or "octopus" wiring connections to wall outlets; no cords under rugs or fabrics.
____ All electrical circuits properly fused: 15 amp for general lighting circuits; 20 amp or more for special circuits.
____ Emergency lighting system operable.
____ Electric motors, fans, heaters, appliances, and fluorescent and other light fixtures free of combustibles; all such equipment easily accessible for replacement.

Heating, Ventilation, Flues, and Vents
____ Natural fireplaces equipped with spark screens.
____ Air-conditioning equipment filters clean.
____ Heating plant checked and serviced by qualified agency (annually).
____ Flues and vents free of dust and obstructions. (See *Kitchen*, below.)
____ Fire door operating in boiler room and incinerator room.
____ No combustible storage in room.

Housekeeping, Storage, and Waste Disposal
____ Brooms, mops, rags, and other cleaning supplies stored properly in metal cabinets or approved cans.
____ Paints, solvents, thinners, and other flammables stored in metal cabinet; oily rags in metal safety containers.
____ Combustibles kept clear of stove, heating appliances, heating plant, and water heater.
____ Dry leaves, shrubbery trimmings, and other combustibles kept away from buildings.
____ No combustibles stored under stairways.

(Figure 30 continued)

Kitchen

____ Hoods, vents, fans, and ducts in good condition and free from grease.

____ Hood filters cleaned regularly; date of last cleaning: _____

____ Hoods equipped with appropriate automatic extinguishing devices.

Surgery and Obstetrics

____ Monthly record readings of conductivity of surgery floor and furnishings, to check degree of insulation resistance.

____ Amount of ether stored in surgery suite. (See *Alcohol, Ether, and Similar Chemicals*, below.)

____ Proper relative humidity (R.H.) maintained; 50 percent R.H. if flammable inhalation anesthetics are used. Otherwise, it must be maintained according to the policy of the medical staff.

____ Mechanical ventilation adequate.

____ Equipment grounded, properly maintained, and tested periodically.

____ Rubber tubes conductive in flammable anesthetizing locations.

____ Rules and regulations posted.

Alcohol, Ether, and Similar Chemicals

____ Properly stored.

____ Properly dispensed.

____ If refrigerator is used for storage of these chemicals, it is provided with explosionproof motor.

____ "No Smoking" signs provided.

Compressed Gases (Nonflammable)

____ Cylinders properly capped and stored in designated area.

____ Cylinders properly secured by chain or strap to wall.

____ Storeroom vented to outside.

____ Fire door operative.

____ "No Smoking" signs provided.

Miscellaneous Hazards

____ Nonsmoking areas equipped with adequate signs.

____ All curtains, draperies, and decorative fabrics in exitways treated with flame retardant.

____ Everyone in every department has been warned never to use flammable fluids for cleaning floors, clothes, or furnishings.

____ Gasoline is kept for use with power mower or generator; is properly located in safety can with self-closing cap.

____ Matches and cigarettes are taken from patients receiving oxygen. Relatives and visitors are warned about smoking and matches in restricted areas; members of the clergy are told not to light candles for religious rites.

____ Target areas such as mechanical equipment rooms, storage and supply rooms, and the laundry receive surveillance beyond routine checks for malfunctions and fire hazards.

Figure 31. All hospital personnel should know the fire hazards and locations of fire extinguishers within their work areas. Some departments, such as maintenance shops, kitchens, and laboratories, are exposed to the hazards of several types of fires. But most departments usually risk only one type. For example, most fires in administrative offices, rest rooms, and lobby areas have been the Class A type. The extinguisher chart that follows is arranged by department, to help the safety surveillance team in comprehensive departmental inspections. However, it is intended only as a guide. Consult with local fire departments and insurance carriers to determine the specific needs of your facility.

Departmental Guide for Fire Extinguisher Locations

Extinguisher Location	Most Likely Class of Fire	Recommended Extinguishers
		(CO_2 is carbon dioxide)

All Areas

Multipurpose (ABC) extinguishers are useful and practical for all types of hospital fires.

Administrative Offices

All areas	A, B, or C	Soda acid, water, or foam and CO_2 or dry chemical
Switchboard	A or C	Foam and CO_2
Accounting	A or C	Water and CO_2 or dry chemical
Admitting	A	Water
Purchasing	A	Water
Payroll	A	Water
Storeroom	A or B	Sprinkler system or water and CO_2 or dry chemical
Medical record room	A	Sprinkler system
Library	A	Sprinkler system

Housekeeping Department

Storeroom	A or B	Sprinkler system or water and CO_2
Janitor closets	A or B	Soda acid and CO_2
Employee restrooms	A	Water
Employee locker room	A	Water
Doctor's lounge	A	Soda acid or water
Main lobby	A	Water

(Figure 31 continued)

Engineering and Maintenance Department

Boiler room	A, B, or C	Water or foam and CO_2 or dry chemical
Carpentry shop	A or C	Water or soda acid and CO_2 or dry chemical
Electrical shop	A or C	Foam and CO_2 or dry chemical
Paint shop	B	CO_2 or dry chemical
Elevator machine room	C	CO_2 or dry chemical
Elevator penthouse	C	CO_2 or dry chemical
Air-conditioning equipment room	C	CO_2 or dry chemical
Machine shop	C	CO_2 or dry chemical

Dietary and Food Service Department

Main kitchen	A, B, or C	Water or soda acid and CO_2 or dry chemical
Dining rooms	A	Water or soda acid
Floor kitchens	A or C	Water or soda acid and CO_2 or dry chemical
Special diet kitchens	A or C	Water or soda acid and CO_2 or dry chemical
Storerooms	A or B	Water or soda acid and CO_2 or dry chemical
Range hoods	B	Fusible link with CO_2 cartridge, steam vent, or dry chemical

Nursing Service

Nurses' stations	A	Water or soda acid
Utility room	A or B	Foam
Solarium or lounge	A	Water or soda acid
Linen room/mattress room	A	Water
Treatment or examining room	A, B, or C	Water
Equipment storage room	B or C	Foam and CO_2 or dry chemical
Outpatient areas	A	Water
Central supply	A, B, or C	Water and CO_2 or dry chemical
Emergency department	A, B, or C	Water and CO_2 or dry chemical
Nursery	A or C	Water and CO_2
Formula room	A	Water
Nurses' home	A or C	Water and CO_2 or dry chemical
Auditorium	A	Soda acid or water
Classroom	A	Soda acid or water

Laundry Department

Laundry workroom	A or B	Water and CO_2
Soiled linen room	A	Water or soda acid
Clean linen room	A	Water or soda acid
Sewing room	A or C	Water and CO_2

Central Service Department

Central station	A	Water or soda acid
Equipment storage room	A, B, or C	Foam and CO_2 or dry chemical

(Figure 31 continued)

Laboratory, Pathology Department

Chemistry, bacteriology, serology, histology	A or B	Water and CO_2 or dry chemical
Basal metabolism room	A	Water
Electrocardiographic room	A or C	Foam and CO_2 or dry chemical
Morgue/museum room	A	Soda acid

Pharmacy

General areas	A or B	Water and CO_2 or dry chemical
Alcohol storage	B	CO_2 or dry chemical

Radiology and Nuclear Medicine

Diagnostic room	A or C	Water and CO_2
Therapy room	A or C	Water and CO_2 or dry chemical
Viewing room	A or C	Water and CO_2 or dry chemical
Film storage room	A	Sprinkler system
Developing room	A	Water

Surgical Suite

Operating room	B or C	Foam and CO_2 or dry chemical
Anesthetic room	A or B	Sprinkler system inside; foam on outside of door
Delivery room	B or C	Foam and CO_2

Special Care Units
(Including intensive care units, intensive cardiac units, hyperbaric pressure chambers, and facilities for renal dialysis)

Special machines, devices of electrical nature	C	CO_2 or dry chemical
Hyperbaric chamber with intensive use of oxygen	B	CO_2 or dry chemical or deluge system

Physical Therapy Department

Physiotherapy	A or C	Water and CO_2
Occupational therapy	A	Soda acid or water

Figure 32. Drills are essential to training employees in combatting fire intelligently and swiftly. Unscheduled drills should be conducted on each shift at least three times a year.

Procedures for a Fire Drill

A blinking lantern and two flags, one marked "Fire Drill" and the other marked "Fire," signify that a fire drill is in progress. When an employee encounters such a setup, he or she should:
1. Respond to the blinking lantern and flags as if to an actual fire.
2. Pull the nearest fire alarm. (The local fire department will have been notified that a fire drill is to be conducted at a specific time.)
3. Telephone the switchboard, identify himself or herself, and tell the operator the location of the fire. The operator then announces the location of the fire over the paging system in code.
4. Close all doors and windows in the area. Alert patients to the fire drill before closing patient room doors.
5. Obtain extinguishers, and return to the fire site.
6. Prepare to disconnect oxygen equipment and tanks in patient rooms. In a drill, this can be simulated by placing a towel over the connections.
7. Secure all patient medical charts in preparation for patient evacuation.
8. Prepare for patient evacuation, but execute evacuation only when such an order is given. Visitors are to be instructed to exit by the nearest stairway immediately upon receiving the evacuation order.

When the alarm is sounded, all hospital fire brigade members on duty should report to the fire area. The hospital fire marshal or safety director should ensure that the surgery department, obstretrics, and intensive and coronary care units are kept informed on the status of the fire. In the event of an actual fire, this communication will be essential to avoid unnecessary disruption of surgical and intensive care activities.

All employees except fire brigade members, key administrative personnel, and those otherwise instructed should remain at their stations. Personnel must refrain from using telephones and elevators during the drill.

At the end of the drill, the switchboard operator announces in code that the drill has been completed.

Figure 33. This sign should be posted in every patient room so that patients will not be distressed when they hear the fire alarm.

Fire Drill Information for Patients

- For your protection, our hospital holds regularly scheduled fire drills so that our employees know exactly what to do in the event of fire.
- Remember, if a drill is conducted during your stay, it will be announced and you will hear the fire bells ring. You will notice the fire and police departments, as well as the hospital fire brigade, responding to our call.
- Relax and cooperate with our able staff. Employees are well trained to help you in any emergency.
- Listen carefully to any instructions.
- Unless there is a real danger, you will not be moved.
- Safety rules comply with recognized standards to protect patients, visitors, and employees.

Figure 34. The safety director, the hospital's fire marshal, or an appointed observer records on a report form the time the bogus fire begins, fills in the form as the drill progresses, and observes employees' reactions. If feasible, a second observer should be stationed at a distance from the drill site to observe response to the emergency. Following the drill, employees should be asked to write their comments and suggestions on a form for this purpose.

Fire Safety Training and Drill Report

Hospital   Date of training/drill: _____
                                                      Hours: _____

Training/Drill: 1 2 3 4 5 6 7 8 9 10 11 12 (Circle number of session)

Response to drill: Excellent   Good   Fair   Poor

Comments:
  Instructor
  _____

  _____

  Staff members
  _____

  _____

  Employees
  _____

  _____

Staff members who attended:
  _____

  _____

Employees who attended:
  _____

  _____

                                          _____
                                          (Signature of instructor)

Chapter 1
Introduction

American Hospital Association. *Security Programs in Health Care Institutions.* Chicago: AHA, 1976.

Joint Commission on Accreditation of Hospitals. *Accreditation Manual for Hospitals.* Chicago: JCAH, published annually.

McGrath, Robert. *Emergency Removal of Patients and First Aid Fire Fighting in Hospitals.* Chicago: American Hospital Association and National Safety Council, 1974.

National Safety Council, *Accident Prevention Manual for Industrial Operations.* Chicago: NSC, 1964.

Chapter 2
The Importance of Safety

American Hospital Association. *Infection Control in the Hospital.* Chicago: AHA, 1979.

Centers for Disease Control. *Guidelines for Prevention and Control of Nosocomial Infections.* Atlanta: CDC, 1981.

Colling, R. *Hospital Security: Complete Protection for Health Care Facilities.* Los Angeles: Security World Publishing Co., Inc., 1976.

DeWitt, C. Is your hospital really secure? *Hospitals.* 55:73-75, Nov. 1, 1981.

Flournoy, D.J., and others. Nosocomial infection linked to handwashing. *Hospitals.* 53:105-7, Aug. 1, 1979.

Hargiss, C.O., and others. Infection control: Guidelines for prevention of hospital acquired infections. *Am. J. Nurs.* 81:2175-83, Dec. 1981.

How to manage violent patients. *Health Care Secur. Saf. Manage.* 2:5-9, May 1981.

Improving your incident reporting system. *Health Care Secur. Saf. Manag.* 1:5-9, Feb. 1981.

Jessee, W.F. Medication errors noted as major source of incident reports. *Hosp. Peer Rev.* 6:141-43, Nov. 1981.

Joint Commission on Accreditation of Hospitals. *Accreditation Manual for Hospitals.* Chicago: JCAH, published annually.

Kaunitz, K.K. What is the status of the law on the use of bed rails and side rails to restrain patients? *Hosp. Med. Staff.* 10:11-14, Dec. 1981.

Keys, P.W. Drug-use review and risk management. *Am. J. Hosp. Pharm.* 38:1533-34, Oct. 1981.

Lanham, G.B., and others. Full coverage of issues reflects importance of risk management. *Hospitals.* 55:165-68, Apr. 1, 1981.

Martin, H. Reduce the risk of liability. *Health Care* 23:16-18, Nov. 1981.

Morse, G.P. Management participation key to successful loss prevention. *Hospitals.* 55:52, 55, Nov. 1, 1981.

Murphy, F.D. *Manual of Model Safety, Environmental, and Infection Control Policies for Hospitals.* Fond du Lac, WI: Health Tech-Service, 1977.

National Fire Protection Association, *Health Care Safety Reports and Articles.* Boston: NFPA, 1975.

Pascal, M.A. *Hospital Security and Safety.* Rockville, MD: Aspen Systems, 1977.

Phillip, M.S. How to handle a hostage-taking incident. *Dimens. Health Serv.* 58:26-27, Apr. 1981.

Quilitch, B., and others. Using an ombudsman and a rights committee to handle client complaints. *Hosp. Community Psychiatry.* 32:127-29, Feb. 1981.

Wear, J.O., and Simmons, D.A. *Hospital Safety Manual.* North Little Rock, AR: Scientific Enterprises, Inc., 1978.

Chapter 3
Safety Planning and Direction

The inspection of hospitals and health services—the approach of the health and safety executive. *Hosp. Eng.* 32:12-14, Sept. 1978.

Joint Commission on Accreditation of Hospitals. *Accreditation Manual for Hospitals.* Chicago: JCAH, published annually.

Kaunitz, K.K. What is the status of the law on the use of bed rails and side rails to restrain patients? *Hosp. Med. Staff.* 10:11-14, Dec. 1981.

McQuade, J. The use and abuse of a safety committee. *Dimens. Health Serv.* 53:14, Feb. 1976.

Night-shift safety. *Hosp. Superv. Bull.* 336:8, May 30, 1979.

Worik, W. *Safety Education.* Englewood Cliffs, NJ: Prentice-Hall, 1979.

Chapter 5
Safety for Patients

American College of Surgeons. *Patient Safety Manual.* Chicago: ACS, 1979.

American Hospital Association, American College of Surgeons, and American Medical Association. *Sharing Responsibility for Patient Safety.* Chicago: AHA, 1979.

DeMars, M.L., and others. Victim-tracking cards in a community disaster drill. *Ann. Emerg. Med.* 9:207-9, Apr. 1980.

Hollis, Margaret. *Safer Lifting for Patient Care.* St. Louis, MO: Blackwell-Mosby, 1981.

Chapter 6
Safety for Employees and Volunteers

American Hospital Association and American Medical Association. *Guiding Principles for an Occupational Health Program in a Health Care Institution.* Chicago: AHA, 1977.

Garratt, D.J., and others. Smoking in hospital: a survey of attitudes of staff, patients, and visitors. *J. Epidemiol. Community Health.* 32:226-28, Sept. 1978.

National Fire Protection Association. *Standard for National Electrical Code* (NFPA no. 56A). Boston: NFPA, 1973.

National Safety Council. *Handbook of Occupational Safety and Health.* Chicago: NSC, 1980.

Night-shift safety. *Home Superv. Bull.,* 336:8, May 30, 1979.

Chapter 7
Safety for Visitors

Shetler, M. Regulations pertaining to seeing eye dogs and/or domestic pets in the hospital. *Hosp. Infect. Control.* 5:76, Apr. 1978.

Chapter 8
Safety for Clinical Services

Bacovsky, R. Disposal of hazardous pharmaceuticals. *Can. J. Hosp. Pharm.* 34:12-13, Jan.-Feb., 1981.

College of American Pathologists. *Fire Regulations for Laboratories.* Skokie, IL: CAP, undated.

Erlick, B.J., and others. *Laboratory Safety: Theory and Practice.* New York City: Academic Press, 1980.

Flury, Patricia A. *Environmental Health and Safety in the Hospital Laboratory.* Springfield, IL: Charles C Thomas, 1978.

Leonard, R.B., and others. Emergency department radiation accident protocol. *Ann. Emerg. Med.* 9:462-70, Sept. 1980.

Norris, F.S., and others. Guidelines for defining and disposing of medical waste. *Aviat. Space Environ. Med.* 49:81-85, Jan. 1978.

Oppman, C. Laboratory safety practices reduce hospital biohazards. *Health Care Newsl.* July-Aug. 1981.

Waldron II, R.L., and others. Radiation decontamination unit for the community hospital. *Amer. J. Roentgenology.* 136:977-81, May 1981.

Walters, Douglas B., American Chemical Society. *Safe Handling of Chemical Carcinogens, Mutagens, and Highly Toxic Substances.* Ann Arbor, MI: Ann Arbor Science, 1980.

Wheeler, W.W. Equipment specifications and performance standards for equipment pertaining to the nuclear medicine department. *Radiol. Manage.* 2:43-48, Summer 1980.

Williams, A. Suggested procedures for disposing hospital solid waste. *Health Care Newsl.* Apr. 1980.

Chapter 9
Safety for Support Services

Blount, R.N. *Housekeeping Procedures for Small Hospitals.* Springfield, IL: Charles C Thomas, 1977.

Gray, M. Infection control in the laundry. *Hosp. Top.* 58:47-48, May-June 1980.

Hargiss, C.O. The patient's environment: haven or hazard. *Nurs. Clin. North Am.* 15:671-88, Dec. 1980.

Mahaffey, Mary J., and others. *Food Service Manual for Health Care Institutions.* Chicago: American Hospital Association, 1981.

Mallison, G.F. CDC expert gives handwashing tips. *Hosp. Infect. Control.* 6:59-61, May 1979.

Oppman, C. Foodborne illnesses: focus on safety. *Hosp. Risk Manage.* 3:89-91, July 1981.

White, D. Fire safety: menace in the kitchen. *Health Soc. Serv. J.* 88:310-11, Mar. 17, 1978.

Zelechowski, G.P. Infection control in housekeeping. *Prof. Sanit. Manage.* 11:32-35, Aug.-Sept. 1979.

Chapter 10
Plant Operation

American Hospital Association. *Compendium of Hospital Electrical Standards.* Chicago: AHA, 1981.

American Hospital Association, *Signs and Graphics for Health Care Institutions.* Chicago: AHA, 1978.

American Society for Hospital Engineering. *Hospital Engineering Handbook.* Chicago: American Hospital Association, 1974.

American Society for Hospital Engineering. *Medical Equipment Management in Hospitals.* Chicago: American Hospital Association, 1978.

American Society of Mechanical Engineers. *Boiler Construction Codes.* New York City: ASME, current edition.

American Welding Society. *Safe Practices for Welding and Cutting Containers That Have Held Combustibles.* New York City: AWS, current edition.

Berger, J. Guidelines for developing an effective electrical safety program. *J. Clin. Eng.* 4:321-27, Oct.-Dec. 1979.

Bond, R.G., and others, eds. University of Minnesota; Division of Environmental Health. *Environmental Health and Safety in Health Care Facilities.* New York City: The MacMillan Co., 1973.

Buchsbaum, W.H., and Goldsmith, B. *Electrical Safety in the Hospital.* Oradell, NJ: Medical Economics, 1975.

Controlling patient-owned appliances. *Hospitals.* 53:57, 61, 64, June 16, 1979.

Koren, H. *Environmental Health and Safety.* New York City: Pergamon Press, 1974.

Luciano, J.R. *Air Contamination Control in Hospitals.* New York City: Plenum Press, 1977.

National Safety Council. *Accident Prevention Manual for Industrial Operations.* Chicago: NSC, 1964.

Neuberg, J., and others. An automated electrical safety and preventive maintenance program. *J. Clin. Eng.* 4:71-75, Jan.-Mar. 1979.

Roth, H.H. *Electrical Safety in Health Care Facilities.* New York City: Academic Press, 1975.

Spooner, R.B. *Hospital Electrical Safety Simplified.* Research Triangle Park, NC: Instrumentation Society of America, 1980.

Stoner, D.L., and others. *Engineering a Safe Hospital Environment.* New York City: John Wiley & Sons, Inc., 1981.

Chapter 11
Disaster Preparedness

American Hospital Association. *Readings in Disaster Preparedness for Hospitals.* Chicago: AHA, 1973.

American Medical Association. *Categorization of Hospital Emergency Capabilities.* Chicago: AMA, 1971.

Baker, F.J. The management of mass casualty disasters. *Topics in Emergency Medicine.* 1:149-57, May 1979.

Bander, K.W. Hospital structures guidelines for coping with snowstorms. *Hospitals.* 52:123-24, Nov. 1, 1978.

Blackouts—what you can do. *Food Management.* 13:38, 41, 72, Feb. 1978.

Colvin, R.J., and others. How to conduct a realistic mock disaster program. *Natl. Saf. News.* 117:75-78, June 1978.

Crooks, L., and others. Disaster planning: a team effort. *AORN J.* 28:395-410, Sept. 1978.

Dildine, D. Disaster planning: are you prepared? *Purchasing Administration.* 2:1, July 1978.

Emergency care in natural disasters. Views of an international seminar. *WHO Chron.* 34:96-100, Mar. 1980.

Establishment of disaster radio response program in the local government radio service for states, territories, and possessions: Federal Communications Commission. Final rule. *Fed. Regist.* 46:52367-74, Oct. 27, 1981.

Fisher, Jr., C.J. Mobile triage team in a community disaster plan. *Amer. J. Roentgenology.* 6:10-12, 1977.

Hill, R.W., and others. Earthquake-resistant hospitals: some cost considerations. *Hospitals.* 51:119-20, Feb. 1, 1977.

Hoenig, S.A. *Medical Instrumentation and Electrical Safety: The View From the Nursing Station.* New York City: John Wiley & Sons, Inc., 1977.

Hoyle, J.D. Tornadoes! Prepare for the unpredictable. *Hospitals.* 51:71-73, Feb. 16, 1977.

Joint Commission on Accreditation of Hospitals. *Accreditation Manual for Hospitals.* Chicago: JCAH, published annually.

Katz, I.B., and others. Planning and developing a community hospital disaster program. *Emerg. Med. Serv.* 7:69-70, 72, 95, Sept.-Oct. 1978.

Klinghoffer, M. A pre-triage plan for mass casualty care. *Occupational Health and Safety.* 47:32-35, Nov.-Dec. 1978.

Melton, R.J., and others. Revising the rural hospital disaster plan: a role for the EMS system in managing the multiple casualty incident. *Ann. Emerg. Med.* 10:39-44, Jan. 1981.

Minimum Requirements of Construction and Equipment for Hospitals and Medical Facilities. Washington, DC: U.S. Bureau of Health Facilities Financing, Compliance, and Conversion, 1979.

Moore, T.D. Administrative approach to disaster preparedness in the pharmacy. *Am. J. Hosp. Pharm.* 36:1337-41, Oct. 1979.

National Fire Protection Association. *Manual on Health Care Emergency Preparedness.* Boston: NFPA, 1981.

Pan American Health Organization. *A Guide to Emergency Health Management After Natural Disaster.* Washington, DC: PAHO Sanitary Bureau, Regional Office of WHO, 1981.

Pittman, S.E. Florida hospital develops a hurricane preparedness plan. *South. Hosp.* 49:6-7, July-Aug. 1981.

Savage, P.E.A. *Disasters: Hospital Planning: A Manual for Doctors, Nurses, and Administrators.* New York City: Pergamon Press, 1979.

Smith, R.S. How to plan for crisis communication. *Public Relations Journal.* 35:17-18, Mar. 1979.

Stanley, G.L. *Hospital Safety and Disaster Policy and Procedure Manual.* Marion, IL: Hospital and Physician Consulting Service, 1977.

Step-by-step emergency plan keeps hospital staff prepared. *Hospitals.* 52:32, Oct. 1978.

Storer, D.L. Disaster planning: communications. *Ohio State Medical Journal.* 75:401-2, June 1979.

Tidemann, C.F. The organization of medical services at the site of a disaster. *World Hospital.* 15:178-80, Aug. 1979.

U.S. Atomic Energy Commission, in cooperation with International Association of Chiefs of Police. *Emergency Handling of Radiation Accident Cases,* series of pamphlets, 1969.

Wiener, P. Setting up an external disaster procedure; and the role of the nursing service supervisor. *Hospital Topics.* 54:22-24, 25, July-Aug. 1976.

Yates, D.W. Major disasters. Surgical triage. *Br. J. Hosp. Med.* 22:323-25, 328, Oct. 1979.

Chapter 12
Fire Safety

American Hospital Association. *Fire Safety Training in Health Care Institutions.* Chicago: AHA, 1975.

Bartels, R.H., and others. *Hospital Fire Brigades: A Training Manual.* Chicago: Camplin, Bartels, and Associates, 1979.

Benedetti, R.P. Understanding fire-retardant and flame-resistant materials. *J. Am. Coll. Health Assoc.* 27:311-14, June 1979.

Factory Mutual Engineering Corporation. *Approved Equipment for Industrial Fire Protection.* Norwood, MA: FMEC, published annually.

Gabriel, S. Fire safety: the struggle to overcome hazards involving textiles. *Health Soc. Serv. J.* 88:314-16, Mar. 17, 1978.

How good is your fire safety training? *Health Care Newsl.* July 1978.

McGrath, Robert. *Emergency Removal of Patients and First Aid Fire Fighting in Hospitals.* Chicago: American Hospital Association and National Safety Council, 1974.

National Fire Protection Association. *Health-Care Safety Reports and Articles: A Compilation of Articles from Fire Journal and Fire Technology.* Boston: NFPA, 1975.

Proposed hospital fire safety system offers choice of protective measures. *Purch. Adm.* 3:1, 36, Sept. 1979.

Quakkelaar, A.J. Firesafety symbols for worldwide communications. *Fire J.* 73:45-47, July 1979.

Robertson, E.V. The invisible fire safety feature—attitude. *Dimens. Health Serv.* 58:21-23, Apr. 1981.

Schmidt, W.A. Smoke detection: part of complete building system. *Specif. Eng.* 41:58-62, May 1979.

Shaikh, A.H. Safety procedures in clinical laboratories. *Am. J. Med. Technol.* 45:793-96, Sept. 1979.

Smoking restrictions help reduce hospital fire hazards. *Health Care Newsl.* Aug. 1980.

Special fire extinguishing systems. *Natl. Saf. News.* 117:57-59, June 1978.

Teague, P.E. *Firesafety in Hospitals.* Boston: National Fire Protection Association, 1977.

for waste disposal, 78–80
See also Hospital safety; Safety
Safety regulations, 7
Safety rules, printed signs for, 30
Security services, 6
Smoking
   hospital policy on, illus., 44
   hospital regulations on, 30
   restrictions on, 37
   rules for visitors, illus., 43
Soldering, safety rules for, 93–94
Special-care units, safety requirements for, 60
Special inspections, 20–21
Sprinkler systems, requirements for, 64
Staff alert in disaster planning, 110
Staff members, specific roles in safety program, 7
Staff safety meetings, 15
Steam-heated equipment, inspection schedules for, 96
Storage areas, periodic inspection of, 19–20
Strikes as internal disasters, 111–12
Support services, safety for, 75–89
Surgical suite
   inspection of, 96–97
   safety guidelines for, 58–59

Thermal and electrical burns and wounds, 35
Training in safety program, 6
Training program for employees, 14–15
Transporting patients, guidelines for, 35, illus., 39, 41

Unfired pressure vessels, inspection schedules for, 96
Unidentified substances, guidelines for handling and
   storage, illus., 72

Union representation, role in safety committee, 12
Unwanted visitors, security guidelines for, 54

Ventilating system, safety requirements for, 63–64
Visitor injury
   hospital investigation and procedures, 54–55
   hospital policy on, 55
Visitor safety
   education for, 53–54
   instructions for, illus., 56
   personal injury incidents and investigations, 54–55
   restricted areas, 54
   unwanted visitors, 54
Volatile liquids, safety in handling, 64
Volunteers, safety for, 50

Waste disposal, safety rules for, 78–80
Water and fuel shortages as internal disasters, 112–13
Welding, safety rules for, 93
Wheelchairs
   lifting patients into, 34
   transporting patients in, guidelines for, illus., 39
Wheeled stretchers, transporting patients on, 35, illus.,
   39
Wood flooring as laboratory hazard, 63
Work environment in employee safety, 46–47
Worker's Compensation Act in occupational injury or
   illness, 4–5

a great bowl of
SOUP

250 Recipes to Prepare, Savor & Share

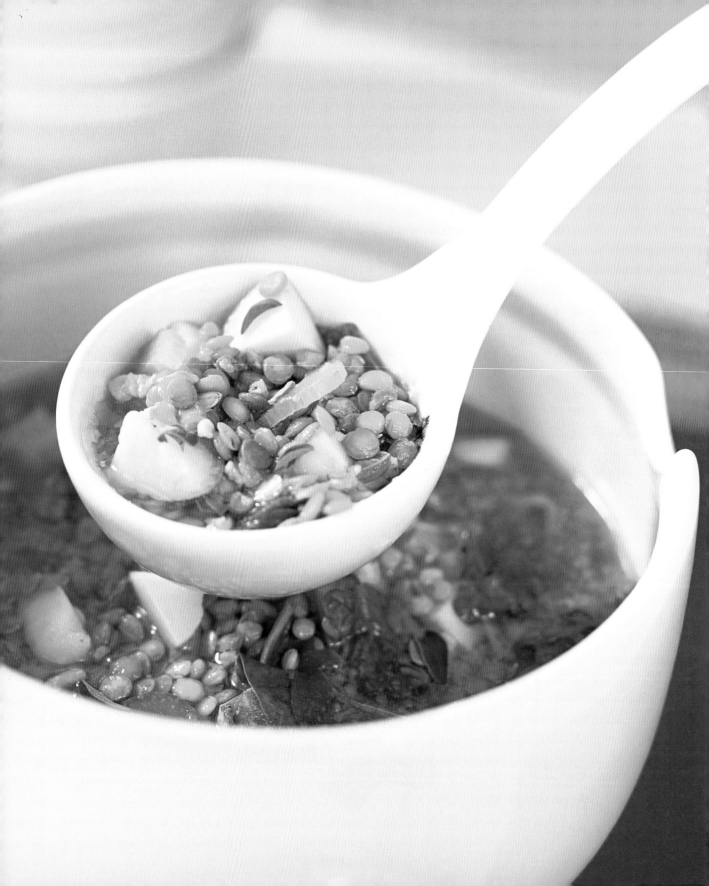

a great bowl of
SOUP

250 Recipes to Prepare, Savor & Share

Edited by Christine Byrnes
Photography by Theresa Raffetto

Main Street
A division of Sterling Publishing Co., Inc.
New York

The Library of Congress has cataloged the paperback edition as follows:

A great bowl of soup : 250 recipes to prepare, savor & share / edited by Christine Byrnes.

   p. cm.

Includes index.

ISBN 1-4027-3364-X

1. Soups. I. Byrnes, Christine.

TX757.G72 2005

641.8'13—dc22

                            2005020298

10 9 8 7 6 5 4 3 2 1

Published by Main Street, a division of Sterling Publishing Co., Inc.
387 Park Avenue South, New York, NY 10016

©2006 by Sterling Publishing Co., Inc.
Photographs ©2004 & 2006 by Theresa Raffetto

This book is comprised of material from the following Sterling titles:
365 Vegetarian Soups ©2002 by Gregg R. Gillespie
Smart Soups ©1998 by Carol Heding Munson
Original recipes provided by Mary B. Johnson

Design by 3+Co.
Photographs by Theresa Raffetto
Food Stylist: Victoria Granof
Prop Stylist: Olivia Mercer
A special thanks to Theo Granof, Ella Harris, and Dunya and Marusya Madubuko.

Distributed in Canada by Sterling Publishing
C/o Canadian Manda Group, 165 Dufferin Street
Toronto, Ontario, Canada M6K 3H6
Distributed in the United Kingdom by GMC Distribution Services
Castle Place, 166 High Street, Lewes, East Sussex, England BN7 1XU
Distributed in Australia by Capricorn Link (Australia) Pty. Ltd.
P.O. Box 704, Windsor, NSW 2756, Australia

Printed in China
All rights reserved

ISBN 13: 978-1-4027-3118-1
ISBN 10: 1-4027-3118-3

For information about custom editions, special sales, premium and
corporate purchases, please contact Sterling Special Sales
Department at 800-805-5489 or specialsales@sterlingpub.com.

Contents

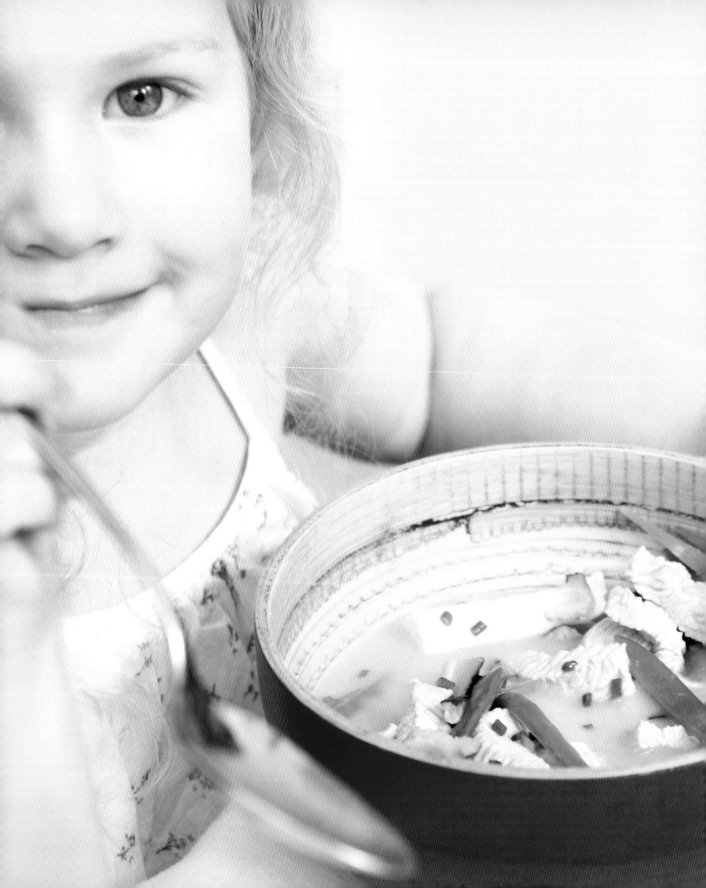

INTRODUCTION

Soup is a wonderful soul-warming food that brims with wholesome ingredients and fantastic flavors. Indeed, soup is the epitome of comfort food. Chicken soup is the elixir of choice when a cold or flu has you feeling down. Soup fills you up, yet can be so healthfully light in fat, carbohydrates, and calories that it may be a dieter's dream. There are endless reasons why soup holds a special place in our menu repertoire. A fragrant and delicate soup can stimulate the appetite, serving as a perfect opener to a dinner. A robust, stick-to-the-ribs soup, served with crusty bread and a salad, makes the perfect one-dish meal.

A Great Bowl of Soup offers 250 recipes chock-full of taste; you are sure to find a recipe for any palate. These soups will remind you how easy and wonderful homemade soup can be, despite the convenience of canned or frozen dinners. Homemade meals allow us not only to know exactly what we are eating, and are often healthier than their canned counterparts, but to create something delicious to share with one another—from a warm, creamy soup sure to warm a cold winter day, to a chilled fruit soup on a hot summer day.

Even with all of its benefits, many people shy away from making soup for one of these reasons: It takes too much time to cook—rumor tells us to set aside about eight hours for simmering! Or, it requires too big a pot—a huge one that must hold ten to twelve quarts, and you must be an expert chef. You'll find that the soups in *A Great Bowl of Soup* debunk such myths—these soups are meant for the busy chef. Serve up one of these soups for the family dinner, or a cozy gathering—they are sure to be a hit without needing too much time or fuss.

In this book, you'll see recipes for a wide variety of soups: some ready to eat in an hour or so, some ready in mere minutes. Some have international origins; some are decidedly domestic. Whether you have time to spend in the kitchen, need a quick dinner fix, or want some super smart cooking tips to help you along—you have chosen the right cookbook.

SOUP LINGO

Bisque: A thick, creamy, rich soup.

Bread Bowl: Hollowed-out round loaf of bread, usually warmed in the oven for 5–10 minutes, used to serve soup in. Hearty, chunky chowders are delicious served up in a bread bowl.

Broth: Liquid made from cooking poultry, meat, fish, or vegetables; it is often used as a base for more involved soups, but can be consumed alone.

Chowder: A chunky soup or stew, usually made with seafood or vegetables.

Dice: To cut into small cubes, each less than half inch.

Garnish: Decorative touch added to food just before serving, usually edible and may add flavor.

Julienne: To cut food into strips about 2" by ½".

Puree: To make food have a thick, creamy liquid texture.

Simmer: To heat below or just at the boiling point of the liquid. Usually done at low to medium-low heat (depending on stovetop).

Stock: Liquid in which meat, poultry, fish, or vegetables have been simmered. It is similar to broth and used as a base for other soups.

SOUP TIPS

Here are some tips to help streamline cooking:

- Use commercial broth and beans. Many store-bought products contain high sodium content, so check for low-sodium products, and rinse your canned beans before cooking. Then you season to taste—that way you are in control of just how salty your dish is. Having said that, we have also provided basic soup stock recipes on pages 14–21. If you ever have the time to cook up some stock, simply freeze 1- and 2-cup quantities for use when the mood hits you. All the recipes will taste good whether you choose homemade or canned stocks.

- Chop your ingredients smaller rather than larger and try for uniformity in the size. This will lend itself to quicker, more even cooking times.

- Most soups are one-pot affairs, so clean up can be a snap, which gives you more time to enjoy your meal.

- Read the recipe from start to finish before beginning your prep. Make sure you understand the directions and reread anything that seems unclear.

- Start by getting all of your ingredients within reach and do all of your prep work before beginning to cook. That way, you can cruise through the instructions and simmer up a great soup.

- If the soup is ready before dinnertime, you can usually simmer it on a very low heat setting until you want to serve it, unless the recipe specifically says not to heat it longer. Egg and cream soups will curdle if left heating for longer than the recipe calls for, so be sure to follow recipe instructions.

- The thickness of your soup can be adjusted. If the soup is too thin, you can add cornstarch or another thickening agent; if it is too thick, add a little bit more liquid (water or broth work well). If you add more liquid, you may need to adjust the seasonings.

- Get creative. If you don't like an ingredient in a recipe, don't use it. And you can always substitute for something you prefer.

- To keep your chilled soups cold, serve in a chilled bowl. Place the bowl in the freezer for up to an hour before placing soup in it.

- Have leftovers? Soups can be safely refrigerated for a couple of days. Make sure to cool it to room temperature before placing it in the refrigerator. If you know you won't eat it within a couple of days, most soups will freeze nicely for up to three months in a sealed container. Soups with eggs and cream shouldn't be frozen, however, since they will curdle during heating.

- To reheat frozen or refrigerated soups, heat on the stovetop over low to medium-low heat until heated through. Be sure to add more liquid if needed, and taste before serving to allow for any seasoning adjustments needed.

- Check out our Soup Pantry section—it's full of delicious breads, crackers, and sauces that go great with your soups. You can cook these up ahead of time, and then you're ready to go when it's soup time.

BASIC FOOD SAFETY

- Defrost frozen ground meat or steaks in the refrigerator, not at room temperature. Allow 12 to 24 hours to defrost 1- to 1½-inch thick steaks or patties.

- Wash hands, the counter, platter, utensils, and containers with hot, soapy water before and after contact with raw meat.

- Do not place cooked meat onto dishes, cutting boards, or platters that have not been cleaned after holding raw meat.

BASIC TOOLS

You can create any of the soups in this book with just a few basic kitchen tools:

Cutting board: At least one board in either wood or plastic is a must-have. Whichever you choose, be sure to get one large enough for unhindered chopping, yet small enough for easy washing. For food safety, remember to use separate boards (or separate sides of one board) for cutting produce and raw meats and to wash the boards thoroughly between uses.

Vegetable peeler: This tool is ideal for peeling thin-skinned root vegetables such as carrots, potatoes, parsnips, and even young butternut squash. Find a peeler with a swivel blade and a comfortable handle.

Paring knife: A paring knife usually comes with a 3- or 4-inch blade and makes short work of trimming mushrooms, peeling fruits, and other similar tasks.

Chef's knife: Select a top-quality knife and keep it sharp for optimum performance. This knife comes in 6-, 8-, 10-, and 12-inch lengths. The 8-inch one gets our vote for versatility. It lets you cut meats, chop vegetables, and mince garlic and herbs in no time flat.

Immersion blender: This handy gadget allows you to purée ingredients directly in the pot. If you don't have one, a blender, food processor, food mill, or potato masher will work.

Measuring cups and spoons: Get a nested set of dry measuring cups for measuring rice, pasta, beans, and frozen peas and corn. Use a liquid measure for broth, tomatoes, and other liquid ingredients. The same set of nested spoons can be used for dry and wet items.

Saucepans and pots: The saucepan is the smaller of the two and has one handle; the pot is larger and has two handles. All of the soups can be made in either vessel. The pot, however, will give you more room for stirring and gentle simmering. Make sure you get a snug-fitting lid for whatever you have. The pot itself should be heavy, and a nonstick interior is not necessary. If making a tomato-based soup, avoid aluminum or iron pans.

Wooden spoons: Wooden spoons are good for most mixing and stirring tasks. They don't scratch pots, pans, or dishes, and their shallow basins are perfectly suited for stirring. Their handles stay cool, and don't melt if you accidentally leave them touching a hot pot.

Large metal spoons: A good-sized spoon with a deep basin is ideal for stirring chunky, hearty soups.

Skimmer: Stainless-steel mesh spoon used to skim foam or fat from the soup. This will help reduce the fat content of the soup.

Ladle: A ladle with a half-cup capacity is great for serving chowders and soups with a lighter base.

Timer: The timer is useful when multitasking—when the broth is simmering for a set amount of time, and you're chopping vegetables, it's easy to forget how long the soup has been simmering. Set the timer, and you'll be assured of simmering the broth the correct amount of time.

NUTRITION NOTE

All the recipes contained in this book have nutritional information based on the smallest serving size recommended, and do not include the nutrition for any serving suggestions such as bread sticks, croutons, crackers. For instance, if the recipe says "makes 4 to 6 servings," and "serve with croutons," our nutrition is based on a four-serving sample size without the croutons. We accounted for adding a pinch of salt to the soups which specify "salt and pepper to taste"; adding more or less, to your taste, will affect the sodium content of the soup. Skimming fat off the top of the soups will lower the fat content, as well as the overall calorie content of the soups. Keep nutrition in mind when making soups; if the recipe says reduced-fat cheese, and you add whole-milk cheese for more flavor, that will affect the nutritional analysis. Our nutrition information is given only as a guideline.

Metric Equivalents

The recipes in this cookbook use the standard United States method for measuring ingredients (teaspoons, tablespoons, and cups). If you need to convert to other measurements, use the charts below. All equivalents are approximate.

Liquid Ingredients by Volume

U.S.				Metric
¼ tsp				1 ml
½ tsp				2 ml
1 tsp				5 ml
3 tsp	1 tbls		½ fl oz	15 ml
	2 tbls	⅛ cup	1 fl oz	30 ml
	4 tbls	¼ cup	2 fl oz	60 ml
	5⅓ tbls	⅓ cup	3 fl oz	80 ml
	8 tbls	½ cup	4 fl oz	120 ml
	10⅔ tbls	⅔ cup	5 fl oz	160 ml
	12 tbls	¾ cup	6 fl oz	180 ml
	16 tbls	1 cup	8 fl oz	240 ml
	1 pt	2 cups	16 fl oz	480 ml
	1 qt	4 cups	32 fl oz	960 ml
			33 fl oz	1000 ml

Cooking/Oven Temperatures

	Fahrenheit	Celsius	Gas Mark
Freeze Water	32° F	0° C	
Room Temp.	68° F	20° C	
Boil Water	212° F	100° C	
Bake	325° F	160° C	3
	350° F	180° C	4
	375° F	190° C	5
	400° F	200° C	6
	425° F	220° C	7
	450° F	230° C	8
Broil			Grill

Dry Ingredients by Weight
(To convert ounces to grams, multiply the number of ounces by 30.)

1 oz	¹⁄₁₆ lb	30 g
4 oz	¼ lb	120 g
8 oz	½ lb	240 g
12 oz	¾ lb	360 g
16 oz	1 lb	480 g

Length
(To convert inches to centimeters, multiply the number of inches by 2.5.)

1 in		2.5 cm	
6 in	½ ft	15 cm	
12 in	1 ft	30 cm	
36 in	3 ft	1 yd	90 cm
40 in		100 cm	1 m

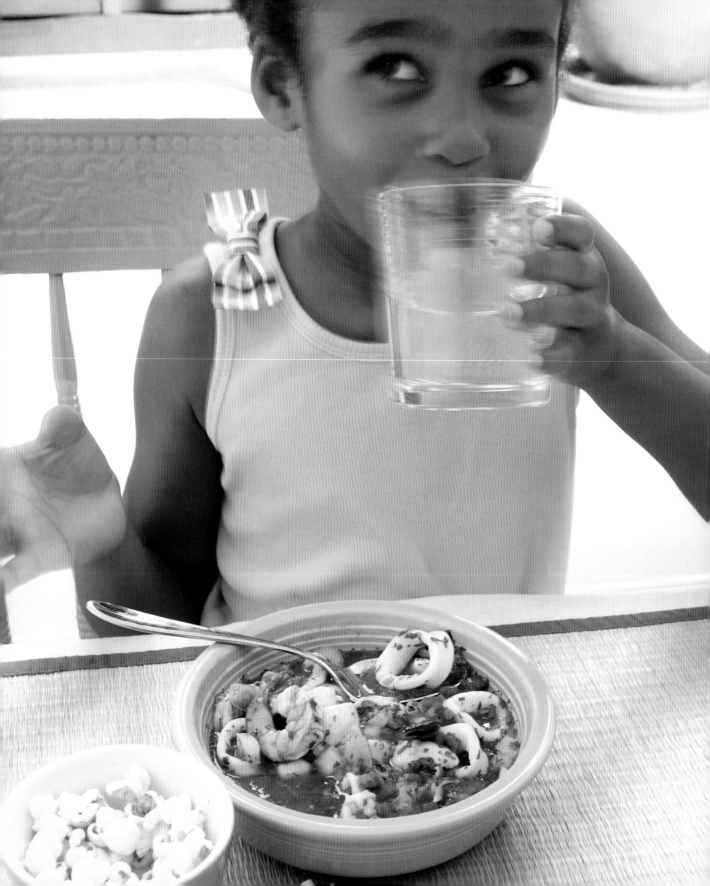

1
SOUP PANTRY

Chicken Stock

PREP TIME: 20 minutes
COOK TIME: 2½ hours

Makes about 6 cups

Like a blank canvas, this very plain stock awaits your artistry. It's perfect for soups because it does not have any salt or sweet ingredients (such as carrots) or seasonings (such as thyme or bay leaf) that may interfere with the flavorings called for in your recipes.

   3-pound mixture of raw chicken carcasses, wings, leg bones, backs, necks, and giblets (not the liver)
   2½ quarts cold water or enough to cover bones
   1 small onion, quartered
   1 small celery rib, chopped
   6 black peppercorns

1. Place the chicken, water, onion, celery, and pepper in a 3-quart saucepan and heat to boiling over medium heat. Skim off any foam. Gently simmer, partially covered, over medium-low heat until the giblets are tender and the bones are falling apart, about 2½ hours.

2. Drain the stock through a colander lined with cheesecloth into another large pot, pressing on the ingredients to extract the juices. Use the stock immediately or cool quickly in an ice bath and store up to 3 days in the refrigerator or 6 months in the freezer.

Each cup: About 39 calories, 5 g protein, 1 g carbohydrate, 1 g total fat (trace saturated), 0 mg cholesterol, 0 mg sodium.

Gingered Chicken Stock

PREP TIME: 15 minutes
COOK TIME: 20 minutes

Makes about 1 quart

Many cultures consider chicken soup to be a panacea for many illnesses or conditions, from a cold to homesickness to a case of the "blues." This fragrant stock will produce soups that restore and renew the spirit.

   5 cups Chicken Stock (at left)
   3 scallions, thinly sliced
   2 star anise
   3-inch piece peeled fresh gingerroot, thinly sliced
   1 teaspoon Chinese peppercorns (optional)

1. Combine the stock, scallions, star anise, ginger, and peppercorns (if using) in a 2-quart saucepan and heat to boiling over medium-high heat. Reduce the heat to low and simmer, covered, 20 minutes.

2. Strain the stock through a fine sieve lined with a double layer of cheesecloth into another saucepan or a heat-safe glass measure. Use stock immediately or cool quickly in an ice bath and store up to 3 days in the refrigerator or 6 months in the freezer.

Each cup: About 40 calories, 5 g protein, 1 g carbohydrate, 1 g total fat (trace saturated), 0 mg cholesterol, 0 mg sodium.

Beef Stock

PREP TIME: 10 minutes
COOK TIME: 2 hours 15 minutes

Makes 9 cups

A lean stock that's rich and flavorful.

    nonstick cooking spray
    2 ribs from roasted beef rib roast
    2 celery stalks, leaves included, halved
    4 large onions, unpeeled, quartered
    4 medium carrots, halved
    2 small turnips, quartered
    2 bay leaves
    8 whole black peppercorns
    1 sprig fresh parsley
    1 sprig fresh rosemary
    10 cups water

1. Coat a nonstick skillet with spray and warm it over medium-high heat for 1 minute. Add the beef ribs and cook them until the pieces are browned on all sides. Transfer the ribs to an 8-quart pot. Add the celery, onions, carrots, turnips, bay leaves, peppercorns, parsley, rosemary, and water. Cover the pot and bring to a boil. Reduce the heat and simmer for 2 hours.

2. Pour the stock through a large strainer into a large bowl or pot. Discard the solids. Chill the stock; then skim and discard the fat that's accumulated on top of the liquid.

Each cup: About 31 calories, 5 g protein, 3 g carbohy-drate, trace total fat (trace saturated), 0 mg cholesterol, 475 mg sodium.

Vegetable Stock

PREP TIME: 5 minutes
COOK TIME: 30 minutes

Makes about 9 cups

This tasty stock is exceptionally easy to make.

    4 large onions, quartered
    4 medium carrots, halved
    4 celery stalks, leaves included, halved
    10 fresh basil leaves
    2 bay leaves
    2 garlic cloves
    8 whole black peppercorns
    1 sprig fresh parsley
    10 cups water

1. Combine the onions, carrots, celery, basil leaves, bay leaves, garlic, peppercorns, parsley, and water in an 8-quart pot. Cover and bring to a boil. Reduce the heat and simmer 25 minutes.

2. Pour the stock through a large strainer into a large bowl or pot. Discard the solids.

Each cup: About 31 calories, 5 g protein, 3 g carbohydrate, 0 g total fat, 0 mg cholesterol, 0 mg sodium.

Basic Fish Stock

PREP TIME: 25 minutes plus soaking
COOK TIME: 30 minutes

Makes about 8 cups

For a more interesting stock, use the bones from several different types of fish. It is essential to let the stock simmer gently and for only 30 minutes or it will develop a bitter flavor. Once the stock has been strained, however, it can be boiled to concentrate the flavor or to reduce the volume for freezing.

2 pounds fish trimmings (heads and bones from scaled and gutted fish) from one or more kinds of non-oily fish such as flounder and halibut
2 quarts cold water or more if needed
½ cup dry white wine or ½ lemon
1 medium onion, sliced
1 large leek, split, well rinsed, and sliced
6 sprigs fresh parsley with stems
2 sprigs fresh thyme
6 black peppercorns

1. Wash fish bones well under running cold water. With kitchen shears, snip off and discard gills from inside head if still attached, and break or cut all the bones into 3-inch pieces. If bones are bloody, soak in a bowl of cold water 30 minutes, changing the water every 10 minutes.

2. Drain the fish bones and place in a 4-quart saucepan. Add 2 quarts water, the wine or lemon, onion, leek, parsley, thyme, and peppercorns. Add more water if needed to barely cover the ingredients. Heat the stock slowly to a boil over medium heat, partially cover, and simmer gently over low heat 30 minutes. Skim off any foam that forms during simmering with a large serving spoon.

3. Strain the stock through a colander lined with cheesecloth into another large pot, pressing gently on the ingredients to extract the juices. Use stock immediately or cool quickly in an ice bath and store up to 3 days in the refrigerator or 6 months in the freezer.

Each cup: About 66 calories, 7 g protein, trace carbohydrate, 3 g total fat (1 g saturated), 3 mg cholesterol, 144 mg sodium.

Fish Stock with Root Vegetables

PREP TIME: 30 minutes plus soaking
COOK TIME: 1 hour

Makes about 6 cups

The complex, earthy flavors and aromas of root vegetables are released by a brief sautéing, which enables them to flow freely and quickly in the short time they simmer with the fish bones.

2 pounds fish trimmings (heads and bones from scaled and gutted fish) from one or more kinds of non-oily fish such as flounder and halibut
4 tablespoons unsalted butter
1 large onion, chopped
1 medium parsnip, peeled and chopped
1 medium carrot, peeled and chopped
1 medium potato, peeled and chopped
1 small celery root (celeriac), peeled and chopped
4 quarts cold water
¼ teaspoon salt
6 black peppercorns
1 bouquet garni (3 sprigs fresh thyme, 1 small bunch Italian parsley, and 1 bay leaf, tied together with cotton string)

1. Wash fish bones well under running cold water. With kitchen shears, snip off and discard gills from inside head if still attached, and break or cut all the bones into 3-inch pieces. If bones are bloody, soak in a bowl of cold water 30 minutes, changing the water every 10 minutes.

2. Drain and rinse the fish bones. Melt the butter in a 4-quart saucepan over medium-high heat and sauté the onion, parsnip, carrot, potato, and celery root until they start to soften, about 7 minutes. Add the water, salt, peppercorns, and bouquet garni and heat to boiling. Reduce the heat to low and simmer gently, partially covered, 30 minutes.

3. Drain the stock through a colander lined with cheesecloth into another large pot, pressing on the ingredients to extract the juices.

4. Wash the original pot and add the strained stock. Return to heat and bring to a boil over medium-high heat. Boil until stock is reduced to about 6 cups, about 20 minutes. Use stock immediately or cool quickly in an ice bath and store up to 3 days in the refrigerator or 6 months in the freezer.

Each cup: About 113 calories, 5 g protein, 1 g carbohydrate, 10 g total fat (5 g saturated), 23 mg cholesterol, 538 mg sodium.

Turkey Stock

PREP TIME: 10 minutes
COOK TIME: 1 hour

Makes 9 cups

A great way to use up leftover turkey wings.

    2 roasted turkey wings, skin included
    2 celery stalks, leaves included, halved
    3 large onions, unpeeled, quartered
    2 medium carrots, halved
    1 small turnip, quartered
    1 parsnip
    2 bay leaves
    8 whole black peppercorns
    1 sprig fresh parsley
    1 sprig sage
    10 cups water

1. Combine the turkey, celery, onions, carrots, turnip, parsnip, bay leaves, peppercorns, parsley, sage, and water in an 8-quart pot. Cover and bring to a boil. Reduce the heat and simmer 1 hour.

2. Pour the stock through a large strainer into a large bowl or pot. Discard the solids. Chill the stock; then skim and discard the fat that's accumulated on top of the liquid.

Each cup: About 64 calories, 6 g protein, 3 g carbohydrate, 3 g total fat (1 g saturated), 7 mg cholesterol, 51 mg sodium.

Game-Bird Stock

PREP TIME: 15 minutes
COOK TIME: 1 hour

Makes 4 cups

Domestic or wild birds are often prized for their breast and leg meat, but there's a treasure left behind in the remaining carcass. The resulting stock makes delicious soup in any recipe calling for chicken stock.

    giblets, wings, and necks of 2 ducks or 4 smaller
        birds (such as pheasant, squab, or quail), rinsed,
        and/or the carcasses of the birds
    1 medium onion, quartered
    1 small celery rib, chopped
    5 cups water

1. Combine the giblets, wings, and necks with the onion, celery, and water in a 3-quart saucepan and heat to boiling over medium heat. Skim off any foam. Simmer over medium-low heat, covered, until the giblets are tender, about 1 hour.

2. Drain the stock through a colander lined with cheesecloth into another large pot, pressing on the ingredients to extract the juices. Use stock immediately or cool quickly in an ice bath and store up to 3 days in the refrigerator or 6 months in the freezer.

Each cup: About 70 calories, 6 g protein, 4 g carbohydrate, 3 g total fat (1 g saturated), 7 mg cholesterol, 70 mg sodium.

Venison Stock

PREP TIME: 20 minutes
COOK TIME: 4 hours

Makes about 3 quarts

Your only source of deer bones and meat may be the family or neighborhood hunter, but chances are you will be the only one who wants the bones and the shank meat. Ask for them in advance as the bones are usually discarded when the meat is butchered and frozen.

4 pounds venison shank bones, cut crosswise into 3-inch pieces
2 pounds venison shank meat
3 carrots, peeled and cut in half lengthwise
1 yellow onion, stuck with 4 whole cloves
1 celery rib, coarsely chopped
5 sprigs fresh thyme or savory
5 sprigs fresh parsley
2 bay leaves
1 tablespoon black peppercorns
3 quarts water or more if needed

1. Rinse the bones and meat well with cold water and place in a 6-quart pot with the carrots, onion, and celery. Tie the thyme, parsley, and bay leaves together in several places with kitchen string so the bundle will not separate during cooking and add to the pot. Add the peppercorns and enough water to cover by 3 inches. Heat to boiling over medium heat, skimming off the foam as it forms, and simmer over medium-low heat until the meat is tender, about 4 hours, adding more water as needed to keep the bones covered by 3 inches of liquid.

2. Pour the stock through a sieve lined with a double layer of cheesecloth into another pot. Cool the stock to room temperature, cover, and refrigerate overnight.

3. Remove the meat from the bones. Shred it and the shank meat and place in a bowl. Cover and refrigerate to use in the soup.

Each cup: About 31 calories, 5 g protein, 3 g carbohydrate, 0 g total fat, 4 mg cholesterol, 0 mg sodium.

Shrimp Stock

PREP TIME: 15 minutes
COOK TIME: 1 hour

Makes about 6 cups

For a more complex stock, use the heads and shells of lobster and crayfish instead of (or in addition) to the shrimp shells and heads. Use any of the shellfish stocks to cook rice, risotto, or polenta, or in sauces for seafood.

- shells and heads from 2 pounds of shrimp (add 1 cup bottled clam juice if you don't have any heads)
- 1 small onion, quartered
- 1 small carrot, coarsely chopped
- 1 bouquet garni (3 sprigs fresh thyme, 1 small bunch Italian parsley, and 1 bay leaf, tied together with cotton string)
- 2 quarts cold water

Combine the shells and heads, onion, carrot, bouquet garni, and water in a 4-quart saucepan and slowly bring to a boil over medium heat. Reduce the heat to low and gently boil, partially covered, 1 hour. Strain through a colander lined with cheesecloth into another large pot, pressing on the ingredients and shaking them gently to extract the juices. Use stock immediately or cool quickly in an ice bath and store up to 3 days in the refrigerator or 6 months in the freezer.

Each cup: About 7 calories, 2 g protein, trace carbohydrate, trace total fat (0 g saturated), 10 mg cholesterol, 95 mg sodium.

Spicy Shrimp Stock

PREP TIME: 15 minutes
COOK TIME: 1 hour

Makes about 6 cups

- shells and heads from 2 pounds of shrimp (add 1 cup bottled clam juice if you don't have any heads)
- 1 small onion, quartered
- 1 small inner celery stalk with leaves, coarsely chopped
- 1 bouquet garni (3 sprigs fresh thyme, 1 small bunch Italian parsley, and 1 bay leaf, tied together with cotton string)
- 2 teaspoons Maryland- or New Orleans–style seafood seasoning
- ¼ teaspoon cayenne pepper
- 2 quarts cold water

Combine the shells and heads, onion, celery, bouquet garni, seasoning, cayenne, and water in a 4-quart saucepan and slowly bring to a boil over medium heat. Reduce the heat to low and gently boil, partially covered, 1 hour. Strain through a colander lined with cheesecloth into another large pot, pressing on the ingredients and shaking them gently to extract the juices. Use stock immediately or cool quickly in an ice bath and store up to 3 days in the refrigerator or 6 months in the freezer.

Each cup: About 7 calories, 2 g protein, trace carbohydrate, trace total fat (0 g saturated), 10 mg cholesterol, 398 mg sodium.

Asian Shrimp Stock

PREP TIME: 15 minutes
COOK TIME: 1 hour

Makes about 6 cups

Soups made from this heady stock are especially soothing and warming from the generous splash of wine and
palate-tingling fresh gingerroot. Chinese Shaoxing rice
wine is the best to use, but Japanese sake is a delicious
choice as well.

> shells and heads from 2 pounds of shrimp (add
>   1 cup bottled clam juice if you don't have
>   any heads)
> 4 scallions, coarsely chopped
> ⅔ cup rice wine or dry sherry
> 2-inch piece peeled fresh gingerroot, sliced
> 2 garlic cloves, crushed
> 2 quarts cold water

Combine the shells and heads, scallions, rice wine,
ginger, garlic, and water in a 4-quart saucepan and
slowly bring to a boil over medium heat. Reduce the
heat to low and gently boil, partially covered, 1 hour.
Strain through a colander lined with cheesecloth into
another large pot, pressing on the ingredients and
shaking them gently to extract the juices. Use stock
immediately or cool quickly in an ice bath and
store up to 3 days in the refrigerator or 6 months
in the freezer.

Each cup: About 51 calories, 1 g protein, 2 g carbohydrate,
trace total fat (0 g saturated), 3 mg cholesterol, 144 mg
sodium.

Vietnamese Spicy Stock

PREP TIME: 15 minutes
COOK TIME: 20 minutes

Makes about 1 quart

> 5 cups Beef or Chicken Stock (pages 15 and 14)
> 2 star anise
> 1 whole clove
> 1-inch piece cinnamon stick
> ½ teaspoon white peppercorns
> 1-inch piece fresh gingerroot (unpeeled is OK), cut
>   into thin slices
> 4 shallots, thinly sliced
> 1 teaspoon sugar

1. Place the stock in a 2-quart saucepan and heat to
   boiling over medium-high heat. While the soup
   heats, crush the anise, clove, cinnamon, and peppercorns on a cutting board with a rolling pin. Crush the
   ginger. Add the spices, ginger, shallots, and sugar to
   the stock and stir to dissolve the sugar.

2. Reduce the heat to low and simmer the stock, covered, 20 minutes. Strain the stock through a fine
   sieve lined with a double layer of cheesecloth into
   another saucepan or a heat-safe glass measure. Use
   stock immediately or cool quickly in an ice bath and
   store up to 3 days in the refrigerator or 6 months in
   the freezer.

Each cup: About 25 calories, 3 g protein, 1 g carbohydrate,
1 g total fat (trace saturated), 0 mg cholesterol, 0 mg sodium.

Basic Fried Croutons

PREP TIME: 10 minutes
COOK TIME: 15 minutes

Makes 8 servings

Homemade croutons are a great way to put leftover bread to good use. The correct role of traditional croutons is to add a crusty, crunchy texture to a spoonful of smooth soup. Croutons should be small enough to fit on a soupspoon, and dried to a crispness (by frying or toasting) so as to remain hard and not soak up the soup. Make them plain, with just salt to season them, or combine one or more flavorings in the variations that follow, whatever you fancy to complement the flavors in your soup.

> 4 to 6 slices firm white, egg, rye, pumpernickel, or other savory bread (you can even use brioche)
> 1 tablespoon unsalted butter
> 2 tablespoons olive oil
> salt and freshly ground pepper to taste (optional)

1. Stack the bread slices on a cutting board and remove the crusts from each side. Cut the stack crosswise in each direction into ½-inch or 1-inch cubes.

2. Melt the butter and the oil in a large skillet over medium heat. Add the bread cubes and sauté until golden and crisp on all sides, about 3 minutes. Transfer to a paper towel–lined plate to drain. Sprinkle with salt and pepper and stir to coat.

Each serving: About 76 calories, 1 g protein, 6 g carbohydrate, 5 g total fat (1 g saturated), 4 mg cholesterol, 67 mg sodium.

Garlic Croutons
Add 1 garlic clove, crushed through a press, to the butter-oil mixture and sauté 1 minute. Then add the bread cubes and continue as recipe directs.

Herb Croutons
Add 1 tablespoon chopped fresh parsley and/or other fresh herbs or mixed herbs or 1 teaspoon dried herb or herbs to the croutons immediately after frying, while they are still in the pan.

Cheese Croutons
Immediately after draining the croutons on paper towels (the croutons should still be hot), sprinkle with ¼ cup finely grated (on a microplane or the small rough side of a box grater) hard cheese such as Parmigiano-Reggiano, Pecorino Romano, Asiago, or Provolone and stir to coat and slightly melt the cheese onto the bread.

Spiced Croutons
Immediately after draining the croutons on paper towels, sprinkle with ¼ teaspoon ground cinnamon, Chinese five-spice powder, curry powder, or Maryland-style seafood seasoning (Old Bay) and stir to coat.

Baked Tuscan Bread Croutons

PREP TIME: 10 minutes
COOK TIME: 15 minutes

Makes 16 servings

These oven-toasted bread cubes are best when tossed into soups that need a little thickening.

  1 round loaf thick crust, sturdy Tuscan Bread (page 29)
  2 tablespoons Italian extravirgin olive oil or more if needed
  1 teaspoon kosher salt
  ½ teaspoon freshly ground black pepper

1. Preheat the oven to 350 degrees. Cut the bread into 1-inch cubes and place in a large bowl. Drizzle 2 tablespoons oil over the bread and toss to coat. Add more oil if needed and sprinkle with the salt and pepper. Toss again to coat.

2. Spread out the croutons on a baking sheet and bake until golden and slightly crisp, about 15 minutes.

Each serving: About 162 calories, 4 g protein, 30 g carbohydrate, 2 g total fat (trace saturated), 0 mg cholesterol, 145 mg sodium.

Soup Puffs

PREP TIME: 25 minutes
COOK TIME: 20 minutes

Makes enough puffs for 8 soup servings

These little crunchy, airy bits of pastry are made from choux pastry, the same dough used to make cream puffs and éclairs. They are spectacular additions to any soup, but they are especially good for glamorizing and supplementing simple broths and stocks. Because they are so rich, they taste best when no other liaison, such as flour or egg yolks, is used to thicken the soup. Although the puffs are solid when they are packed into cookie tins or plastic food-storage bags, they get soft. Freeze them and add, almost frozen, to cold soups, if you want crisp puffs in warm weather.

  ½ cup water
  4 tablespoons unsalted butter, cut into small
    pieces
  pinch salt
  ½ cup unbleached all-purpose flour
  2 large eggs, beaten, at room temperature

1. Preheat the oven to 375 degrees. Line a large baking sheet with parchment.

2. Combine the water, butter, and salt in a 1-quart saucepan over medium heat and cook until the butter melts and the water boils. Immediately remove the pan from the heat and add the flour all at once. Beat vigorously with a wooden spoon to blend the mixture into a dough. Cook the dough, over medium heat, stirring constantly, until the water evaporates and the dough forms a thick mass that pulls away from the sides of the pan. Remove the pan from the heat and cool 5 minutes.

3. Add 2 tablespoons beaten egg to the dough and beat vigorously. Add the remaining egg, 2 tablespoons at a time, beating until it is incorporated.

4. Place the dough in a pastry bag fitted with a star or plain tip and pipe small (½-inch diameter) dots onto the prepared baking sheet about 1 inch apart. Pull up on the dots as you pipe them out so they have a whimsical tip in the center. Bake the puffs until crisp and golden brown, 15 to 20 minutes.

5. Turn off the oven. Prick each puff with a skewer to release the steam and let dry in the oven 5 to 10 minutes. Store the puffs in an airtight container for up to 24 hours. The puffs can be frozen. To recrisp the puffs, reheat (or thaw and reheat) on a baking sheet in a 350-degree oven for about 5 minutes.

Each serving: About 98 calories, 2 g protein, 6 g carbohydrate, 7 g total fat (4 g saturated), 69 mg cholesterol, 53 mg sodium.

Cheese Puffs
Beat ¾ cup grated Gruyère, Parmigiano-Reggiano or Pecorino Romano, or other flavorful grating cheese into the dough after adding the eggs.

Puff Pastry Croutons

PREP TIME: 15 minutes
COOK TIME: 15 to 20 minutes

Makes enough croutons for 8 soup servings

1 sheet prepared puff pastry (half of a
    17-ounce package), thawed according to
    package directions
1 egg yolk beaten with 2 teaspoons heavy cream
chopped mixed herbs such as rosemary, thyme,
    and Italian parsley
1 teaspoon kosher salt or shards of fine sea salt,
    such as Maldon sea salt

1. Preheat the oven to 425 degrees. Line a half-sheet
   pan or heavy baking sheet with parchment.

2. Place pastry on a cutting board and cut crosswise
   and lengthwise with a very sharp knife (clean cuts
   will ensure the pastry layers separate and rise) to
   make 1-inch croutons (or any size you wish).

3. Brush top only of pastry with the egg yolk, being careful not to let any mixture drip down the sides or it will
   prevent pastry from rising evenly, and prick all over
   with a fork. Mix herbs and salt and sprinkle over pastry. Place the croutons on the prepared baking sheet
   and bake until the croutons are puffed, browned, and
   crisp, 15 to 20 minutes (the time depends on the type
   of pastry). If croutons brown too quickly before they
   are fully puffed, reduce the heat to 350 degrees.
   Transfer to a wire rack to cool until using.

Each serving: About 175 calories, 3 g protein, 14 g carbohydrate, 12 g total fat (3 g saturated), 27 mg cholesterol,
365 mg sodium.

Hardtack Pilot Crackers

HARD "OYSTER" CRACKERS

PREP TIME: 15 minutes
COOK TIME: 20 to 30 minutes

Makes about 4 dozen

There are dozens of bite-size breads that are made to
complement seafood soups. The traditional staple of
early mariners went by a variety of names—oyster
crackers, pilot biscuits, pilot crackers, ship bread, ship
biscuit, sea bread, hardtack, hardbread.

2 cups all-purpose flour plus more for rolling out
    the crackers
1½ teaspoons brown sugar
1½ teaspoons salt
¾ cup milk
2 tablespoons unsalted butter, melted

Preheat the oven to 400 degrees. Line a baking sheet
with parchment. Combine the flour, brown sugar,
and salt in a medium bowl and mix. Make a well in
the center and add the milk and butter. Stir with a
fork until a dough forms; turn out on a lightly floured
work surface. Roll out to a ½- to ¾-inch thickness
and cut into bite-size squares or pieces. Stick a fork
down into the top but not through the crackers and
place forked side up on the prepared baking sheet.
Bake until golden brown and firm, 20 to 30 minutes.

Each cracker: About 28 calories, 1 g protein, 5 g carbohydrate, 1 g total fat (trace saturated), 2 mg cholesterol,
79 mg sodium.

Gremolata

PREP TIME: 5 minutes

Makes about 1¼ cups, about 8 servings

This spritely sprinkle of fresh lemon zest, garlic, and parsley breaks up the intense concentration of cooked flavors in foods such as osso buco and rich soups. There are infinite variations using other herbs and cheeses, so feel free to play with the recipe to match it to your soup.

> ½ bunch fresh parsley, rinsed, dried, stemmed,
>   leaves minced (about 1 cup)
> finely chopped zest of 1 lemon
> 2 garlic cloves, minced

Combine the parsley, zest, and garlic in a medium bowl and toss with a fork to mix well.

Each serving: About 5 calories, trace protein, 1 g carbohydrate, trace total fat (0 g saturated), 0 mg cholesterol, 5 mg sodium.

Basil Gremolata
Add 5 tablespoons chopped fresh basil along with the parsley.

Cheese Gremolata
Add 1¼ cups freshly grated Parmigiano-Reggiano, Pecorino Romano, aged Monterey Jack, Asiago, or other hard grating cheese to the mixture.

Herbed Garlic Bread

PREP TIME: 10 minutes
COOK TIME: 10 minutes

Makes 16 servings

The store-bought versions are delicious, but an artisanal loaf combined with home-applied seasonings will make even the homeliest soup a beauty queen.

> 1 large loaf French or Italian bread
> 8 tablespoons (1 stick) unsalted butter,
>   at room temperature
> 2 large garlic cloves, crushed through a press
> 2 tablespoons chopped fresh parsley
> 1 tablespoon finely snipped fresh chives
> 1 teaspoon minced fresh thyme or oregano leaves
>   (no stems) or a mixture of both
> ½ teaspoon kosher salt
> ¼ teaspoon freshly ground pepper

1. Preheat the oven to 375 degrees. Cut the bread crosswise into 1-inch-thick slices but do not cut all the way through the bottom of the loaf. Place lengthwise on a sheet of foil long enough to fold over in the center.

2. In a small bowl, combine the butter, garlic, herbs, salt, and pepper and mix well. Spread about 1 teaspoon of the mixture over the cut sides of the bread. Seal the foil around the bread and bake on the center oven rack until the butter melts and the loaf is hot, about 10 minutes.

Each serving: About 129 calories, 3 g protein, 14 g carbohydrate, 7 g total fat (4 g saturated), 16 mg cholesterol, 239 mg sodium.

Garlic Croûtes

PREP TIME: 5 minutes
COOK TIME: 5 to 10 minutes

Makes 8 croûtes

These bread slices are visual bonuses to bowls of soup.
You can make them hours in advance and just pop them
into the oven to warm a few minutes before serving.

    8 (½-inch-thick) slices French or Italian
      bread (slice on a diagonal)
    4 teaspoons extravirgin olive oil (you may need a
      little more)
    4 small cloves garlic, cut in half lengthwise

**Preheat the broiler. Line a baking sheet with foil.
Place the bread slices on the baking sheet and brush
bread on both sides with olive oil. Broil on both sides
until lightly golden. Rub cut side of garlic over one or
both sides of the toasted bread.**

Each croûte: About 108 calories, 3 g protein, 17 g carbohydrate, 3 g total fat (1 g saturated), 0 mg cholesterol, 192 mg
sodium.

Cheese Croûtes

Omit the olive oil and garlic. Mix ½ cup grated cheese
(such as sharp Cheddar or Pecorino-Romano) and
2 tablespoons softened butter together until smooth in
a small bowl. Season with salt, pepper, powdered mustard, and cayenne pepper so the mixture is spicy. Broil
the bread, as above, on one side until toasted. Turn the
slices over, spread the top with cheese butter, dividing
evenly, and broil again until the tops are golden brown.

Fried Bread Triangles

PREP TIME: 5 minutes
COOK TIME: 5 minutes per batch

Makes 4 servings

When serving hot soups, it is essential to serve a hot
bread to eat alongside the soup. Here's an addictive
cracker to set into a fresh tomato soup—or any other
vegetable soup.

    4 slices homemade-type white bread
    ⅓ cup olive oil or vegetable oil or more if needed

**Cut each slice of bread diagonally into 2 triangles.
Heat the oil in a 10- or 12-inch skillet over medium
heat, add the bread, and fry until browned on both
sides. Transfer to paper towels to drain.**

Each serving: About 87 calories, 2 g protein, 12 g carbohydrate, 3 g total fat (trace saturated), trace cholesterol,
135 mg sodium.

French Peasant Flat Bread

PREP TIME: 25 minutes plus standing
COOK TIME: 25 minutes

Makes about 30 servings

These easy bread squares are best served right out of the oven.

4 to 4½ cups unsifted all-purpose flour plus
   more for the plate
2 cups warm water (110 to 115 degrees)
1 envelope active dry yeast
1 tablespoon sugar
2 teaspoons coarse sea salt or kosher salt
7 tablespoons extravirgin olive oil
cornmeal for dusting the pan
2 tablespoons finely chopped fresh rosemary or
   sage leaves
1 tablespoon freshly ground black pepper
water in a spray bottle for misting

1. Sprinkle a dinner plate with flour. Combine the water, yeast, sugar, and 1 teaspoon salt in a warm, large mixing bowl and stir with a wooden spoon until the yeast, sugar, and salt dissolve. Stir in enough flour to form a loose dough and scrape out onto the prepared plate with a rubber spatula. Immediately slide the dough back into the bowl, flour side down. Cover the bowl with plastic wrap and let rise in a warm place, such as on a running clothes dryer or kitchen counter over a running dishwasher, for 45 minutes.

2. Grease a rimmed baking sheet with 3 tablespoons olive oil and sprinkle lightly with cornmeal. Spread the dough over the pan, flattening it and pressing it down with the fingertips of both hands, rather than pushing and stretching it, to entirely cover the bottom of the pan. Work from above so the angle of your fingers hits the dough at 90 degrees to create an evenly dimpled surface.

3. Brush or sprinkle the dough with 3 tablespoons olive oil, then sprinkle evenly with the rosemary, pepper, and remaining 1 teaspoon salt. Loosely cover the dough with plastic wrap and let rise about 45 minutes, depending on how thick you want the cooked bread to be. (Make it once, letting it rise 45 minutes, and decide how much more or less thick you'd like it next time.)

4. Preheat the oven to 425 degrees. Bake the dough 10 minutes, remove from the oven, and drizzle with the remaining 1 tablespoon oil. Mist lightly with water in a spray bottle and return to the oven. Reduce the heat to 375 degrees and bake the bread until the crust is crisp and sizzling on the underside, about 15 minutes. When the bread is cool enough to handle, slide it onto a cutting board and cut it into pieces as desired with kitchen shears, a chef's knife, or a cleaver.

Each serving: About 92 calories, 2 g protein, 14 g carbohydrate, 3 g total fat (1 g saturated), 0 mg cholesterol, 155 mg sodium.

Tuscan Bread

PREP TIME: 30 minutes plus standing
COOK TIME: 40 minutes

Makes about 16 servings

1 teaspoon active dry yeast
2 cups warm water (110 to 115 degrees)
5 cups unbleached all-purpose flour plus more for kneading
oil for greasing the bowl
cornmeal for dusting the pan
water in a spray bottle for misting

1. The day before baking: Dissolve ¼ teaspoon yeast in ⅔ cup warm water in a medium bowl and let stand until foamy, about 10 minutes. Stir in 1⅓ cups flour and mix until blended. Cover with plastic wrap and let stand at room temperature overnight.

2. The next day, dissolve ¾ teaspoon yeast in ⅓ cup water in a medium bowl and let stand until foamy, about 10 minutes. Add the first yeast mixture and remaining 1 cup water and mix well. Stir in the remaining 3⅔ cups flour, about 1 cup at a time, until a dough forms; turn it out onto a floured surface. Knead the dough until smooth and elastic, about 10 minutes, sprinkling just enough extra flour over the dough to keep it from sticking to your hands and the work surface.

3. Lightly grease a large bowl with oil and add the dough. Turn the dough over so it is oiled on all sides. Cover with plastic wrap and let stand until doubled in bulk, about 1 hour.

4. Gently turn out the dough onto a work surface and pull the edges under to form a large ball with a smooth top. If you have a pizza stone or quarry tiles to line the oven rack, place in the oven and place the dough on a sheet of parchment. If you don't have a pizza stone/tiles, sprinkle a heavy baking sheet with cornmeal and gently place the dough on top. Cover the dough with a clean kitchen towel and set aside to rise until doubled in bulk, about 1 hour.

5. To bake the bread: Preheat the oven to 450 degrees. (Leave the pizza stone/tiles in the oven to preheat.) With a clean razor blade or sharp knife, slash a tic-tac-toe grid in the top of the dough. Slide the bread and parchment onto the pizza stone/tiles with a bread or pizza peel or place the baking sheet with the bread into the oven. Bake the bread 15 minutes, misting the loaf every 5 minutes with water from a spray bottle. Reduce the heat to 400 degrees and bake the bread until crusty and cooked through, about 25 minutes longer. Remove the bread and let cool completely on a wire rack before slicing.

Each serving: About 147 calories, 4 g protein, 30 g carbohydrate, 1 g total fat (trace saturated), 0 mg cholesterol, 1 mg sodium.

Potato and Mixed-Herb Focaccia

PREP TIME: 15 minutes
COOK TIME: 20 minutes

Makes 15 (3-inch) squares

flour for dusting
1 pound frozen bread dough, thawed, at
    room temperature
extravirgin olive oil as needed
12 ounces baking potatoes, skin on, very thinly sliced
¾ teaspoon coarse sea salt or kosher salt
½ teaspoon chopped fresh rosemary leaves
½ teaspoon chopped fresh thyme leaves (no stems)
½ teaspoon dried oregano, crushed
¼ teaspoon freshly ground pepper
6 fresh basil leaves, stacked and finely shredded

1. Preheat the oven to 400 degrees. Grease an 18" by
   13" baking sheet with oil.

2. On a lightly floured work surface, roll out the dough
   to the size of the pan, place the dough into the pan,
   and press and stretch it to fit to all the corners.
   Brush the dough liberally with oil and arrange the
   potato slices, overlapping by about ¼ inch, on the
   dough. Brush the potatoes liberally with oil.

3. Mix the salt, rosemary, thyme, oregano, and
   pepper in a small bowl and sprinkle over the
   potatoes. Bake until the potatoes are tender, their
   edges are browned and curled, and the dough is
   golden brown, 15 to 20 minutes.

4. Slide the focaccia onto a cooling rack to cool until
   the steam is released, about 2 minutes. Slide the

bread onto a cutting board and sprinkle with the
basil. Cut into 3-inch squares or as desired.

Each serving: About 63 calories, 2 g protein, 11 g carbohydrate, 1 g total fat (trace saturated), 0 mg cholesterol, 55 mg
sodium.

Focaccia with Gorgonzola-Walnut Cream
Preheat the oven, prepare the pan, and spread the
dough over the pan, flattening it and pressing it down
with the fingertips of both hands, rather than pushing
and stretching it, to entirely cover the bottom of the pan.
Work from above so the angle of your fingers hits the
dough at 90 degrees to create an evenly dimpled
surface. Brush the dough with olive oil. Mash together
8 ounces Gorgonzola cheese, crumbled, ½ cup chopped
walnuts, and ¼ cup heavy cream in a bowl and spread
over the dough. Bake at 425 degrees for 10 minutes,
reduce the heat to 375 degrees, and bake until the topping is golden, about 10 minutes.

Sweet Onion Focaccia
Peel and very thinly slice 12 ounces of sweet onions
such as Vidalia, Maui, or Walla-Walla. Preheat the oven,
prepare the pan, and spread the dough over the pan,
flattening it and pressing it down with the fingertips of
both hands, rather than pushing and stretching it, to
entirely cover the bottom of the pan. Work from above so
the angle of your fingers hits the dough at 90 degrees to
create an evenly dimpled surface. Brush the dough with
olive oil. Spread the onions on top and sprinkle with 3
tablespoons extravirgin olive oil, a little bit of fine sea
salt or kosher salt, and a generous grinding of black
peppercorns. Bake as directed for the Potato and Mixed-
Herb Focaccia.

Sopaipillas

PREP TIME: 30 minutes
COOK TIME: 5 minutes

Makes 8 servings

These are tasty, crisp breads that will add glamour to soups flavored with tomato or cilantro. They are said to have originated in New Mexico over 200 years ago.

> 2 cups unsifted all-purpose flour plus more for rolling out the dough
> 1 teaspoon salt
> ¾ teaspoon baking powder
> ½ teaspoon sugar
> ½ cup warm water
> 2 tablespoons vegetable oil plus more for frying
> 2 tablespoons milk
> warmed honey (optional)
> ground cinnamon (optional)
> fine sea salt (optional)

1. Mix the flour, salt, baking powder, and sugar in a medium bowl. Stir in the water, 2 tablespoons oil, and the milk with a wooden spoon, mixing until a dough forms. Turn out the dough onto a lightly floured surface and knead until smooth, about 3 minutes. Cover dough with a bowl and let rest 15 minutes.

2. Heat 2 inches vegetable oil in a deep large saucepan over medium-high heat until the oil registers 375 degrees on a deep-fat thermometer. Divide the dough into 8 equal pieces and roll each out on a lightly floured surface to a 5-inch round. Fry the sopaipillas, two at a time, until puffed and golden, about 30 seconds. Turn each over and fry until golden. Drain on paper towels. While hot, drizzle with honey or sprinkle with cinnamon or salt. Serve warm.

Each serving (without honey or seasoning): About 164 calories, 3 g protein, 24 g carbohydrate, 6 g total fat (1 g saturated), 1 mg cholesterol, 337 mg sodium.

Nothing-but-Cheese Crisps

PREP TIME: 5 minutes
COOK TIME: about 10 minutes

Makes 6 servings

> 1 tablespoon olive oil
> ¾ cup shredded cheese (one kind or a mix)
> salt and freshly ground black pepper to taste

Heat the oil in a 10-inch nonstick skillet over medium-low heat. For each crisp, sprinkle 2 tablespoons of cheese in a 3-inch round in the pan and sprinkle lightly with salt and pepper. Cook until the cheese melts and is crisp. Gently flip over each crisp to cook lightly on the other side. Transfer to a paper towel–lined plate to drain. Serve immediately.

Each serving: About 62 calories, 4 g protein, trace carbohydrate, 5 g total fat (2 g saturated), 7 mg cholesterol, 220 mg sodium.

Scallion Pancakes

PREP TIME: 50 minutes
COOK TIME: 20 minutes

Makes 6 pancakes, 6 to 12 servings

   3 cups sifted all-purpose flour, plus more
      for kneading
   1 cup water
   2 tablespoons dark sesame oil
   10 to 15 scallions, finely chopped
   1½ teaspoons salt
   peanut oil for frying

1. Place the flour in a medium bowl and make a well in the center. Add the water and stir until a dough forms. Cover with plastic wrap and let rest 30 minutes.

2. Knead the dough on a lightly floured surface for 2 minutes. Cut the dough into 6 equal pieces, place one piece of dough on a lightly floured work surface, and roll to a 10" by 6" rectangle that is ⅛-inch thick. With the long side of the dough rectangle facing you, brush 1 teaspoon sesame oil over the dough and sprinkle with one-sixth of the scallions and then ¼ teaspoon salt. Roll up the dough to form a fairly loose roll, and pinch the ends and along the side seam to seal. Coil the roll into a round, gently press to flatten and join the pieces of the coil, and roll it gently with a rolling pin to form a 6-inch patty that is about ¼ inch thick. Cover with a clean kitchen towel and repeat with the remaining dough, scallions, sesame oil, and salt.

3. Preheat the oven to low. Heat 2 teaspoons oil in an 8-inch nonstick skillet over medium heat and fry the pancake, covered, until browned about 2 minutes.

Turn the pancake over and fry until browned on the second side. Transfer to a paper towel–lined baking sheet and keep warm in the oven while frying the remaining pancakes. To serve, cut each pancake crosswise into quarters.

Each pancake: About 321 calories, 7 g protein, 51 g carbohydrate, 10 g total fat (2 g saturated), 0 mg cholesterol, 585 mg sodium.

Rice-Paper Crisps

PREP TIME: 5 minutes
COOK TIME: about 10 minutes

Makes 6 servings

   peanut oil or vegetable oil for frying
   6 wedges Vietnamese rice-paper wrappers
   Chinese five-spice powder, curry powder, or
      ground cinnamon for dusting

Heat about ¼ inch oil in an 8-inch skillet over medium-high heat. Add a rice-paper wedge and fry until puffed all the way through. Immediately transfer with tongs to a paper towel–lined plate and sprinkle with Chinese five-spice powder, curry powder, or ground cinnamon. Repeat with remaining wrappers.

Each serving: About 47 calories, 1 g protein, 7 g carbohydrate, 2 g total fat (trace saturated), 0 mg cholesterol, 13 mg sodium.

Buttery Cheese Straws

PREP TIME: 20 minutes
COOK TIME: about 15 minutes

Makes about 42 straws

1 cup sifted unbleached all-purpose flour plus
more for rolling
½ teaspoon baking powder
⅛ teaspoon cayenne pepper or more to taste
8 tablespoons (1 stick) cold unsalted butter
in pieces
1 cup finely grated (on a microplane) Parmigiano-
Reggiano cheese or extra-sharp Cheddar cheese
3 tablespoons ice water
coarse sea salt and paprika or minced walnuts

1. Preheat the oven to 375 degrees. Line a baking sheet
with parchment. Place the flour, baking powder, and
pepper in a medium bowl and mix well. Add the
butter and cheese and mix until blended as for
piecrust dough, with a pastry blender, two knives, or
your fingertips. Stir in the water just until blended.
Pack the dough into a cookie press fitted with a star
tip and screw on the plunger and cap.

2. Press out long straws onto the parchment and sprinkle
lightly with salt and paprika, or the nuts. Cut into 2½-
inch lengths and separate slightly. Bake until the straws
are firm and golden, about 8 minutes. Remove from the
pan immediately and cool on wire racks.

Each straw without toppings: About 41 calories, 1 g protein,
2 g carbohydrate, 3 g total fat (2 g saturated), 8 mg cholesterol, 51 mg sodium.

Sesame Seed Crackers

PREP TIME: 20 minutes
COOK TIME: 20 minutes

Makes 30 to 40 crackers

¼ cup corn oil plus more for greasing
1 cup whole-wheat flour
½ cup unbleached all-purpose flour
¼ cup soy flour
¼ cup sesame seeds
1 teaspoon salt
⅓ cup cold water or more if needed

1. Preheat the oven to 350 degrees. Lightly oil a large
rimless baking sheet. Place the flours, sesame
seeds, and salt into a large bowl and mix well. Make
a well in the center and pour the oil and water into
the well. Stir with a fork until blended, adding more
water if necessary to make a smooth but not sticky
dough that forms a firm ball.

2. Place the dough in the center of the baking sheet
and roll out to an ⅛-inch rectangle. Score the dough
into 1½- to 2-inch squares with a knife, but do not
cut completely through the dough. (The lines will
allow the dough to break cleanly into squares after
baking but the crackers would brown too much if
they cook as separate pieces.) Bake until crisp and
golden, about 20 minutes. Watch the crackers carefully as the seeds easily scorch.

Each serving of 30 cracker batch: About 47 calories, 1 g protein, 5 g carbohydrate, 3 g total fat (trace saturated), 0 mg
cholesterol, 78 mg sodium.

Matzoh

PREP TIME: 20 minutes
COOK TIME: 18 minutes

Makes 4 matzohs

> 2 cups unbleached all-purpose flour and more
>   for rolling
> ½ to ¾ cup cold water

1. Preheat the oven to 500 degrees. Place the flour in a pile on a work surface or in a bowl and make a well in the center. Pour ½ cup water into the well and stir it with a fork, dragging the flour into the water from inside the pile. Add more water if needed until all the flour is mixed in and the dough is soft and pliable but not sticky.

2. Divide the dough into 4 equal pieces and knead each about 10 times, using a little flour to keep the dough from sticking. Scrape the work surface to remove any particles of dough and dust with clean flour. Roll one piece of dough into a 7-inch round that is less than ⅛ inch thick. Pierce the round completely through with a fork to keep the matzoh from buckling as it bakes. Lift the dough onto the rolling pin for support and place it on a heavy, ungreased baking sheet. If there is room on a baking sheet for 2 rounds, repeat with another piece of dough. If space is limited, do not roll out the dough until it can go directly into the oven.

3. Bake the matzoh until it curls, looks very dry, and shows some patches and edges, about 10 minutes, and turn it over. Bake until it is golden brown on the second side, 5 to 8 minutes longer. (Some very dark blisters are desirable because they add a special flavor.) Transfer to a wire rack to cool. Repeat with remaining dough.

Each serving: About 227 calories, 7 g protein, 48 g carbohydrate, 1 g total fat (trace saturated), 0 mg cholesterol, 2 mg sodium.

Whole-Wheat Matzoh
Use whole-wheat flour instead of the all-purpose flour in the above recipe. You will need to add more water, about ¼ cup to get the dough to form. The whole-wheat version will be a little thicker than the plain matzoh.

Seasoned Matzoh
Rub one side of the baked matzoh with the cut side of an onion or garlic clove (or both) and slightly mist the flavored side with water from a spray bottle. Sprinkle with kosher salt or fine sea salt and freshly ground black pepper and bake on a baking sheet in a 375-degree oven until dry and crisp, 5 to 7 minutes.

Brittle Bread

PREP TIME: 15 minutes
COOK TIME: 5 minutes

Makes about 40 servings

2¾ cups unbleached all-purpose flour plus more
    for rolling
1 to 2 tablespoons sugar
½ teaspoon baking soda
½ teaspoon salt
8 tablespoons unsalted butter (1 stick), in ½-inch
    pieces, frozen if using a food processor
1 cup (8 ounces) plain yogurt
water in a spray bottle for misting
chopped dried herbs, spices, kosher salt, freshly
    ground black pepper, and/or seeds (such as
    mustard, fennel, cumin, sesame) as desired

1. Preheat the oven to 400 degrees. Place the flour,
   sugar, baking soda, and salt into a large bowl and
   mix well. Add the butter and cut in as for piecrust
   with a pastry blender or 2 knives until the mixture
   resembles cornmeal. Add the yogurt and stir with a
   fork until the mixture forms a dough.

2. Break off marble-size pieces of dough and roll out
   on a lightly floured surface to 7-inch rounds that are
   less than ⅛-inch thick, even paper-thin. Place on
   ungreased baking sheets and mist with water.
   Sprinkle with any combination of seasoning, or any
   single seasoning. Bake until crisp and golden brown,
   3 to 5 minutes. Transfer to wire racks to cool.

Each serving: About 57 calories, 1 g protein, 7 g carbohydrate, 3 g total fat (2 g saturated), 7 mg cholesterol, 71 mg
sodium.

Graham Crackers

PREP TIME: 1 hour
COOK TIME: 20 minutes per batch

Makes about 3 dozen

Serve these with any fruit soup to provide a sweet but
earthy counterpoint to the sweetness of the soup.

2¾ cups whole-wheat (graham) flour plus more
    for rolling
½ teaspoon baking powder
½ teaspoon salt
⅛ teaspoon ground cinnamon
8 tablespoons unsalted butter, softened
⅔ cup packed brown sugar
½ cup water
corn oil for greasing the pan (optional)

1. Mix the flour with the baking powder, salt, and cinnamon in a medium bowl. Combine the butter and sugar
   in a large bowl and beat until fluffy and no longer
   gritty. Stir in one-fourth of the flour mixture at a time,
   alternating with one-third of the water, until blended.
   Cover with plastic wrap and let rest 30 minutes.

2. Preheat the oven to 350 degrees. Grease 2 baking
   sheets with oil or line with parchment. Roll out the
   dough on a lightly floured surface to an 1/8-inch-thick
   rectangle. Cut into 2-inch squares with a pizza cutter
   or knife or use a 2-inch cookie cutter to cut out
   rounds. Place crackers on the prepared baking sheet
   and bake until lightly browned, about 20 minutes.

Each cracker: About 64 calories, 1 g protein, 9 g carbohydrate, 3 g total fat (2 g saturated), 7 mg cholesterol, 66 mg
sodium.

Lavash

ARMENIAN THIN BREAD

PREP TIME: 45 minutes plus standing
COOK TIME: 5 minutes per batch

Makes about 14 crackers

2 tablespoons plus 1 cup warm water (110 to
    115 degrees)
1½ teaspoons sugar
1½ envelopes active dry yeast
3½ cups unbleached all-purpose flour and more
    for kneading and rolling
1½ teaspoons salt
4 tablespoons unsalted butter, melted and cooled
vegetable oil for greasing the bowl
water in a spray bottle for misting

1. Place 2 tablespoons warm water and ½ teaspoon
   sugar in a small bowl and stir until the sugar
   dissolves. Sprinkle the yeast on top and let stand until
   the yeast is dissolved and foamy, about 10 minutes.

2. Place the flour and salt in a large bowl and mix well.
   Make a well in the center and pour the remaining
   1 cup warm water into the well. Add the yeast
   mixture, remaining 1 teaspoon sugar, and the butter
   and stir with a spoon until blended and a dough
   forms. Turn out the dough onto a lightly floured
   surface and knead until smooth and elastic, about
   10 minutes. Add more flour as needed to keep the
   dough from sticking. Shape the dough into a
   smooth ball.

3. Clean the mixing bowl and grease with oil. Place the
   dough in the bowl and turn to grease all sides. Cover
   with plastic wrap and let rise in a warm place until
   doubled in bulk, about 3 hours.

4. Preheat the oven to 450 degrees. Punch down the
   dough and separate into 4 or more equal-size pieces
   with your hands. Place a piece of dough on a lightly
   floured surface, and cover the remaining pieces with
   plastic wrap. Lightly flour the dough piece and roll it
   out with light strokes from the center, rotating the
   dough a little after each stroke. Shape the dough as
   desired, into a long, very thin, irregular, free-form
   strip or a neat rectangle. Cut the rectangle into triangles with a pizza cutter. Place the triangles or the
   irregular strip on an ungreased baking sheet. Mist
   the dough with water and prick all over with a fork.

5. Repeat with another piece of dough and bake until
   golden brown, 3 to 5 minutes. Turn the crackers over
   if they are not cooked through (it will depend on how
   thick they are) and bake 1 to 2 minutes longer.
   Transfer to wire racks to cool. Repeat with remaining
   dough. While the crackers bake, roll out remaining
   dough, making only enough crackers to bake immediately after rolling.

Each cracker: About 151 calories, 4 g protein, 25 g carbohydrate, 4 g total fat (2 g saturated), 9 mg cholesterol, 282 mg
sodium.

Quick Pepper-Parmesan Crisps

PREP TIME: 25 minutes plus standing
COOK TIME: 6 minutes per batch

Makes 6 servings

1¾ cups unbleached all-purpose flour plus more
   for kneading and rolling
⅓ cup freshly grated (with a microplane)
   Parmigiano-Reggiano cheese
¾ teaspoon salt
½ teaspoon freshly ground black pepper
⅔ cup warm water
1 tablespoon olive oil
water in a spray bottle for misting

1. Place the flour, cheese, salt, and pepper in a bowl
   and gradually stir in the water and oil until a firm but
   not sticky dough forms. Turn out the dough onto a
   lightly floured surface and knead until smooth, about
   3 minutes. Separate into 6 equal pieces of dough,
   shape into balls, and lightly dust with flour. Place on
   a cutting board, cover with plastic wrap, and let rest
   at least 20 minutes or up to 12 hours.

2. Preheat the oven to 450 degrees. Place a heavy large
   baking sheet on the middle rack of the oven to preheat. Meanwhile, roll out a piece of dough on a lightly
   floured surface to a paper-thin round about 8 inches
   in diameter.

3. Remove the hot baking sheet from the oven, drape
   the round over the rolling pin, and transfer the dough
   to the hot pan. Mist lightly with water. Bake until
   golden, 2 to 3 minutes, turn the round over, mist it
   again, and bake until crisp and browned around the
   edges, 2 to 3 minutes longer. Remove the bread
   from the pan (it should be crisp enough to stay flat;
   return it to the oven to bake a minute or so longer if
   it bends). Cool on a wire rack. Repeat with the
   remaining dough.

Each serving: About 178 calories, 6 g protein, 28 g carbohydrate, 4 g total fat (1 g saturated), 4 mg cholesterol, 392 mg
sodium.

Aioli

PREP TIME: 10 minutes

Makes about 1½ cups, about 24 servings

This classic French garlic mayonnaise is a wonderful spread on sandwiches
and as a binder in salads, but it's also a traditional thickener for soup. Just
be sure not to simmer or boil the soup once the sauce goes in, or the egg
will curdle.

> 1 large egg or 2 egg yolks
> 1 large garlic clove, peeled
> 1 tablespoon fresh lemon juice or more to taste
> 1 to 1½ cups extravirgin olive oil or more if needed
> salt and pepper to taste

**Combine the egg, garlic, lemon juice, and 2 tablespoons oil in a food
processor and blend until smooth, about 1 minute. With the machine
running, pour in enough of the remaining oil through the feed tube in a
thin, steady stream to a make creamy and smooth sauce that is thick but
not stiff. Stop the machine and scrape the sides. Taste the sauce and
season with salt and pepper and more lemon juice if needed.**

Each serving: About 83 calories, trace protein, trace carbohydrate, 9 g total fat
(1 g saturated), 9 mg cholesterol, 27 mg sodium.

Saffron Aioli

A dollop of this is traditional in fish soups. Combine ¼ teaspoon saffron
threads and 1 tablespoon hot water in a small bowl and let soak 20 minutes.
Whisk the saffron and water into 1 to 2 cups mayonnaise.

Saffron-Orange Aioli

Add 1 teaspoon grated orange zest and 1 tablespoon fresh orange juice to
Saffron Aioli.

Bread Aioli

PREP TIME: 15 minutes

Makes about 1¾ cups, about 28 servings

The addition of a slice of bread makes for a bit more substantial mayonnaise.

  1 (½-inch-thick) slice French bread
  3 tablespoons half-and-half
  2 egg yolks
  2 large garlic cloves, peeled
  1 tablespoon fresh lemon juice or more to taste
  1¼ to 1½ cups extravirgin olive oil or more if needed
  salt and pepper to taste

1. Combine the bread and half-and-half in a small bowl and let soak
   5 minutes. Hold the bread in your fingers and squeeze out the
   half-and-half.

2. Combine the squeezed bread, egg yolks, garlic, lemon juice, and
   2 tablespoons oil in a food processor and blend until smooth, about
   1 minute. With the machine running, pour in enough of the remaining oil
   through the feed tube in a thin, steady stream to a make a creamy and
   smooth sauce that is thick but not stiff. Stop the machine and scrape the
   sides. Taste the sauce and season with salt and pepper and more lemon
   juice if needed.

Each serving: About 94 calories, trace protein, 1 g carbohydrate, 10 g total fat
(2 g saturated), 16 mg cholesterol, 27 mg sodium.

Potato Aioli
Instead of the soaked bread, use 2 tablespoons mashed potato (without milk
or butter).

Bean or Legume Aioli

PREP TIME: 10 minutes

Makes 1½ cups, about 24 servings

You can use beans or lentils to thicken an aioli. Mix and match the beans' flavor and color to the soup and vary the flavor of the aioli by using different herbs.

½ cup cooked beans or lentils (from dried beans or drained, rinsed canned beans)
½ cup fresh mint, cilantro, or Italian parsley leaves
juice of 1 lemon
1 large egg
1 garlic clove, peeled
1 cup extravirgin olive oil
salt and pepper to taste

Combine the beans, herbs, lemon juice, egg, garlic, and ½ cup oil in a food processor and blend until smooth, about 1 minute. With the machine running, pour in the remaining oil through the feed tube in a thin, steady stream and to make a creamy and smooth sauce. Stop the machine and scrape the sides. Taste the sauce and season with salt and pepper.

Each serving: About 89 calories, 1 g protein, 1 g carbohydrate, 9 g total fat (1 g saturated), 9 mg cholesterol, 27 mg sodium.

Romesco Sauce

PREP TIME: 25 minutes
COOK TIME: 1 hour 15 minutes

Makes about 2 cups, about 16 servings

Spanish Romesco sauce is a many splendored, multi-versioned thing. To summarize the sauce at best, most interpretations contain roasted, dried, or raw red piquillo pepper (the Spanish ñora bell pepper, which is sweet but with a little heat), roasted or raw garlic, and toasted almonds and/or hazelnuts. Some contain tomatoes and/or bread. See the following recipes for two other versions. Stir Romesco into fish soups, use it as a dip for grilled vegetables, or spread it over toasted slices of French bread.

¼ cup blanched Spanish Marcona almonds or other almonds
¼ cup hazelnuts
12 garlic cloves, unpeeled
6 large ripe plum tomatoes, cored, halved, and seeded
1 cup extravirgin olive oil, preferably Arbequina olive oil or other Spanish olive oil, plus more for drizzling and finishing
sea salt
1 dried ancho chile, soaked in hot water 20 minutes
1 can or jar (about 150 grams) imported Spanish piquillo peppers or 1 jar (8 ounces) roasted red peppers and ¼ teaspoon cayenne pepper
1 to 2 tablespoons aged sherry vinegar or red-wine vinegar or to taste
1 to 2 tablespoons red wine, preferably Spanish, such as Priorato or Rioja, or to taste

1. Preheat the oven to 400 degrees and line a baking pan with foil. Spread the almonds and hazelnuts in a rimmed baking sheet and roast until toasted, about 8 minutes, stirring every 2 minutes. Place the almonds in a food processor and the hazelnuts on a clean kitchen towel. Rub the skins off the hazelnuts with the towel and add to the food processor; set aside to cool.

2. While the nuts cool, place the garlic cloves and tomatoes in the baking sheet, drizzle with about 1 tablespoon oil, and sprinkle the tomatoes with salt. Toss to coat and arrange the tomatoes cut sides up in the sheet. Bake 15 minutes, reduce the heat to 350 degrees, and bake until the garlic is soft and golden brown but not burned, about 20 minutes. Remove the garlic from the pan and set aside. Continue cooking the tomatoes until roasted, about 40 minutes. Let cool.

3. Drain the ancho chile, cut in half lengthwise, and remove the seeds. With a sharp knife, scrape the flesh from the skin, chop coarsely, and add it to the nuts in the food processor. Squeeze the garlic pulp from the skins into the food processor. Remove the skins from the tomatoes, coarsely chop the flesh, and place in the food processor. Add the piquillo peppers. Pulse several times to mix. Process until a paste forms. With the machine running, pour in about 1 cup oil in a thin stream until the texture resembles yogurt. Season with salt, vinegar, and wine.

Each serving: About 280 calories, 1 g protein, 4 g carbohydrate, 30 g total fat (4 g saturated), 0 mg cholesterol, 270 mg sodium.

Romesco Sauce with Bread and Raw Garlic

PREP TIME: 10 minutes
COOK TIME: 5 minutes

Makes about 1¼ cups, about 10 servings

Maybe you have lived your whole life without Romesco sauce and now you have more choices than you imagined. Spoon it into soups, or onto croûtes to add to soups. Experiment with this variation of the basic sauce to elevate the flavor of soups without overpowering the basic ingredients.

½ cup extravirgin olive oil, preferably Arbequina olive oil or other Spanish olive oil plus more for drizzling and finishing
2 (½-inch-thick) slices French bread with the crusts, torn into 1-inch pieces
½ cup blanched Spanish Marcona almonds or ¼ cup blanched almonds and ¼ cup skinned toasted hazelnuts
1 can or jar (about 150 grams) imported Spanish piquillo peppers or 1 jar (8 ounces) roasted red peppers and ¼ teaspoon cayenne pepper
3 large garlic cloves, minced
1 small jalapeño pepper, seeded and minced
1 to 2 tablespoons red-wine vinegar
sea salt to taste

1. Heat ¼ cup oil in a small skillet over medium heat and gently fry the bread and almonds until the bread is crisp and golden brown (do not let the heat get too high or it will destroy the delicate flavor of the oil). Pour the contents of the skillet into a food processor and pulse until the nuts are finely ground. Place in a bowl.

2. Place the piquillo peppers in the food processor and pulse until mixed. With the machine running, pour the remaining ¼ cup olive oil through the feed tube in a thin, steady stream and process until smooth; pour into the bowl with the nut mixture. Add the garlic and jalapeño and mix well. Season with vinegar and salt.

Each serving: About 157 calories, 2 g protein, 5 g carbohydrate, 15 g total fat (2 g saturated), 0 mg cholesterol, 460 mg sodium.

Romesco Sauce with Spanish Paprika

PREP TIME: 10 minutes
COOK TIME: 5 minutes

Makes about 1 cup, about 4 servings

¼ cup red wine, preferably Spanish, such as Priorato or Rioja
2 tablespoons pimentón (sweet or bittersweet Spanish paprika) or
    other paprika
2 tablespoons hot water
pinch crushed saffron threads
2 tablespoons extravirgin olive oil, preferably Spanish
3 garlic cloves, sliced
½ cup fresh breadcrumbs
¼ cup blanched almonds or skinned, toasted hazelnuts
⅓ cup Fish Stock or Vegetable Stock (pages 16 or 15), or water
1 tablespoon white-wine vinegar
sea salt to taste

1. Mix the wine and pimentón in a small bowl until blended to a paste; set
   aside. Combine the hot water and saffron in another small bowl and
   set aside.

2. Heat the oil in a small skillet over medium heat and gently sauté the
   garlic, breadcrumbs, and almonds until the bread is crisp and golden
   brown (do not let the heat get too high or it will destroy the delicate
   flavor of the oil). Pour the contents of the skillet into a food processor,
   add the pimentón paste, saffron infusion, stock, and vinegar and pulse
   until smooth. Place in a bowl and season with salt.

Each serving: About 78 calories, 2 g protein, 4 g carbohydrate, 6 g total fat
(1 g saturated), trace cholesterol, 107 mg sodium.

Rouille

PREP TIME: 20 minutes

Makes about 6 servings

Note the similarities in this vibrant Provençal sauce and the dynamic Romesco Sauce with Bread and Raw Garlic (page 42). The word *rouille* is French for "rust" and is appropriate because of the brownish-red color from the roasted peppers. It is traditionally stirred into bouillabaisse or other fish or vegetable soups or served with boiled fish or octopus.

  1 cup 1-inch pieces of crusts from a French baguette
  ¼ cup cold water
  2 freshly roasted, peeled, and seeded red bell peppers or jarred
     roasted red peppers or Spanish piquillo peppers
  2 small garlic cloves, halved
  ¼ cup extravirgin olive oil
  1 tablespoon fresh lemon juice
  sea salt to taste
  cayenne pepper to taste
  1 tablespoon hot water plus more if needed

1. Place the crust pieces in a small food processor and drizzle with the water. Pulse until evenly dampened. Let stand 10 minutes.

2. Add the peppers and garlic to the bread and process until smooth. With the machine running, pour in the oil through the feed tube in a thin, steady stream and process until the sauce is creamy and smooth. Pulse in the lemon juice. Scrape the sauce into a bowl and season with sea salt and a pinch of cayenne or more to taste. (The sauce should be fiery.) If the sauce is too stiff, thin with a little hot water.

Each serving: About 113 calories, 1 g protein, 7 g carbohydrate, 10 g total fat (1 g saturated), trace cholesterol, 780 mg sodium.

Skordalia

PREP TIME: 15 minutes
COOK TIME: 20 to 30 minutes

Makes 2 cups, about 8 servings

Also called *Skorthaliá*, this rich sauce is used as a flavorful finish to fish soups (and is also served with grilled vegetables, meat, chicken, and fish). The pungent mixture is best stirred by dollops into the broth of a soup or stew. Note that the flavor is enhanced if the sauce is refrigerated overnight.

1 pound waxy potatoes, all the same size, unpeeled
2 teaspoons salt or more to taste
4 large garlic cloves, crushed through a press
½ cup extravirgin olive oil, preferably Greek
¼ cup fresh lemon juice, white-wine vinegar, or
   mild white vinegar
freshly ground white pepper to taste

1. Place the potatoes into a 2-quart saucepan, add enough water to cover, and swirl in 1 teaspoon salt. Cover and heat to boiling over medium-high heat. Reduce the heat to medium and simmer until the potatoes are easily pierced to the center with a paring knife, 20 to 30 minutes. (Do not test before 20 minutes to keep the skin from splitting.)

2. Drain the potatoes and when they are cool enough to handle, remove the skins. Place the potatoes into a bowl and mash them until smooth with the garlic and remaining 1 teaspoon salt. When the potatoes are smooth, gradually mash in the oil and lemon juice. Season with pepper and additional salt if necessary.

Each serving: About 168 calories, 1 g protein, 11 g carbohydrate, 14 g total fat (2 g saturated), 0 mg cholesterol, 293 mg sodium.

Skordalia with Breadcrumbs

This is a lighter sauce, perfect in the summer with chilled soups and fried vegetables such as eggplant, zucchini, and green tomatoes. Instead of using the potatoes, remove the crusts from 8 ounces of day-old bread, tear up the bread, and place in a bowl. Drizzle with water and toss until evenly soaked. Squeeze out the water and place the bread in a food processor. Add the garlic and 1 teaspoon salt and pulse to mix. With the machine running, add the oil and then the lemon juice in a thin stream through the feed tube until blended to a smooth puree. Season with pepper and more salt to taste. Makes about 1 cup, about 8 servings.

Classic Pesto

PREP TIME: 10 minutes

Makes about 2 cups, about 16 servings

This world-embraced condiment is a gift from Genoa. The concentrated mixture of basil, garlic, pine nuts, cheese, and olive oil quickly spreads its intensity into soup, perking up bland beans or hearty but monotonous meats such as turkey. The word *pesto* is derived from the Italian *pestare*, which means to pound, for the sauce is traditionally made in a mortar and pounded with a pestle.

2 large garlic cloves, halved
2 cups firmly packed stemmed fresh basil leaves
¾ cup grated Parmigiano-Reggiano cheese
2 tablespoons pine nuts
¾ cup extravirgin Italian olive oil or more if needed

Place the garlic, basil, cheese, and nuts in food processor or blender. Cover and blend until smooth. With the machine running, pour in the oil through the feed tube in a thin, steady stream and process into a thick, smooth paste, adding a little more oil if the mixture is stiff and stopping to scrape the sides.

Each serving: About 118 calories, 2 g protein, 1 g carbohydrate, 12 g total fat (2 g saturated), 4 mg cholesterol, 88 mg sodium.

Variations:
You can create all kinds of pesto by varying the leafy part and the nut part. Try spinach leaves with walnuts or parsley with pistachios.

Olive Pesto

PREP TIME: 10 minutes

Makes about 2 cups, about 16 servings

Here, olives replace cheese and basil in an exotic variation on Italy's ubiquitous sauce. Imported but not brine-packed olives are best—use French, Italian, Spanish, Greek, or Moroccan olives, spicy mixed olives, or even almond-stuffed olives.

1 garlic clove, diced
½ red onion
15 cups pitted olives
¼ cup pine nuts
½ cup extravirgin olive oil or more if needed

Combine the garlic, onion, olives, and pine nuts in a food processor and blend until evenly chopped, about 1 minute. With the machine running, pour the ½ cup oil through the feed tube in a thin, steady stream and process until a thick, smooth paste forms, adding a little more oil if the mixture is stiff.

Each serving: About 87 calories, trace protein, 2 g carbohydrate, 9 g total fat (1 g saturated), 0 mg cholesterol, 111 mg sodium.

Pistou

PREP TIME: 10 minutes

Makes about 1¼ cups, 8 servings

This pungent sauce, France's parry to Italy's pesto, is obviously similar but characteristically Provençal because of the addition of tomatoes.

 2 very ripe plum tomatoes, skinned and seeded
 2 large garlic cloves, halved
 ¾ cup freshly grated Parmigiano-Reggiano cheese
 ¼ cup packed stemmed fresh basil leaves
 ¼ to ⅓ cup extravirgin olive oil
 salt and freshly ground pepper to taste

Combine the tomatoes, garlic, cheese, and basil in a food processor or blender and blend until they form a paste. With the machine running, pour in enough of the oil through the feed tube in a thin, steady stream to make a smooth and thick but not stiff texture. Scrape into a bowl and season with salt and pepper.

Each serving: About 107 calories, 4 g protein, 1 g carbohydrate, 10 g total fat (3 g saturated), 7 mg cholesterol, 248 mg sodium.

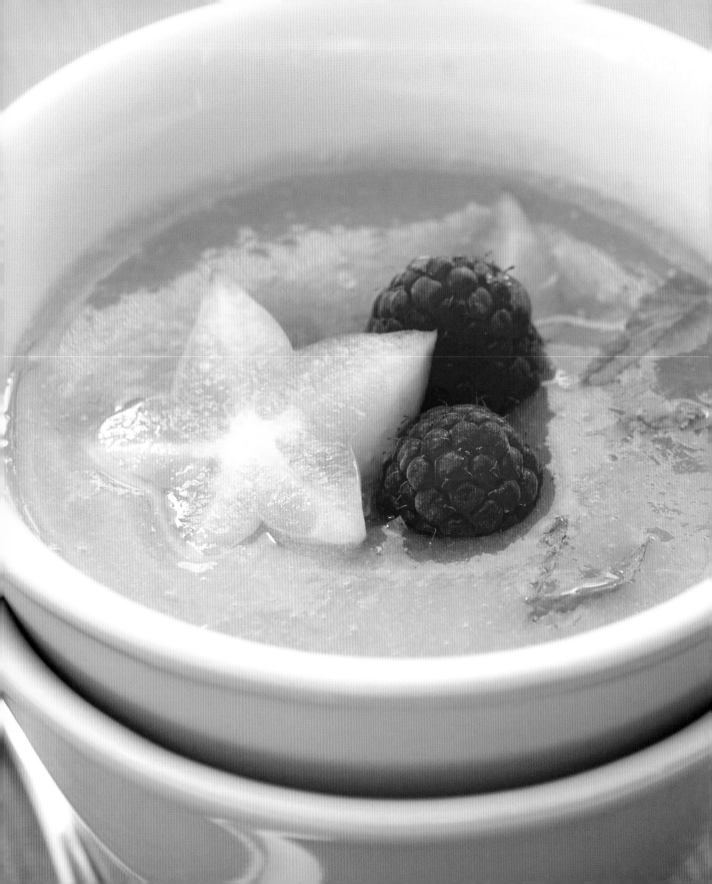

2
FRUIT SOUPS

Spiced Mixed Fruit Soup

PREP TIME: 10 minutes
COOK TIME: 15 minutes, plus 30 minutes to chill

Makes 4 servings

For bright, fresh-looking pears and nectarines, cut them right before adding to the soup.

    2 cups apple juice
    1 cinnamon stick
    2 whole allspice berries
    2 lemon tea bags
    2 cups vanilla low-fat yogurt
    1 Bartlett pear, cored and chopped
    1 cup cubed watermelon
    1 cup white grapes
    1 cup red grapes
    1 nectarine, pitted and chopped

1. Combine the apple juice, cinnamon, allspice, and tea bags in a 2-quart saucepan. Cover and bring to a boil. Reduce the heat and simmer 5 minutes. With a slotted spoon, discard the cinnamon, allspice, and tea. Chill for 30 minutes.

2. In a serving bowl, whisk together the yogurt and 1½ to 2 cups of the juice mixture. Determine how much juice mixture to use by the consistency of the soup. Stir in the pears, watermelon, white grapes, red grapes, and nectarine.

Each serving: About 266 calories, 7 g protein, 58 g carbohydrate, 2 g total fat (1 g saturated), 6 mg cholesterol, 87 mg sodium.

Chilled Blueberry Soup

PREP TIME: 10 minutes
COOK TIME: 1 hour to chill

Makes 4 servings

    1 pint fresh blueberries
    1 cup fresh orange juice
    ½ cup plus 1 tablespoon sour cream
    1 tablespoon granulated sugar
    1 tablespoon packed light brown sugar
    ¾ teaspoon ground nutmeg

1. In a blender or food processor, puree the blueberries, orange juice, ½ cup sour cream, granulated sugar, brown sugar, and nutmeg until smooth. Pour into a large bowl, cover, and chill for at least an hour.

2. In a small bowl, using a wire whisk, beat the remaining 1 tablespoon sour cream until smooth. Spoon into a pastry bag fitted with a fine round tip.

3. Pour the soup into chilled bowls, and squeeze the sour cream from the pastry bag onto the top of the soup in a design.

Each serving: About 170 calories, 2 g protein, 29 g carbohydrate, 6 g total fat (4 g saturated), 13 mg cholesterol, 19 mg sodium.

Classic Strawberry Soup

PREP TIME: 10 minutes
COOK TIME: 15 minutes, plus 2 hours to chill

Makes 6 servings

Strawberry soup is an old standard and thought to be one of the first cold berry soups created.

  ½ teaspoon instant tapioca
  1 cup fresh unsweetened orange juice
  2 pints fresh strawberries
  1 tablespoon fresh lemon juice
  cinnamon to taste
  allspice to taste
  ½ cup granulated sugar plus more if needed
  1 teaspoon lemon zest
  1 cup buttermilk
  1 lime, thinly sliced, for garnish
  additional sliced strawberries for garnish

1. In a bowl, combine the tapioca and orange juice and set aside for 5 minutes. In a blender or food processor, puree the strawberries until smooth.

2. In a saucepan, combine the tapioca mixture and strawberries. Stir in the lemon juice, cinnamon, and allspice. Bring to a boil; reduce to a simmer, and cook, stirring constantly, until thickened. Turn off the heat and stir in the sugar. Cool slightly, cover tightly, and refrigerate for about 2 hours, or until completely chilled.

3. To serve, stir in the lemon zest and buttermilk. With a wire whisk, stir vigorously. Taste and add sugar if needed. Ladle into well-chilled bowls, garnish with lime and strawberry slices, and serve.

Each serving: About 150 calories, 3 g protein, 34 g carbohydrate, 1 g total fat (1 g saturated), 3 mg cholesterol, 37 mg sodium.

Red, White, and Blue Soup

PREP TIME: 1 hour, 10 minutes
COOK TIME: 5 minutes, plus 1 hour to chill

Makes 4 servings

Refreshingly tart flavors. Smooth, creamy texture. Vibrant red, white, and blue colors. All make this soup of blueberries, raspberries, and lemon yogurt a winner.

  2 cups blueberries
  2 tablespoons honey
  ½ cup white grape juice
  1¼ cups buttermilk
  1 cup red raspberries plus more for garnish
  ½ cup vanilla low-fat yogurt for serving
  1 teaspoon grated lemon zest

1. Combine the blueberries, honey, and ¼ cup grape juice in a microwave-safe bowl. Microwave on High for 3 minutes. Transfer the blueberry mixture to a blender and add ¾ cup buttermilk. Puree the mixture, and transfer to a medium-size bowl. Chill for 1 hour.

2. Combine the raspberries and remaining ¼ cup grape juice in a microwave-safe bowl. Microwave on High for 2 minutes. Transfer the raspberry mixture to a clean blender. Puree the mixture, and transfer to a small bowl. Chill for 1 hour.

3. To serve: Whisk together the yogurt and lemon zest. Whisk the remaining ½ cup buttermilk into the blueberry mixture. Divide the mixture among 4 serving bowls. Swirl some of the raspberry puree into each bowl of soup. Top each serving with a dollop of yogurt and raspberries.

Each serving: About 170 calories, 6 g protein, 34 g carbohydrate, 2 g total fat (1 g saturated), 8 mg cholesterol, 88 mg sodium.

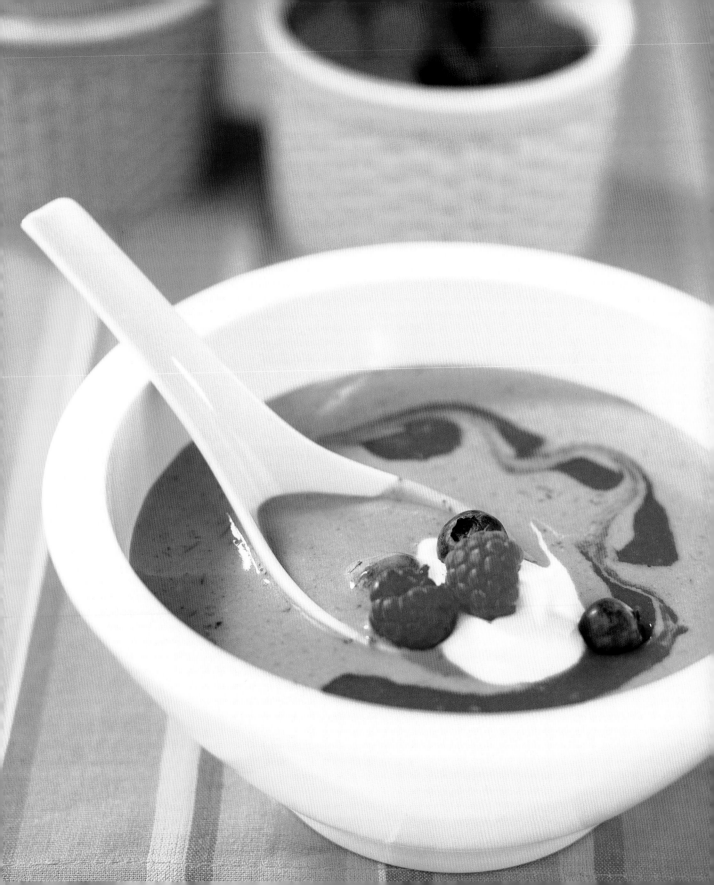

Chilled Raspberry Soup

PREP TIME: 5 minutes
COOK TIME: 25 minutes, plus 8 hours to chill

Makes about 4 servings

Simmering the wine cooks off most of the alcohol in the soup.

    2 packages (10 ounces each) frozen raspberries, thawed
    2 cups burgundy wine
    2½ cups water
    3-inch cinnamon stick
    2 teaspoons cornstarch or arrowroot combined with
       2 tablespoons water
    1 cup heavy cream blended with 2 tablespoons confectioners' sugar

1. In a 6-quart pot, combine the raspberries, wine, water, and cinnamon.
   Bring to a boil. Reduce to a simmer, cover lightly, and cook, stirring
   occasionally, 15 minutes. Remove from heat.

2. In a blender or food processor, puree the soup in batches until smooth.
   Strain through a sieve, discarding any seeds, and return the mixture to
   the pan.

3. Stir to mix the cornstarch mixture, then stir into the soup. Return to a
   boil and cook, stirring frequently, for 2 to 3 minutes or until slightly
   thickened. Remove from the heat, cool a little, cover tightly, and refrigerate for at least 8 hours.

4. To serve: Ladle the soup into chilled bowls and drizzle with the cream.
   With a knife, make several swirls in the soup, and serve immediately.

Each serving: About 489 calories, 3 g protein, 40 g carbohydrate, 23 g total fat
(14 g saturated), 82 mg cholesterol, 35 mg sodium.

Cold Sweet-Cherry Soup with Limoncello

PREP TIME: 1 hour 15 minutes plus chilling
COOK TIME: 5 minutes

Makes 4 to 6 servings

If you don't have limoncello, use another liqueur, such as amaretto or cassis. Stir in 1 tablespoon first and taste. The concentrated flavor and sweetness of the liqueur should support—not overpower—the cherries.

2 pounds fresh sweet cherries
½ cup sugar
2 tablespoons limoncello (Italian lemon-flavored liqueur) or more to taste
2 cups water
3-inch cinnamon stick
½ cup mascarpone or crème fraîche
long thin shavings of lemon zest for garnish

1. Rinse the cherries and discard the stems and pits. Place in a stainless-steel 2-quart heavy saucepan and sprinkle with the sugar and limoncello. Toss to coat. Cover and set aside to macerate for 1 hour.

2. Set aside 1 cup cherries with a little of their juice. Add the water and cinnamon stick to the remaining cherries; heat to boiling over medium heat, stirring. Remove from the heat and let stand 30 minutes.

3. Drain the cherries, reserving the liquid. Discard the cinnamon stick. Puree the cherries through a food mill into a bowl or puree in a food processor and press through a fine sieve into a bowl. Stir in the cooking liquid and season to taste with additional limoncello if needed. Cover and refrigerate until cold.

4. To serve: Ladle the soup into shallow bowls. Cut the reserved cherries in half and place in a bowl. Add the mascarpone, stir to mix, and add a dollop to each bowl. Sprinkle with lemon-zest shavings.

Each of 4 servings: About 343 calories, 4 g protein, 67 g carbohydrate, 7 g total fat (4 g saturated), 11 mg cholesterol, 12 mg sodium.

Cold Tart-Cherry Soup

PREP TIME: 15 minutes plus chilling
COOK TIME: 20 to 45 minutes

Makes 6 servings

If using canned cherries, use their liquid in step 1 to replace an equal amount of water. Use less sugar if the cherries are packed in heavy or light syrup.

3 cups plus 2 tablespoons cold water
1 cup sugar
3-inch cinnamon stick
4 cups pitted fresh sour cherries or drained
   canned sour cherries
1 tablespoon arrowroot
¾ cup dry red wine, chilled
¼ cup heavy cream
pinch freshly grated nutmeg
chunk bittersweet chocolate for shaving

1. Combine 3 cups water, the sugar, and cinnamon stick in a 2-quart saucepan and heat to boiling over medium-high heat, stirring to dissolve the sugar. Add the cherries, reduce the heat to low, and simmer, partially covered, until the cherries are tender, about 35 minutes for fresh cherries and 10 minutes for canned cherries.

2. Discard the cinnamon stick. Mix the arrowroot with the remaining 2 tablespoons water in a cup until blended; stir into the soup. Cook, stirring, until the soup has thickened and the broth is clear, 2 minutes. Pour the soup into a heat-safe 2-quart glass measure and cool to room temperature. Cover and refrigerate until cold.

3. To serve: Stir the wine into the soup and ladle into bowls. Whip the cream and nutmeg just until it is slightly thickened and barely mounds on itself (it will not float on the soup if it is too stiff). Spoon some cream over the soup in each bowl. With a vegetable peeler, shave some chocolate over each serving.

Each serving: About 236 calories, 2 g protein, 50 g carbohydrate, 3 g total fat (2 g saturated), 4 mg cholesterol, 10 mg sodium.

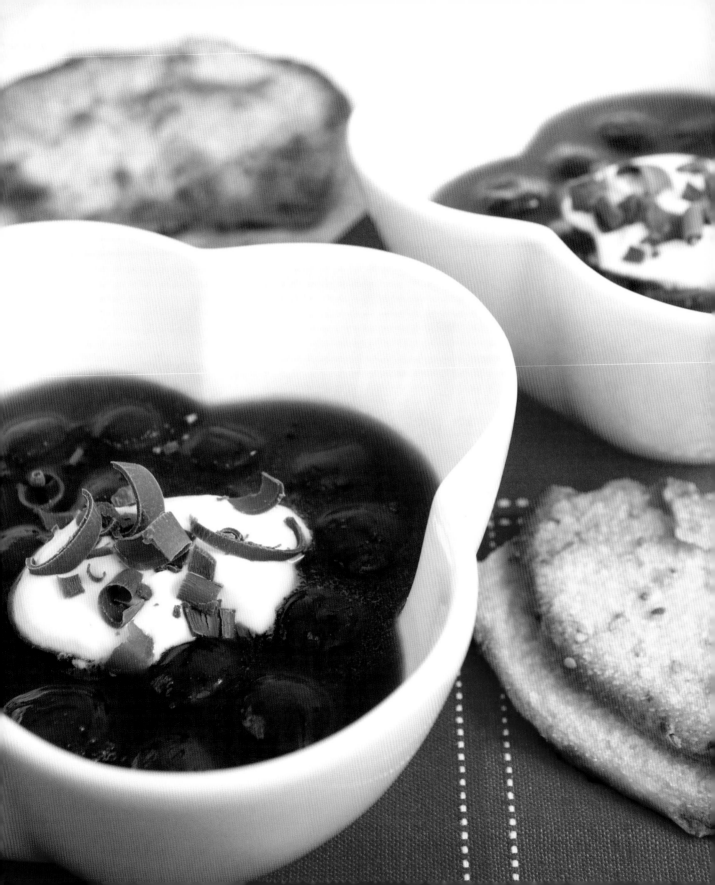

Chilled Cranberry Soup

PREP TIME: 15 minutes
COOK TIME: 25 minutes, plus 30 minutes to chill

Makes 4 servings

This would be great served at Thanksgiving.

  1 package (12 ounces) fresh cranberries
  3 cups water
  1 cup granulated sugar plus more if needed
  ¾ cup packed light brown sugar
  2 cinnamon sticks
  2 allspice berries
  2 whole cloves
  4 black peppercorns
  1 tablespoon cornstarch mixed with 2 tablespoons cold water
  ¾ cup heavy cream, whipped to soft peaks
  ½ cup dry red wine or to taste

1. Thoroughly rinse the cranberries under running water, shaking to remove
   excess water.

2. In a 6-quart pot, combine the water, granulated and brown sugars, the
   cinnamon, allspice, cloves, and peppercorns. Bring to a boil. Reduce to a
   simmer, add the cranberries, and cook, stirring occasionally, for about
   15 minutes, or until the berries are tender.

3. Stir to mix the cornstarch mixture and add to the soup; bring to a boil.
   Cook, stirring constantly, until thickened. Let cool and then refrigerate
   until ready to serve.

4. To serve: Stir in the whipped cream and wine. Taste and add sugar if needed.

Each serving: About 571 calories, 1 g protein, 104 g carbohydrate, 17 g total fat
(10 g saturated), 61 mg cholesterol, 36 mg sodium.

Apple Raisin Soup

PREP TIME: 5 minutes
COOK TIME: 25 minutes, plus 20 minutes to chill

Makes 3 to 4 servings

Apples and raisins are a tried-and-true pairing. They've been used in everything from cookies to bread to poultry stuffing—they're a natural for soup.

   2 cups unsweetened apple juice or cider
   2 large McIntosh apples, peeled, cored, and diced
   ¾ cup seedless raisins
   2-inch cinnamon stick
   1 tablespoon packed light brown sugar
   1 tablespoon brandy or rum

1. In a soup kettle or Dutch oven, combine the apple juice, apples, raisins, and cinnamon. Bring to a boil, then reduce the heat, cover, and simmer for about 15 minutes, or until the apples are fork tender.

2. Remove from heat, stir in the brown sugar and brandy, cover tightly, and chill until ready to serve. Discard the cinnamon stick before serving.

Each of 3 servings: About 253 calories, 1 g protein, 62 g carbohydrate, 1 g total fat (trace saturated), 0 mg cholesterol, 10 mg sodium.

Cold Papaya Soup

PREP TIME: 15 minutes
COOK TIME: 4 hours to chill

Makes 2 servings

   1 medium (6-inch) ripe papaya
   sugar to taste
   2 tablespoons fresh lime juice
   water or unsweetened apple juice

1. Peel and seed the papaya; cut into chunks. Reserve the seeds in the refrigerator.

2. In a blender or food processor, puree the papaya until very smooth. Pour into a bowl, and add sugar to taste. Stir in the lime juice. If the mixture is too thick, add water or apple juice, 1 teaspoonful at a time. This soup is supposed to be very thick.

3. Cover and chill in the refrigerator for at least 4 hours. Serve in chilled fruit cups with a small spoonful of the reserved seeds in the center.

Each serving: About 84 calories, 1 g protein, 21 g carbohydrate, trace total fat (trace saturated), 0 mg cholesterol, 8 mg sodium.

Orange-Mango Soup

PREP TIME: 10 minutes, plus 1 hour to chill
COOK TIME: 2 days to chill

Makes about 4 servings

    1 tablespoon orange zest
    3 large very ripe mangoes, pared
    1½ cups buttermilk or more if needed
    1½ cups fresh orange juice
    3 teaspoons honey, or to taste, warmed
    1 tablespoon lemon or lime juice
    1 large navel orange, peeled and cut into ½-inch slices, for serving
    8 small fresh mint leaves for garnish (optional)

1. In a blender or food processor, puree the orange zest and mangoes together until smooth. Strain through a sieve, pressing with the back of a spoon. Pour the liquid into a bowl, cover tightly, and refrigerate for at least 1 hour. Discard the solids in the sieve.

2. Stir the buttermilk, orange juice, and 2 teaspoons honey into the soup. (If it appears too thick, add more buttermilk.) Cover tightly and chill in the refrigerator for about 2 days.

3. To serve: Add the lemon juice and remaining 1 teaspoon honey. Pour into chilled bowls and float slices of orange on top. Garnish with mint and serve immediately.

Each serving: About 226 calories, 6 g protein, 49 g carbohydrate, 2 g total fat (1 g saturated), 7 mg cholesterol, 84 mg sodium.

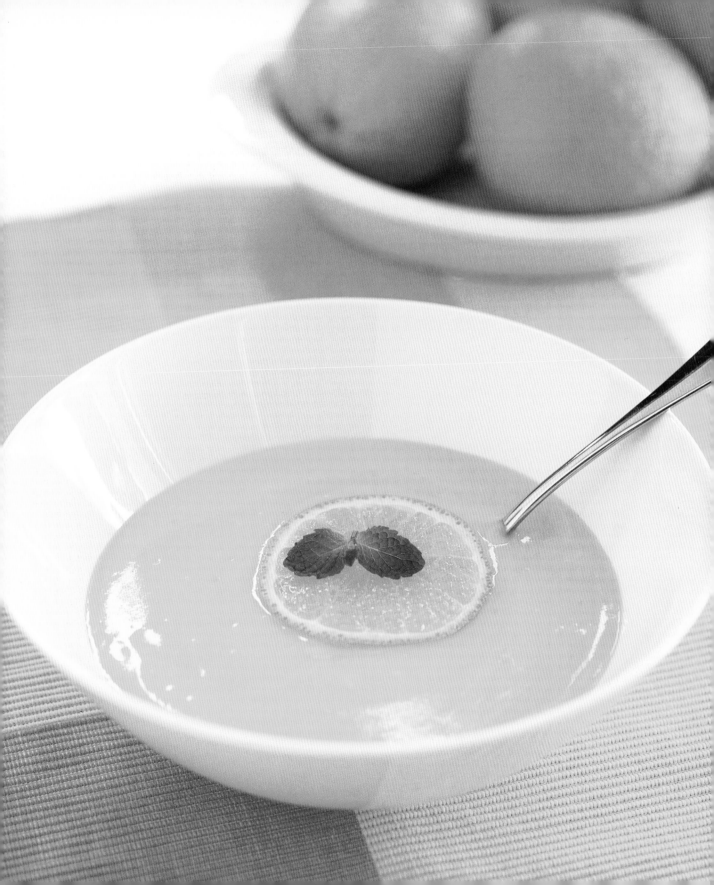

Blood-Orange and Mixed-Melon Soup

PREP TIME: 10 minutes plus chilling
COOK TIME: about 10 minutes

Makes 6 servings

The dramatically crimson flesh and juice of blood oranges never fails to astound. An assortment of other colorful fruits creates an energetic mélange of flavors, textures, and forms.

1 cup water
½ cup sugar
3 cups blood orange juice
1 cup small balls cantaloupe
1 cup small balls honeydew melon
1 cup small balls seedless watermelon
1 cup blueberries
½ cup halved red seedless grapes
½ cup halved green seedless grapes
2 tablespoons fresh lemon juice
¼ teaspoon salt

1. Combine the water and sugar in a small saucepan and heat to boiling over medium heat, stirring until the sugar dissolves. Boil 1 minute; pour into a heat-safe bowl to cool.

2. Heat the orange juice in the same saucepan to boiling over medium-high heat. Reduce the heat to medium and simmer until reduced to 2 cups. Add to the sugar syrup and cool completely.

3. In a large serving bowl, combine the orange juice mixture, cantaloupe, honeydew, watermelon, blueberries, grapes, lemon juice, and salt. Stir gently to mix. Cover with plastic wrap and refrigerate until serving.

4. To serve: Ladle into chilled shallow soup bowls so the fruits make a colorful pattern in the brilliant soup.

Each serving: About 166 calories, 2 g protein, 41 g carbohydrate, 1 g total fat (trace saturated), 0 mg cholesterol, 107 mg sodium.

Jellied Citrus Trio Consommé

PREP TIME: 25 minutes plus chilling
COOK TIME: 5 minutes

Makes 6 servings

This is a palate-refreshing soup that can easily stand in for a sorbet between courses.

1 quart water
grated zest of 1 grapefruit
grated zest of 1 orange
grated zest of 1 lime
2 envelopes unflavored gelatin
2 egg whites, beaten to a froth
shells of 2 clean eggs, lightly crushed
2 cups strained fresh grapefruit juice
1 cup strained fresh orange juice
2 tablespoons strained fresh lime juice
dash Angostura bitters
salt to taste
slivers of preserved lemon zest or candied orange
    peel for garnish (optional)
candied violets for garnish (optional)
mint sprigs for garnish

1. Pour the water into a heavy 3-quart saucepan and stir in the grated zests. Sprinkle the gelatin on top and let stand until softened, about 5 minutes. Add the egg whites and shells and heat over medium-high heat until boiling, whisking constantly, not in a circle but always away from you, until the mixture boils.

2. When the citrus broth begins to foam and rise, remove the pan from the heat. Let the mixture stand 5 minutes. Meanwhile, line a large sieve with a generous double layer of dampened cheesecloth (or a dampened linen or other non-terry-cloth tea towel). Place over a large heat-safe 2-quart glass measure or bowl that is deep enough so that the bottom of the sieve is about 4 inches from the bottom of the bowl.

3. Gently pour the citrus broth, zest, and shells into the sieve and let drain without disturbing or the consommé will be cloudy. Stir the fruit juices and bitters into the broth. Season with salt and pour into a shallow glass baking dish. Cover with plastic wrap and refrigerate 4 to 6 hours, until it is firm enough to hold its shape in a spoon.

4. To serve: Cut the consommé into cubes and transfer to chilled compote dishes or glass soup plates with a flat metal spatula. Garnish with preserved lemon zest slivers, candied violets, and mint sprigs.

Each serving: About 63 calories, 4 g protein, 12 g carbohydrate, trace total fat (0 g saturated), 0 mg cholesterol, 73 mg sodium.

Chinese Orange Soup with Rice-Flour Pearls

PREP TIME: 10 minutes
COOK TIME: about 10 minutes

Makes 4 to 6 servings

You can use tapioca—the large fish-eye size or the smaller pearl size—instead of making the pearls from the glutinous rice flour. Soak the tapioca as directed on the package and cook it in the syrup.

2 large navel oranges
2 cups plus 3 tablespoons water or more if needed
¼ cup sugar
½ cup glutinous rice flour (not regular rice flour) or Japanese sweet rice flour

1. Cut off the rind and white pith of the oranges and, working over a bowl to catch the juices, cut out the segments and place in the juice. Squeeze the inside "network" of the orange to extract all the juice. Cut the segments crosswise in half and set aside.

2. In a small saucepan, combine 2 cups water and the sugar and heat to boiling, stirring to dissolve the sugar. Boil 1 minute. Set aside.

3. Place the glutinous rice flour in a small bowl and stir in 3 tablespoons water or enough to form a soft dough. Break off tiny pieces of dough and roll each between the palms of your hand to form a pea-size ball. When you have them all made, reheat the syrup to boiling over medium heat and add the balls. Boil until they float to the surface, about 1 minute. Add the oranges and their juice and heat through. Serve hot.

Each of 4 servings: About 147 calories, 2 g protein, 34 g carbohydrate, 1 g total fat (trace saturated), 0 mg cholesterol, 2 mg sodium.

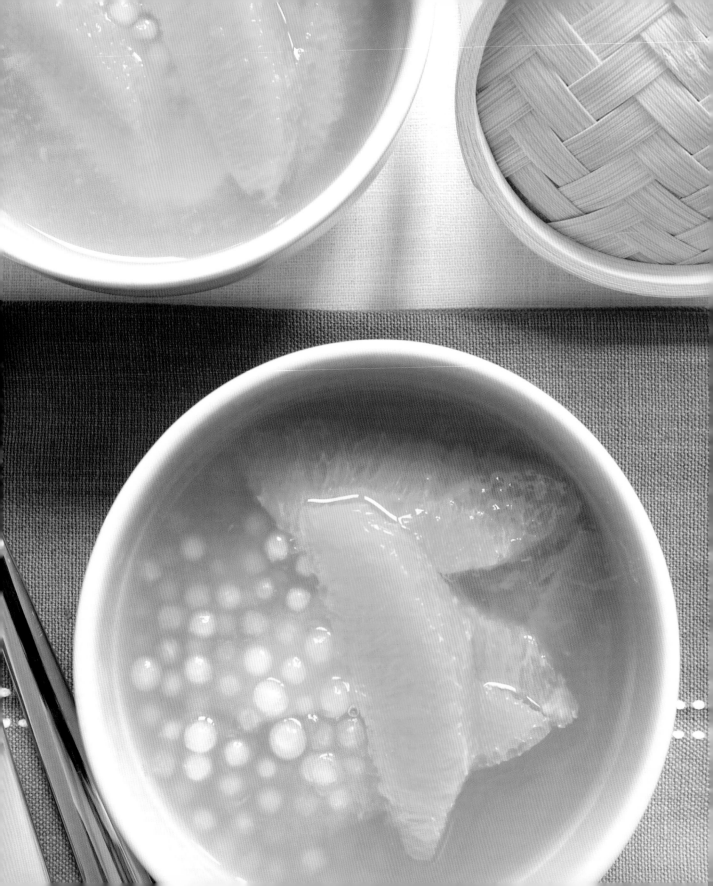

Cinnamon Peach Soup

PREP TIME: 5 minutes
COOK TIME: 15 minutes, plus 4 hours to chill

Makes 4 to 6 servings

The blend of cinnamon and good, ripe peaches is heavenly.

    3 whole cloves
    3 allspice berries
    3 cardamom pods
    2 pounds ripe peaches, pared and diced
    2 cups fresh orange juice
    3 tablespoons fresh lime juice
    3 to 4 tablespoons warmed honey
    1 teaspoon ground cinnamon
    1 teaspoon ground ginger
    1 cup unflavored yogurt or sour cream
    1 tablespoon diced candied ginger
    salt and pepper
    fresh sprigs mint for garnish

1. Tie up the cloves, allspice, and cardamom in a 4-inch square of cheesecloth. In a soup kettle or Dutch oven, combine the spice bag, peaches, orange juice, lime juice, honey, cinnamon, and ginger. Simmer 5 to 10 minutes, or until the fruit is well softened. Remove from the heat, discard the spice bundle, and cool the soup slightly.

2. In a blender or food processor, puree the soup in batches until smooth. Place in a bowl, cover tightly, and chill for at least 4 hours.

3. Just before serving, with a wire whisk, beat in the yogurt; stir in the candied ginger. Add salt and pepper to taste, garnish with mint sprigs, and serve immediately.

Each serving: About 243 calories, 5 g protein, 54 g carbohydrate, 3 g total fat (1 g saturated), 8 mg cholesterol, 31 mg sodium.

Quick Peach-Schnapps Soup

PREP TIME: 10 minutes
COOK TIME: 20 minutes

Makes 4 servings

Keep a can of peaches in the pantry to make this soup for a quick starter or dessert.

    1 can (about 29 ounces) sliced peaches in light syrup
    1 cup dry or sweet white wine
    2 star anise
    1 tablespoon grated peeled fresh gingerroot
    ¼ teaspoon freshly ground white pepper
    2 tablespoons cornstarch
    ½ cup water
    ½ cup sour cream
    2 tablespoon peach schnapps, brandy, or peach nectar, or more
        to taste
    1 tablespoons fresh lemon juice

1. Drain the peaches, reserving the juice. Puree the peaches in a blender or food processor and pour into a 2-quart saucepan. Add the reserved juice. Add the wine, star anise, ginger, and pepper and heat to simmering over medium heat. Simmer 10 minutes.

2. Mix the cornstarch and water in a small cup until blended. Pour the cornstarch mixture into the soup and whisk over medium-high heat until thickened and clear.

3. Mix the sour cream, schnapps, and lemon juice in a small bowl. Pour mixture into the soup. Discard the star anise. Serve the soup hot or cold.

Each serving: About 236 calories, 2 g protein, 36 g carbohydrate, 5 g total fat (3 g saturated), 11 mg cholesterol, 27 mg sodium.

> ### FLAVORFUL GARNISH
> - Frozen sliced peach have a wonderful flavor. Remove enough of them from a bag and let thaw just until softened and use them as an icy-cold garnish.

Peach and Cherry Soup with Raisins

PREP TIME: 25 minutes plus chilling
COOK TIME: 35 minutes

Makes 6 servings

Plan ahead to make sure the peaches you use in this soup are thoroughly ripe, a tough order since most peaches are sent to market underripe to lengthen their shelf life. To ripen peaches, poke some holes in a paper bag and add the peaches (and an apple, if you like, for quicker ripening). Set the bag aside at room temperature for a few days.

5 cups plus 2 tablespoons water
6 ripe peaches
1 orange, thinly sliced
1 lemon, thinly sliced
1 lime, thinly sliced
3-inch cinnamon stick
½ cup sugar or more to taste
½ cup seedless golden raisins
¼ cup fresh lemon juice
1 cup pitted tart cherries
1 cup pitted sweet cherries
¼ cup sweet red vermouth
1½ tablespoons cornstarch
softly whipped cream for serving

1. Heat 5 cups water to boiling in a 3-quart saucepan; add the peaches and cook 4 minutes. With a slotted spoon, transfer the peaches to a colander and rinse with cold water until cool enough to handle. (Reserve the water in the saucepan.)

2. Meanwhile, add the orange, lemon, lime, cinnamon stick, sugar, raisins, and lemon juice to the peach cooking water. Stir to dissolve the sugar and simmer 20 minutes.

3. Skin the peaches, cut in half, discard the pits, and thinly slice. Add the peaches and cherries to the soup and return to a boil. Add the vermouth. Mix the cornstarch with the remaining 2 tablespoons water until blended; stir into the soup. Cook, stirring, until the soup is clear and thickened, about 1 minute. Pour the soup into a heat-safe bowl and cool. Cover and refrigerate until thoroughly chilled.

4. To serve: Ladle the soup into chilled soup bowls and garnish each with a dollop of whipped cream.

Each serving with ½ cup whipped heavy cream: About 239 calories, 3 g protein, 54 g carbohydrate, 3 g total fat (2 g saturated), 7 mg cholesterol, 13 mg sodium.

Swedish Dried-Fruit Soup

PREP TIME: 45 minutes plus chilling
COOK TIME: 20 minutes

Makes 6 servings

Once the dried fruits soften, they release their concentrated flavors and juices in abundance.

¾ cup dried apricots
¾ cup dried plums
6 cups cold water
1 lemon
1 Golden Delicious apple, peeled, cored, and sliced
    crosswise into 6 rings
¾ cup sugar
3 tablespoons quick-cooking tapioca
3-inch cinnamon stick
3 tablespoons dried cranberries or cherries
2 tablespoons dried currants or raisins
mint sprigs for garnish

1. Quarter the apricots and plums with kitchen shears and place in a 3-quart saucepan. Add the water and let soak 30 minutes.

2. Peel the zest from the lemon in one strip if possible with a vegetable peeler; add to the saucepan with the apricot/plum mixture. Cut the lemon in half and squeeze 2 tablespoons juice. Add the apple to the juice and toss to coat so the flesh will not brown. Set the apple aside.

3. Add the sugar, tapioca, and cinnamon stick to the soup and heat to boiling over medium-high heat, stirring to dissolve the sugar. Reduce the heat to low, cover the pan, and simmer 10 minutes, stirring well every 4 minutes. Add the cranberries, currants, and apple with lemon juice to the soup and simmer 5 minutes, until the apple is tender when pierced with a paring knife (try not to split the apple rings).

4. Pour the soup into a large heat-safe bowl and cool to room temperature. Discard the lemon peel and cinnamon stick and cover the bowl with plastic wrap. Refrigerate the soup until cold. Serve the soup in chilled bowls, including an apple slice in each serving, and garnish each serving with a mint sprig.

Each serving: About 243 calories, 2 g protein, 63 g carbohydrate, trace total fat (0 g saturated), 0 mg cholesterol, 3 mg sodium.

Warm Mocha Soup with Orange Sabayon and Tropical Fruits

PREP TIME: 30 minutes
COOK TIME: 10 minutes

Makes 6 servings

This is an extravaganza, but then when you serve a warm, chocolate-based soup, it's time to pull out all the stops! For ease, you can use lightly sweetened and softly whipped heavy cream instead of the sabayon.

   1 cup heavy cream
   2 tablespoons sugar
   ⅔ cup sweet wine such as Beaumes-de-Venise or
      Vin Santo
   ¼ cup espresso coffee or double-strength brewed
      coffee
   2 tablespoons vanilla syrup
   6 ounces best-quality bittersweet chocolate (such
      as Valrhona Guanaja 70%), chopped

Sabayon
   4 sugar cubes
   1 small orange
   3 egg yolks
   ½ cup sugar
   ¼ cup fresh orange juice

VANILLA SYRUP
   • Vanilla syrup is available at Italian grocery
     stores or you can make a sugar syrup by mixing ½
     cup water with ¼ cup sugar and boiling it for
     1 minute. Stir in ½ teaspoon pure vanilla extract.

Fruits
   6 lychees, fresh or canned
   2 rings (½-inch thick) fresh pineapple, cut into
      1-inch pieces
   1 passion fruit, halved and seeds scraped out into a
      small cup
   ½ cup diced mango
   shavings of fresh coconut for garnish

1. Combine the cream and sugar in a heavy 2-quart saucepan and heat to simmering over medium heat. Remove from the heat and add the wine, coffee, and vanilla syrup. Return to medium heat and bring to a simmer. Remove the pan from the heat, add the chocolate, and cover. Let stand 5 minutes; stir until the chocolate is melted. Cover and set aside.

2. For the sabayon: Scrape the sugar cubes over the orange until coated with zest. Combine the sugar cubes, egg yolks, and sugar in a heat-safe bowl set over (not in) simmering water. With a portable electric mixer at medium speed, beat until mixture is thick and falls from the beaters in a thick ribbon, about 10 minutes. Add the orange juice and, with mixer at high speed, beat sauce until frothy and thick. Serve immediately.

3. To serve: Ladle soup into wide shallow soup or pasta bowls. Drizzle sabayon over the soup. Arrange fruits on top and sprinkle with coconut shavings.

Each serving: About 377 calories, 4 g protein, 52 g carbohydrate, 17 g total fat (9 g saturated), 121 mg cholesterol, 28 mg sodium.

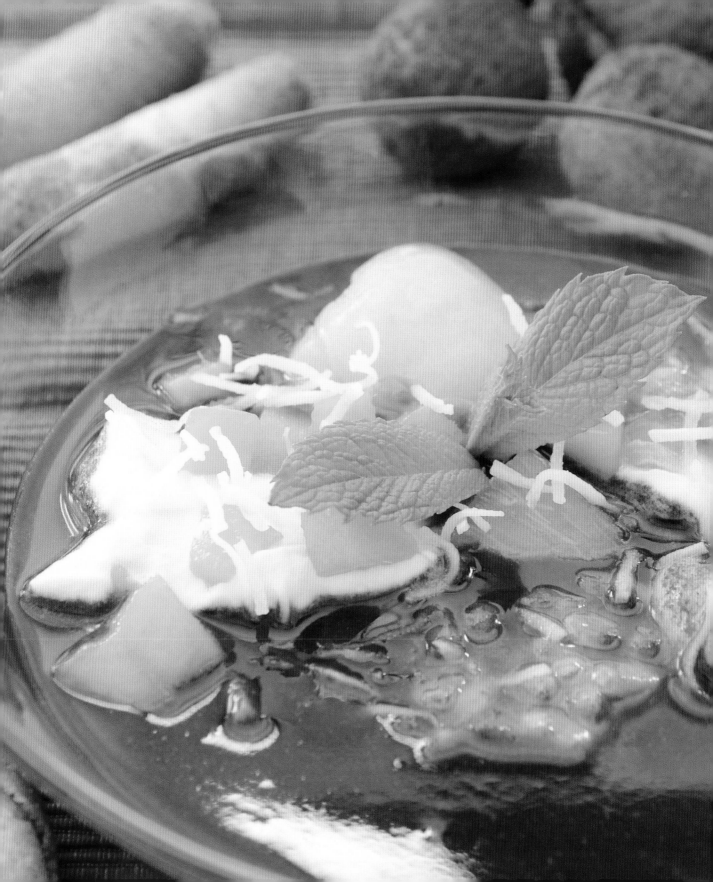

Watermelon Soup with Blackberries, Peaches, and Pistachios

PREP TIME: 25 minutes plus chilling

Makes 6 servings

With year 'round availability, watermelon can add a touch of summer during winter's shortest days. Adjust the other fruits according to the freshest flavors available. Or, add melon-ball scoopfuls of colorful sorbets or toasted pound-cake "croutons."

4 pounds watermelon
½ cup sugar
½ cup fresh lime juice
¾ cup shelled lightly salted natural pistachios, toasted
1 ripe peach
1 cup small blackberries
15 fresh mint leaves

1. Remove the rind from the watermelon and cut the flesh into chunks. Discard the seeds. Place the flesh in a blender or juicer and puree. Pour the puree into a bowl, add the sugar and lime juice, and stir until the sugar is dissolved. Cover and refrigerate until chilled.

2. To serve: Chop ½ cup pistachios and place in a bowl. Halve the peach and discard the pit. Cut into ½-inch dice; add to the chopped pistachios. Stir in the blackberries. Spoon the mixture into the centers of flat soup bowls. Ladle the soup around and sprinkle with the remaining ¼ cup whole pistachios. Stack the mint leaves on a cutting board and cut lengthwise into fine shreds; sprinkle over the soup.

Each serving: About 227 calories, 5 g protein, 39 g carbohydrate, 8 g total fat (1 g saturated), 0 mg cholesterol, 4 mg sodium.

Cantaloupe Soup

PREP TIME: 25 minutes plus chilling

Makes 4 servings

This mostly melon soup makes a good first course because it is not too sweet.

1 ripe cantaloupe (about 2 pounds)
¼ cup Pineau des Charentes or other semisweet aperitif or dessert
   wine or white grape juice and more if needed
16 fresh mint or lemon verbena leaves for garnish
nasturtium flowers (optional)

1. Cut the melon in half and scoop out the seeds. Cut each half into 6 wedges and discard the rind. Cut the flesh into 1-inch cubes. In batches, puree the melon in a food processor. Strain the puree through a fine sieve into a 2-quart glass measure. Whisk in the wine; refrigerate until chilled.

2. To serve: Rewhisk the soup and add more wine if needed to make a nice texture. Stack the mint leaves on a cutting board and cut lengthwise into fine shreds. Ladle the soup into soup bowls and sprinkle the mint leaves on top. Garnish with nasturtium flowers if you like.

Each serving: About 59 calories, 1 g protein, 10 g carbohydrate, trace total fat (trace saturated), 0 mg cholesterol, 12 mg sodium.

REFRIGERATING THE SOUP

- Because cantaloupe absorbs other odors, store the soup in a tightly covered container, not just in a bowl covered with plastic wrap.

Ginger Mango Soup with Radishes and Jalapeños

PREP TIME: 25 minutes

Makes 4 servings

Ripe mangoes are lip-smacking sweet, but are easily balanced with savory ingredients to make salsas and first-course soups such as this eye- and palate-pleasing starter.

3 ripe mangoes, pitted and diced into ½-inch chunks
¼ cup fresh lemon juice
½ teaspoon salt
2 (3-inch) pieces fresh gingerroot, peeled
4 large jalapeño peppers, seeded and finely chopped into ¼-inch squares (use rubber gloves when handling hot peppers)
2 bunches chilled small radishes, trimmed and quartered
juice of 1 lime

1. Press 1 cup mango pieces through a sieve into a bowl (puree first in a blender or food processor if they aren't soft enough to squish). Stir in the lemon juice and salt. Grate the ginger on a microplane. Press half of it through a fine sieve into the mango puree, pinching the ginger with your fingers to extract the juice. Stir the puree and set aside.

2. In a medium bowl, combine the remaining mango pieces, the jalapeños, radishes, and lime juice. Press out the juice of the remaining grated ginger into the radish mixture as you did for the puree. Mix well.

3. To serve: Spoon the radish mixture into piles in the centers of flat soup bowls. Spoon the mango puree around each pile, dividing evenly.

Each serving: About 126 calories, 2 g protein, 32 g carbohydrate, 1 g total fat (trace saturated), 0 mg cholesterol, 307 mg sodium.

MAKE AHEAD
- If you want to prepare the soup ahead of time, cut up the vegetables and make the puree through step 1, but do not mix them together. Cover and refrigerate separately until serving; then finish the soup starting with step 2.

Chilled Buttermilk Soup with Stilton and Pears

PREP TIME: 20 minutes plus chilling

Makes 4 to 6 servings

This soup can be served either as an appetizer or a dessert. The sweetness of the pears are countered by salty nuggets of Stilton, and the walnuts add a diverting crunch.

2 ripe pears, peeled and cored
2 tablespoons fresh lemon juice
1 tablespoon sugar
1 quart buttermilk
6 ounces Stilton cheese, crumbled into
   ½-inch pieces
freshly ground pepper to taste
½ cup toasted walnut pieces or toasted skinned
   hazelnuts for serving
4 fresh basil leaves, slivered, for serving

1. Dice pears into ½-inch pieces and place in a bowl. Add the lemon juice and sugar and toss to coat and dissolve the sugar. Cover and refrigerate at least 30 minutes or up to several hours before serving.

2. Place half of the pears and all of their juice in a blender and add 1 cup buttermilk. Pulse and then blend until smooth. Pour into a 2-quart glass measure or bowl. Add 1 cup buttermilk to the blender and pulse to blend any pear bits and juice into the buttermilk. Add to the pear mixture; stir in the remaining buttermilk, the remaining diced pears, and the Stilton. Season with pepper to taste. Serve immediately or cover and refrigerate until serving.

3. To serve: Ladle the soup into bowls and sprinkle with walnuts and basil.

Each of 4 servings: About 400 calories, 20 g protein, 31 g carbohydrate, 24 g total fat (10 g saturated), 48 mg cholesterol, 1,027 mg sodium.

Apricot Soup with Gingered Fruit Salsa

PREP TIME: 15 minutes
COOK TIME: 20 minutes

Makes 4 to 6 servings

Although apricot season is brief, it is cause for celebration. Because there's not a lot of sugar in this recipe, the apricot flavor remains characteristically tangy, and the tartness of the salsa enables the soup to be served either as a first course or a dessert.

3 cups water
2 pounds ripe apricots
¼ cup sugar
¼ cup fresh lemon juice

Gingered Fruit Salsa
1 star fruit, thinly sliced crosswise
1 kiwifruit, peeled, thinly sliced crosswise
½ cup fresh raspberries
1 tablespoon finely grated peeled fresh gingerroot
1 tablespoon slivered fresh mint leaves
1 tablespoon fresh lemon juice

1. Heat the water to boiling in a 2-quart saucepan. In batches, cook the apricots for 3 minutes, transferring each batch with a slotted spoon to a colander placed in the sink. (Reserve the water in the pan.) Rinse the apricots with cold water and remove the skins with a paring knife. Cut the apricots in half lengthwise and discard the pits.

2. Return the apricots to the water and add the sugar. Heat to boiling over medium-high heat, stirring until the sugar dissolves. Reduce the heat to low and simmer, partially covered, until the apricots are tender, about 8 minutes.

3. Transfer the apricots to a food processor with a slotted spoon; puree. Scrape the puree back into the apricot cooking liquid and stir in the lemon juice. To serve the soup cold, transfer to a bowl and cool; cover and refrigerate until chilled. To serve hot, gently heat the soup just before serving.

4. For the Salsa: Mix the star fruit, kiwifruit, raspberries, ginger, mint, and lemon juice in a large bowl.

5. To serve: Ladle the soup into shallow bowls and scatter the salsa over the top so the different fruits and mint add contrast to the apricot base.

Each of 4 servings: About 190 calories, 4 g protein, 46 g carbohydrate, 1 g total fat (trace saturated), 0 mg cholesterol, 4 mg sodium.

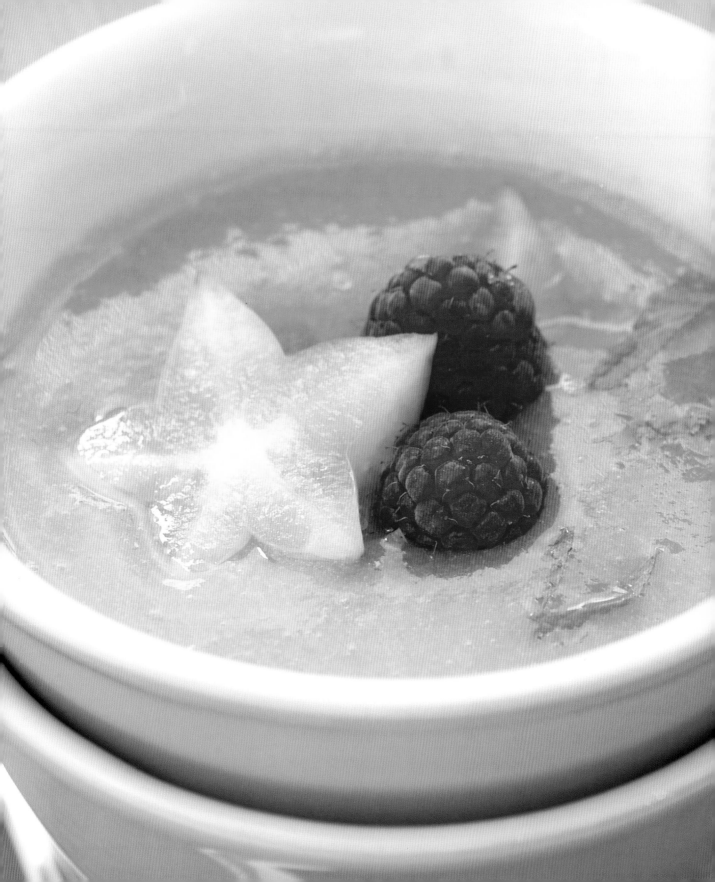

Chayote and Honey–Lemon Verbena Soup

PREP TIME: 15 minutes plus chilling
COOK TIME: 35 minutes

Makes 4 servings

Also known as *mirliton* and *christophene*, the delicately flavored chayote is a potassium-rich fruit that was once the principal food of the Aztecs and Mayas.

    3 cups water
    ¼ cup honey or more if needed
    1 bunch lemon verbena
    2 chayote
    1 cup lemon yogurt
    ground cinnamon for dusting
    1 cup wild blueberries

1. Combine the water and honey in a 2-quart saucepan. Heat to boiling, stirring to dissolve the honey. Reserve 12 lemon verbena leaves in a cup of water. Add the remaining lemon verbena to the honey-water and cover. Simmer over low heat while preparing the chayote.

2. Peel the chayote with a vegetable peeler and cut in half. Discard the pits and slice the fruits crosswise into ½-inch-thick slices. (Your hands will need rinsing as the flesh exudes a tacky juice.) Add the slices to the lemon-verbena infusion; cover and heat to boiling over medium-high heat. Reduce the heat to low and simmer until tender, about 20 minutes.

3. Transfer the chayote slices to a food processor with a slotted spoon and puree. Strain the cooking liquid through a sieve into a 2-quart heat-safe glass measure. Scrape the puree into a bowl. Add 2 cups cooking liquid and whisk until blended. Add enough of the remaining cooking liquid to make a thin but not watery soup; taste and sweeten with more honey if necessary. Chill the soup or gently reheat over medium-low heat.

4. To serve: Ladle the soup into shallow bowls. Stir the yogurt to thin it evenly; add a spoonful to each bowl. Dust the yogurt with cinnamon and sprinkle the berries around the yogurt. Drain the reserved lemon verbena leaves and stack on a cutting board. Cut lengthwise into slivers and sprinkle among the berries.

Each serving: About 141 calories, 3 g protein, 30 g carbohydrate, 2 g total fat (1 g saturated), 8 mg cholesterol, 33 mg sodium.

Caramelized Pineapple and Banana in Spiced Rum Soup with Toasted Coconut

PREP TIME: 10 minutes
COOK TIME: 20 minutes

Makes 8 servings

Tropical fruits are especially appreciated in cold weather, when it seems like those days at the beach never happened. Perk up your spirits with this rum-splashed dessert.

    4 tablespoons unsalted butter
    ½ cup sugar
    1 pound ½-inch cubes pineapple (fresh or drained canned)
    2 firm barely green bananas, cut into rough ½-inch cubes
    ½ cup spiced rum
    1 quart unsweetened pineapple juice
    ¼ cup fresh lemon juice
    1 cup grated fresh coconut, toasted, for garnish

1. Melt the butter in a 3-quart saucepan over medium-high heat. Add the sugar and stir until melted. Add the pineapple and banana and stir until coated. Cook over medium heat until softened, about 5 minutes. Add the rum and cook until the liquid has almost evaporated, about 2 minutes. Add the pineapple juice and lemon juice and heat to boiling. Simmer over low heat until the pineapple and banana is softened, about 2 minutes.

2. To serve: Ladle the soup into warmed soup bowls and sprinkle with the toasted coconut.

Each serving: About 294 calories, 2 g protein, 46 g carbohydrate, 10 g total fat (7 g saturated), 16 mg cholesterol, 5 mg sodium.

White Grape Gazpacho

PREP TIME: 25 minutes
COOK TIME: 5 minutes, plus 8 hours to chill

Makes about 6 servings

¼ cup blanched almonds
2 garlic cloves
salt and pepper to taste
4 slices stale white bread, crusts removed
4 cups ice water
6 tablespoons canola oil
3 tablespoons white wine vinegar
2 tablespoons sherry wine vinegar
Garlic Croutons (page 22) for serving
1½ cups seedless green grapes for serving

1. In a blender, combine the almonds, garlic, and salt and pepper to taste. Process on high until smooth. Place the bread in a bowl and add 1 cup ice water. Soak through, squeeze out the water, and put the bread in the blender with the garlic mixture.

2. With the processor running on low, add the canola oil and 1 cup ice water. Add the white wine and sherry wine vinegars and blend on high speed until smooth. Add 1 cup of water, and process on high for about 1 minute. Pour into a bowl, and add the remaining 1 cup of water. Add salt and pepper to taste, cover tightly, and refrigerate for at least 8 hours.

3. To serve: Ladle the cold soup into chilled bowls and sprinkle the croutons and green grapes on top.

Each serving: About 277 calories, 3 g protein, 19 g carbohydrate, 22 g total fat (3 g saturated), 5 mg cholesterol, 111 mg sodium.

> TIP
> • Try freezing any fruit you plan to use as a garnish while you are chilling the soup in the refrigerator. This is a great way to keep a chilled soup cool during the meal.

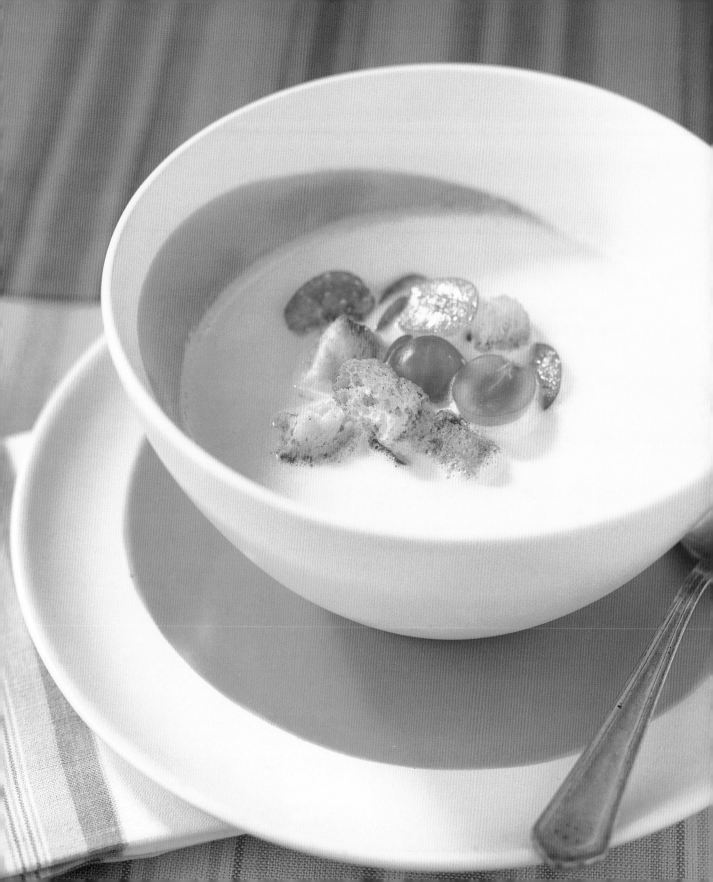

Beulah's Peeled Grapes in Muscat-Grappa Broth

PREP TIME: 5 minutes
COOK TIME: 10 minutes

Makes 6 servings

Your prep time will be well spent when your guests discover the joys of the juicy tenderness of the naked grape.

1 quart Muscat grape juice or white grape juice
½ cup peeled seedless green grapes, halved
½ cup peeled seedless red grapes, halved
½ cup peeled seedless purple grapes, halved
2 tablespoons finely chopped raisins
2 tablespoons grappa (Italian eau de vie) or more to taste
½ cup toasted slivered almonds, warmed, for serving

Combine the grape juice, grapes, raisins, and grappa in a 2-quart saucepan and heat to simmering over medium heat. Ladle into warmed soup bowls and sprinkle with the almonds.

Each serving: About 242 calories, 4 g protein, 46 g carbohydrate, 5 g total fat (1 g saturated), 0 mg cholesterol, 7 mg sodium.

Black Plum, Red Wine, and Star Anise Soup with Goat Cheese

PREP TIME: 15 minutes plus chilling
COOK TIME: 1 hour 30 minutes

Makes 4 to 6 servings

This soup is not sweet enough to make a dessert soup, but shines as an appetizer.

2 cups water
1 cup full-bodied red wine
½ cup sugar
4 whole star anise
pinch sea salt and more to taste
1½ pounds very ripe black plums (approximately 6 plums)
4 ounces fresh goat cheese for serving
¼ cup chopped toasted hazelnuts or almonds for serving

1. Combine the water, wine, and sugar in a 2-quart saucepan and heat to boiling, stirring. Boil 1 minute; add the star anise and salt. Remove from heat, cover, and steep for 1 hour.

2. Place the plums in the wine mixture, cover, and heat to boiling over medium heat. Cook plums until tender, about 15 minutes. Transfer the plums to a bowl with a slotted spoon. When they are cool enough to handle, discard the skins, cut in half, and discard the pits. Cut into 1-inch chunks, place in a food processor, and puree. Scrape the puree into a bowl. Add 2 cups cooking liquid and whisk until blended. Add enough of the remaining cooking liquid to make a thin but not watery soup; taste and season with more salt if necessary. Chill the soup or gently reheat over medium-low heat.

3. To serve: Ladle the soup into shallow bowls and sprinkle with small clumps of crumbled goat cheese and the hazelnuts.

Each of 4 servings: About 406 calories, 11 g protein, 50 g carbohydrate, 16 g total fat (7 g saturated), 30 mg cholesterol, 174 mg sodium.

Wine and Raspberry-Custard Soup

PREP TIME: 10 minutes
COOK TIME: about 15 minutes

Makes 6 servings

You can use strawberries instead of the raspberries in this dessert soup and add some sliced fresh berries to each bowl for a garnish.

1 package (10 to 12 ounces) frozen raspberries in light syrup, thawed
1 cup mascarpone cheese
6 egg yolks
1 tablespoon finely grated lemon zest
1 bottle (about 3 cups) muscatel or other sweet white or rose wine
½ pint fresh raspberries for garnish
fresh mint leaves for garnish

1. Press the thawed raspberries and their juice through a fine sieve into the top of a double boiler or a stainless-steel bowl placed over simmering water. Add the cheese, egg yolks, and lemon zest and cook over medium heat, whisking constantly, until the custard is hot and thick.

2. Heat the wine in a 2-quart saucepan until simmering; remove from the heat. Whisk a ladleful of the hot wine into the custard and then whisk the custard into the saucepan of wine. Keep whisking until the soup is cooled enough and the custard does not curdle.

3. To serve: Serve the soup immediately in warmed bowls or chill the soup and serve in chilled bowls; garnish with berries and mint.

Each serving: About 305 calories, 5 g protein, 19 g carbohydrate, 12 g total fat (6 g saturated), 227 mg cholesterol, 33 mg sodium.

Baked Rhubarb Soup with Honey Croutons

PREP TIME: 10 minutes
COOK TIME: 30 minutes

Makes 8 servings

It takes a lot of sugar to sweeten the sourness of rhubarb, but note that
even a dessert soup can be too sweet to enjoy. Here the natural sweetness
of apple juice helps to stretch the sugar and balance the broth without
making it cloyingly sweet. Honey-glazed croutons will make the perfect
match for the rhubarb chunks on each spoonful

  1 pound fresh rhubarb, trimmed and cut crosswise into ½-inch slices
    (about 4 cups)
  ¼ cup sugar
  2 tablespoons all-purpose flour
  1 teaspoon freshly grated nutmeg
  dash salt
  1 quart apple cider or juice
  6 tablespoons unsalted butter, melted
  ½ cup honey
  5 slices bread, cut into ½-inch cubes (about 4 cups)

1. Preheat the oven to 375 degrees. Combine the rhubarb, sugar, flour,
   nutmeg, and salt in a deep 3-quart casserole and mix well. Stir in the
   apple juice until blended.

2. Combine the butter and honey in a medium bowl and whisk until blended.
   Add the bread cubes and stir until coated. Spoon the bread mixture over
   the rhubarb mixture. Bake until the topping is golden brown, about
   30 minutes.

Each serving: About 285 calories, 2 g protein, 50 g carbohydrate, 10 g total fat
(6 g saturated), 24 mg cholesterol, 179 mg sodium.

Plantain Soup with Mango Salsa

PREP TIME: 15 minutes
COOK TIME: 40 minutes

Makes 4 servings

Although plantain soup is often used to cure bellyaches in the tropics, it is a delicious starter in the best of times.

1 green plantain
2 tablespoons extravirgin olive oil
1 small onion, finely chopped
1 carrot, peeled and finely chopped
2 garlic cloves, minced
1 red bell pepper, seeded and finely chopped
1 teaspoon ground cumin
2 plum tomatoes, diced
4 cups Chicken or Vegetable Stock (Chapter 1) or more if needed
2 tablespoons cilantro leaves
¼ teaspoon cayenne pepper
salt and freshly ground pepper to taste

Mango Salsa
1 mango, peeled, pitted, and diced
1 cup finely diced fresh pineapple
1 jalapeño pepper, seeded and minced (use rubber gloves when handling hot peppers)
1 scallion, trimmed and minced
2 tablespoons minced fresh cilantro
2 tablespoons fresh lime juice
salt and freshly ground pepper to taste

1. Cut off and discard the ends of the plantain; cut the remaining plantain crosswise in thirds. Slice the skin of each third lengthwise to the flesh and pry back and remove the skin with your thumb. Coarsely grate the plantain into a bowl and set aside.

2. Heat the oil in a 3-quart saucepan over medium-high heat. Add the onion, carrot, and garlic. Sauté until softened but not browned, about 4 minutes. Add the bell pepper and cumin and sauté 1 minute. Add the tomatoes and sauté 1 minute. Add the stock, cilantro, and cayenne and heat to boiling. Add the grated plantain and simmer over medium-low heat until the plantain is tender, about 25 minutes.

3. Meanwhile, make the salsa: Combine the mango, pineapple, jalapeño, scallion, cilantro, lime juice, salt, and pepper in a bowl and mix well. Set aside.

4. Puree the soup through a food mill placed over a 2-quart saucepan. Add more stock if needed; taste and season with salt and pepper. Heat through and ladle into warmed shallow soup bowls. Scatter spoonfuls of the salsa over the soup in each bowl.

Each serving: About 282 calories, 8 g protein, 39 g carbohydrate, 12 g total fat (2 g saturated), 0 mg cholesterol, 312 mg sodium.

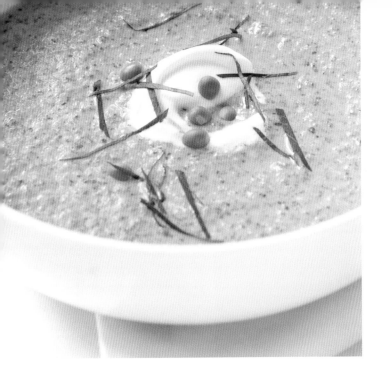

3

CHILLED
VEGETABLE
SOUPS

Fast Gazpacho

PREP TIME: 15 minutes
COOK TIME: 30 minutes to chill

Makes 4 servings

Hailing from Spain, gazpacho is an intriguing chilled soup of tomatoes, cucumbers, and other summertime vegetables. This version, which gets its zest from garlic and dried chile, is ready with the whirl of a blender's blade.

 2 cans (15 ounces each) diced tomatoes
 1½ cups reduced-sodium tomato juice
 1 medium cucumber, chopped
 1 green bell pepper, seeded and chopped
 1 medium onion, chopped
 1 ancho chile pepper, seeded and chopped
 4 garlic cloves, chopped
 2 teaspoons red wine vinegar
 2 teaspoons olive oil
 salt and pepper to taste
 2 cups Plain Croutons (page 22) for serving

ANCHO PEPPERS
• Ancho peppers, which are dried poblano peppers, give this recipe just the right zip. If you can't find them, use ¼ to ½ of a minced, seeded cayenne pepper.

Combine the tomatoes, tomato juice, cucumber, bell pepper, onion, chile pepper, garlic, vinegar, and olive oil in a blender. Process the mixture until the vegetables are partially pureed. Chill the soup until cold, 30 to 40 minutes. Taste and season with salt and pepper if needed. Top each serving with croutons.

Each serving: About 146 calories, 4 g protein, 25 g carbohydrate, 4 g total fat (1 g saturated), 0 mg cholesterol, 238 mg sodium.

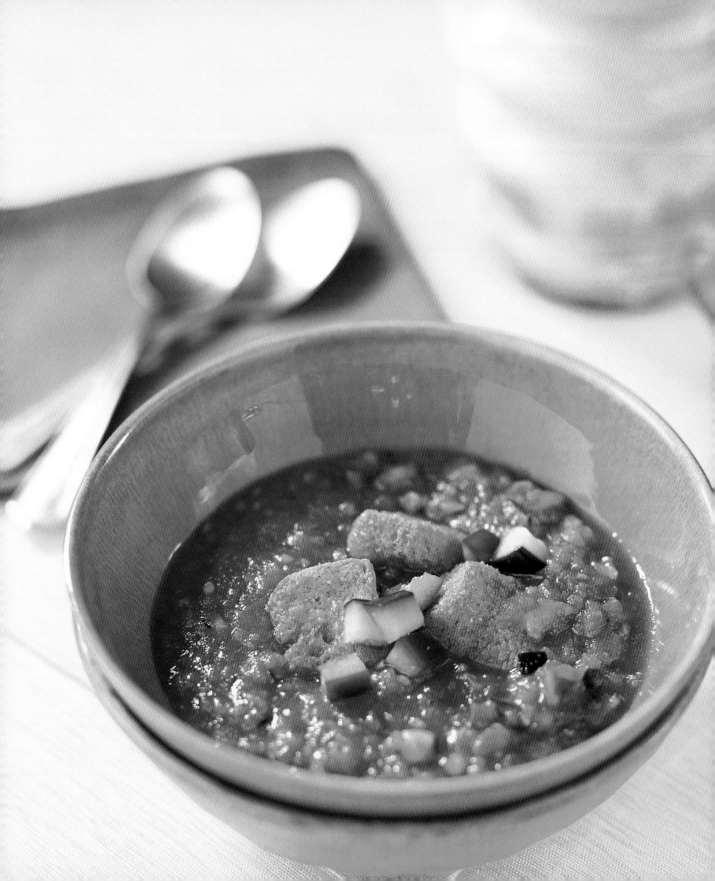

Chilled Tomato Basil Soup

PREP TIME: 10 minutes
COOK TIME: 50 minutes, plus 4 hours to chill

Makes 4 servings

3 tablespoons margarine
1 tablespoon vegetable oil
1 medium yellow onion, finely chopped
1 medium leek (white only), finely chopped
1 medium carrot, peeled and finely chopped
1 medium celery stalk, finely chopped
2 tablespoons chopped fresh basil plus leaves
   for garnish
2 cans (16 ounces each) diced tomatoes
3 tablespoons tomato paste
2 tablespoons all-purpose flour
2½ cups Vegetable Stock (page 15)
½ cup light cream
salt and pepper to taste
¼ cup sour cream or unflavored yogurt
   for serving

1. Heat the margarine and oil together in a medium saucepan, and sauté the onion, leek, carrot, celery, and basil until the onion is transparent. Add the tomatoes and tomato paste, and cook, stirring occasionally, for about 5 minutes. Stir in the flour until incorporated, and add the stock. Bring to a boil, then reduce to a simmer, cover lightly, and cook without stirring for about 20 minutes. Remove from heat.

2. In a blender or food processor, puree the mixture in batches, until smooth. Strain and press through a fine sieve, and return the mixture to the pot. Bring to a boil, then reduce to a simmer, and cook for 3 to 4 minutes.

3. Turn off the heat, stir in the cream, and add salt and pepper to taste. Cool slightly. Cover tightly and refrigerate for at least 4 hours.

4. Using a wire whisk, stir the soup vigorously. Ladle into chilled bowls, and garnish with basil leaves and dollops of sour cream.

Each serving: About 340 calories, 8 g protein, 37 g carbohydrate, 21 g total fat (7 g saturated), 26 mg cholesterol, 818 mg sodium.

Cold Dilled Tomato Soup

PREP TIME: 10 minutes
COOK TIME: 15 minutes, plus 45 minutes to chill

Makes 4 servings

3 cups low-sodium tomato juice
1 celery stalk, chopped
1 medium onion, chopped
¼ teaspoon red pepper flakes
½ teaspoon curry powder
¼ teaspoon ginger
1 teaspoon grated lemon zest
1 cup nonfat or reduced-fat sour cream
salt and pepper to taste
2 tablespoons snipped fresh dill or chives
   for garnish

1. In a 3-quart pot, bring 1 cup tomato juice to a boil. Add the celery, onion, and pepper flakes, and simmer for 10 minutes. Remove from the heat. Stir in the curry, ginger, lemon zest, and remaining 2 cups of tomato juice. Transfer the mixture to a blender and puree. Chill for 45 minutes.

2. Stir in the sour cream. Taste and season with salt and pepper if needed. Top each serving with dill.

Each serving: About 107 calories, 4 g protein, 23 g carbohydrate, 1 g total fat (trace saturated), 5 mg cholesterol, 218 mg sodium.

Vichyssoise with Roasted Peppers

PREP TIME: 20 minutes
COOK TIME: 20 minutes, plus 1 hour to chill

Makes 6 servings

2 teaspoons unsalted butter
2 large leeks, white part only, chopped
2 large waxy potatoes, peeled and diced
1¾ cups Chicken Stock (page 15)
¼ teaspoon white pepper
¼ teaspoon celery seeds
1 teaspoon white wine vinegar
2 cups 2% milk
salt to taste
¼ cup chopped roasted red peppers

1. Melt the butter in a 6-quart pot over medium-high heat. Add the leeks, and cook until they are translucent, about 5 minutes. Stir in the potatoes, stock, pepper, celery seeds, and vinegar. Cover and bring to a boil. Reduce the heat and simmer 15 minutes. Remove pot from heat; let the mixture cool, uncovered, for 2 minutes. Transfer the mixture to a blender jar. Process until pureed.

2. Pour the mixture into a large bowl, stir in the milk, and chill the soup thoroughly, about 1 hour. Taste and season with salt if needed. Top each serving with peppers.

Each serving: About 110 calories, 5 g protein, 16 g carbohydrate, 3 g total fat (2 g saturated), 10 mg cholesterol, 399 mg sodium.

Heirloom-Tomato Aspic with Basil Oil

PREP TIME: 40 minutes plus standing
COOK TIME: 10 minutes

Makes 6 servings

2 pounds very ripe heirloom tomatoes (all one variety), hard stem part cut out

2 cups tightly packed basil leaves plus small sprigs for garnish

1 teaspoon salt or more to taste

3 gelatin sheets or 1½ envelopes unflavored gelatin

⅓ cup olive oil

freshly ground black pepper

1. Make the tomato juice up to a day before serving: Roughly chop the tomatoes and place in a bowl. Gently tear 1 cup basil leaves into pieces and mix with the chopped tomatoes. Sprinkle with 1 teaspoon salt. Pass through a juicer or puree in a blender; strain through a sieve lined with a double layer of cheesecloth. (You might have to do this in more than one batch.) Taste the juice and adjust the seasoning with salt if necessary.

2. Pour 3 cups tomato juice into a glass measure and set aside. Place 1 cup of the remaining tomato juice in a small saucepan and add the gelatin; let stand 10 minutes, until the gelatin is completely soft. Slowly heat this mixture, stirring constantly, until the gelatin is dissolved. Stir the gelatin mixture into the 3 cups reserved tomato juice, cover with plastic wrap, and refrigerate overnight or until set. (The aspic will set more quickly if you pour it into a shallow glass baking dish to set.)

3. While the aspic sets, make the basil oil: Have a bowl of ice and water ready. Heat a small saucepan of salted water to boiling and add the remaining 1 cup basil leaves. Cook 10 seconds and pour through a sieve. Immediately plunge the basil into the ice water and chill completely. Drain the basil and squeeze to dry as much as possible. Place the basil on a cutting board and cut into slivers. Place slivers in a blender, place the lid on with the center removed, and turn the machine on low. Add the oil gradually through the lid and blend until smooth, about 2 minutes. Pour the basil through a sieve lined with a coffee filter and set over a small deep bowl. Set aside to drain into a clear green liquid; do not press down on the leaves or it may cause the liquid to cloud.

4. To serve: Have ready 6 classic martini glasses. Uncover the aspic and test its firmness; it should be spoonable. If it isn't, gently stir it to break it into even pieces. Spoon a tablespoon of basil oil into each glass and gently spoon the tomato aspic on top of the oil so there is a circle of green around the glass. Season the top with a generous grind of pepper and garnish with a small basil sprig.

Each serving: About 137 calories, 4 g protein, 4 g carbohydrate, 12 g total fat (2 g saturated), 0 mg cholesterol, 400 mg sodium.

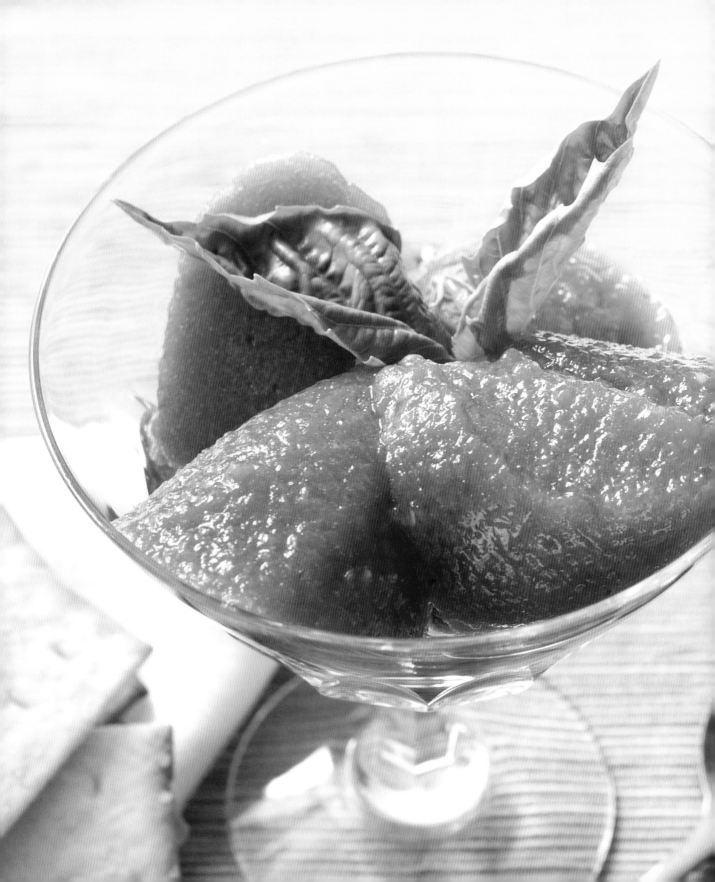

Cucumber-Parsley Soup

PREP TIME: 10 minutes
COOK TIME: 20 minutes, plus 1 hour and 10 minutes to chill

Makes 4 servings

This low-fat summertime refresher is truly "cool as a cucumber." Fresh parsley and dill make it extraordinary. Peel the cucumber only if it is waxed.

  2 teaspoons canola oil
  ½ cup chopped onion
  2 cups Chicken Stock (page 14)
  2 cups diced cucumber
  1 cup diced peeled potato
  1 cup fresh parsley leaves
  ½ teaspoon dry mustard
  ½ teaspoon freshly ground black pepper
  1 cup 2% milk
  salt and pepper to taste
  ¼ cup snipped fresh dill for garnish

1. Warm the oil in a 6-quart pot over medium-high heat for 1 minute. Add the chopped onion and sauté until transparent. Stir in the stock, cucumber, potato, parsley, and mustard. Cover and bring to a boil. Reduce the heat, and simmer until the potatoes are tender, about 15 minutes. Remove from the heat, and let cool for 10 minutes.

2. Transfer the mixture to a blender jar. Process until pureed, and stir in the black pepper. Chill for 1 hour.

Stir in the milk. Taste and season with salt and pepper if needed. Top each serving with dill.

Each serving: About 86 calories, 3 g protein, 10 g carbohydrate, 4 g total fat (1 g saturated), 5 mg cholesterol, 274 mg sodium.

Spring Pea Soup with Mint and Chives

PREP TIME: 15 minutes
COOK TIME: 10 minutes plus chilling

Makes 6 servings

The French often cook their fresh peas with lettuce and serve the resulting dish as a separate course. This soup takes that classic combination to the blender, and adds two other seasonal flavors as fresh accents.

  2 cups water
  ½ teaspoon salt or more to taste
  3 cups shelled fresh peas (3 pounds unshelled)
  2 cups shredded Romaine lettuce
  2 tablespoons finely shredded mint leaves
  ¼ cup heavy cream or more if needed
  1 to 2 tablespoons snipped fresh chives
  chive blossoms for garnish

1. Have ready a large bowl with ice and a little water with a smaller (at least 2-quart), preferably stainless-steel bowl inside, resting on the ice. Place 2 cups ice in the stainless-steel bowl.

Chilled Guacamole Soup

PREP TIME: 10 minutes
COOK TIME: 45 minutes to chill

Makes 4 servings

Holy guacamole! This is a subtly delightful soup. Its flavors—creamy avocado and sour cream—are mild and pleasing. Its color—pale green—is quiet and soothing. And it all comes together with the pulse of a blender.

3½ cups Chicken Stock (page 14)
1 Florida avocado, cut into ½-inch cubes
1 cup nonfat sour cream
1 medium onion, chopped
2 tablespoons lemon juice
2 garlic cloves, crushed through a press
½ teaspoon chili powder
salt and pepper to taste
1 teaspoon paprika for garnish

Combine the stock, avocado, sour cream, onion, lemon juice, garlic, and chili powder in a blender jar. Process until pureed. Chill for 45 minutes. Taste and season with salt and pepper if needed. Top each serving with the paprika.

2. Heat 2 cups water to boiling with ½ teaspoon salt in a 2-quart saucepan. Add the peas and simmer until tender, about 5 minutes. Add the lettuce and mint and stir until the lettuce is wilted, about 1 minute. Pour the mixture over the ice in the stainless-steel bowl and stir to chill the soup rapidly, until the ice melts. Remove the stainless-steel bowl from the larger bowl; empty and dry the larger bowl.

3. In batches, puree the soup in a blender, pouring the puree into the larger, chilled bowl. Stir in the cream and more ice water if soup is too thick. Taste, and add more cream or salt if needed. Cover the soup and store in the refrigerator until ready to serve. To serve: Ladle soup into chilled bowls. Sprinkle with chives and garnish with chive blossoms.

Each serving: About 97 calories, 5 g protein, 11 g carbohydrate, 4 g total fat (2 g saturated), 14 mg cholesterol, 202 mg sodium.

Each serving: About 156 calories, 5 g protein, 19 g carbohydrate, 8 g total fat (2 g saturated), 5 mg cholesterol, 518 mg sodium.

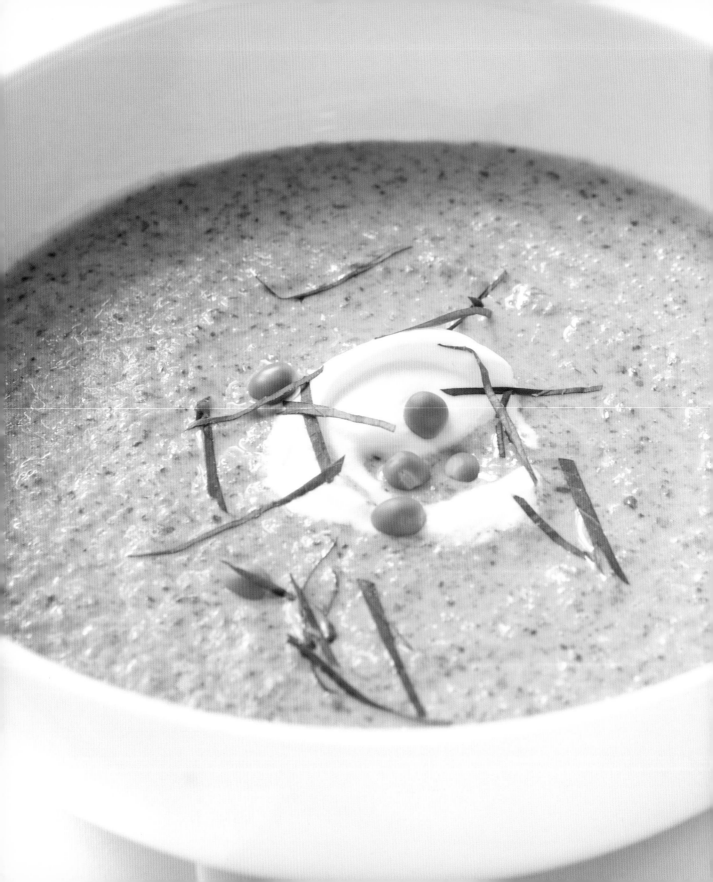

Cream of Lettuce Soup

PREP TIME: 20 minutes
COOK TIME: 30 minutes plus chilling

Makes 6 to 8 servings

Try diced unpeeled Kirby cucumbers or chilled cooked fresh peas as tasty and colorful garnishes (in addition to the mint). Boston and romaine lettuce are good choices, but even Iceberg is delish! This soup is nice hot, too, with a sprinkle of Croutons (page 22).

 2 large heads of lettuce
 2 tablespoons unsalted butter
 1 medium onion, thinly sliced
 2 tablespoons flour
 3 cups whole milk
 salt and ground white pepper to taste
 1 cup heavy cream
 15 fresh mint leaves, stacked and shredded just
  before using

1. Separate the leaves from the lettuce heads and rinse well. Drain and coarsely shred.

2. Melt the butter in a 2-quart saucepan over medium heat. Add the lettuce and onion and cover. Cook until the lettuce is translucent, about 5 minutes. Remove the pan from the heat and stir in the flour until blended.

3. Heat the milk until hot and gradually stir into the lettuce mixture. Cook, stirring, over medium-high heat, until bubbly, about 1 minute. Simmer over low heat 20 minutes.

4. Cool soup slightly and blend in a blender until smooth. Or, drain the solids through a sieve placed over a heat-safe glass measure and puree them in a food processor. Pour the blended soup into a bowl or combine the puree and the liquid in a bowl. Season to taste with salt and pepper. Cover and refrigerate until thoroughly chilled.

5. Whip the cream lightly, just enough to hold its shape (it will sink if it is whipped to a firm texture). Ladle the soup into shallow bowls and gently spoon the cream on top. Sprinkle with the mint and serve.

Each serving: About 275 calories, 6 g protein, 13 g carbohydrate, 23 g total fat (14 g saturated), 82 mg cholesterol, 317 mg sodium.

Curried Apple and Carrot Soup

PREP TIME: 10 minutes
COOK TIME: 25 minutes, plus 4 hours to chill

Makes about 3 cups

This sweet soup has just enough of a bite to make your guests come back
for a second taste.

  1¼ cups unsweetened apple juice
  1 medium McIntosh apple, peeled, cored, and chopped
  1 cup cooked sliced carrots (about 2 medium carrots)
  ¼ cup shredded Gouda cheese
  1 package (3 ounces) cream cheese
  1 tablespoon honey
  2 teaspoons lime juice or lemon juice
  ½ teaspoon curry powder
  salt and pepper to taste
  ½ cup chopped toasted walnuts for garnish

1. In a saucepan, combine the apple juice, chopped apple, and carrots.
   Bring to a boil, and stir in the Gouda cheese. Cook, stirring constantly,
   until the cheese has melted. Remove from heat.

2. In a blender, puree the soup in batches until smooth. Pour half the mixture back into the blender, and add the cream cheese, honey, lime juice,
   and curry powder. Process on high until smooth. Pour all of the mixture
   into a bowl, cover tightly, and chill for at least 4 hours.

3. Taste and season with salt and pepper if needed. Serve in chilled bowls
   topped with nuts.

Each cup: About 269 calories, 7 g protein, 27 g carbohydrate, 15 g total fat (10 g
saturated), 52 mg cholesterol, 336 mg sodium.

Chilled Yogurt Soup with Spinach and Herbs

PREP TIME: 15 minutes
COOK TIME: 15 minutes plus chilling

Makes 4 to 6 servings

For easier blending, whisk the yogurt in a bowl until it is looks like softly whipped cream before blending into the soup.

2 tablespoons olive oil

1 medium onion, chopped

3 scallions, tender green and white portions finely chopped

3 garlic cloves, chopped

1 cup chopped fresh Italian parsley plus more for garnish

⅓ cup snipped fresh dill plus more for garnish

1 large bunch spinach, washed, drained, and stemmed

1 teaspoon salt plus more to taste

¼ teaspoon freshly ground pepper plus more to taste

5 cups Vegetable Stock (page 15)

1½ cups plain yogurt plus more for serving

1 cup chickpeas, cooked from dried or use rinsed canned chickpeas

fresh lemon juice to taste

1 Kirby cucumber, peeled, seeded, and finely diced, for serving

1. Heat the oil in a 3-quart saucepan over medium heat and sauté the onion until softened but not brown, about 7 minutes. Add the scallions, garlic, parsley, and dill and sauté until softened, about 3 minutes. Add the spinach, salt, and pepper and sauté until the spinach wilts, about 2 minutes. Add the stock and heat to boiling over medium-high heat.

2. Drain the soup through a fine sieve placed over a 2-quart heat-safe glass measure or bowl. Puree the solids in a food processor or blender, adding enough stock to puree easily. Stir the puree into the remaining stock; whisk in the yogurt until blended. Cover and refrigerate until chilled.

3. To serve: Stir the chickpeas into the soup and season with salt, pepper, and lemon juice. Ladle the soup into chilled shallow soup bowls and garnish each with a dollop of yogurt, a sprinkle of cucumber, and a dusting of parsley and dill.

Each of 4 servings: About 231 calories, 11 g protein, 25 g carbohydrate, 11 g total fat (3 g saturated), 12 mg cholesterol, 704 mg sodium.

Chilled Cream-of-Vegetable Soup

PREP TIME: 15 minutes
COOK TIME: 50 minutes, plus 1 hour and 10 minutes to chill

Makes 6 servings

3 fresh parsley sprigs plus minced parsley
   for garnish
1 bay leaf
½ teaspoon crushed dried thyme
2 whole cloves
1 small garlic clove, crushed through a press
1 cup chopped celery leaves
1 medium carrot, peeled and diced
1 small green bell pepper, seeded and diced
1 cup finely chopped spinach leaves
1 large white onion, chopped
4 cups Vegetable Stock (page 15)
¼ cup rice
2 egg yolks
2 cups half-and-half
salt and pepper to taste
sour cream for serving
minced chives for garnish
2 medium tomatoes, peeled and chopped,
   for garnish

1. Tie the parsley, bay leaf, thyme, cloves, and garlic in a square of cheesecloth to make an herb bundle.

2. In a 6-quart pot, combine the herb bundle, celery leaves, carrot, green pepper, spinach, onion, stock, and rice. Bring to a boil. Reduce to a simmer, cover lightly, and cook, stirring occasionally, for about 30 minutes, or until the rice is tender. Discard the herb bundle and remove from heat.

3. In a blender or food processor, puree the soup in batches, processing until smooth. Return to the pot, and reheat.

4. In a small bowl, whisk together the egg yolks and several tablespoons of soup until smooth. Stir this mixture back into the hot soup mix until incorporated. (Do not allow to boil.) Add the half-and-half, heat through, remove from heat, and add salt and pepper to taste. Cool to room temperature. Chill in the refrigerator for about 1 hour.

5. When ready to serve, whisk the soup vigorously and ladle into chilled soup bowls. Dollop with sour cream and garnish with chopped parsley, chives, and tomatoes.

Each serving: About 330 calories, 10 g protein, 47 g carbohydrate, 12 g total fat (7 g saturated), 100 mg cholesterol, 1,018 mg sodium.

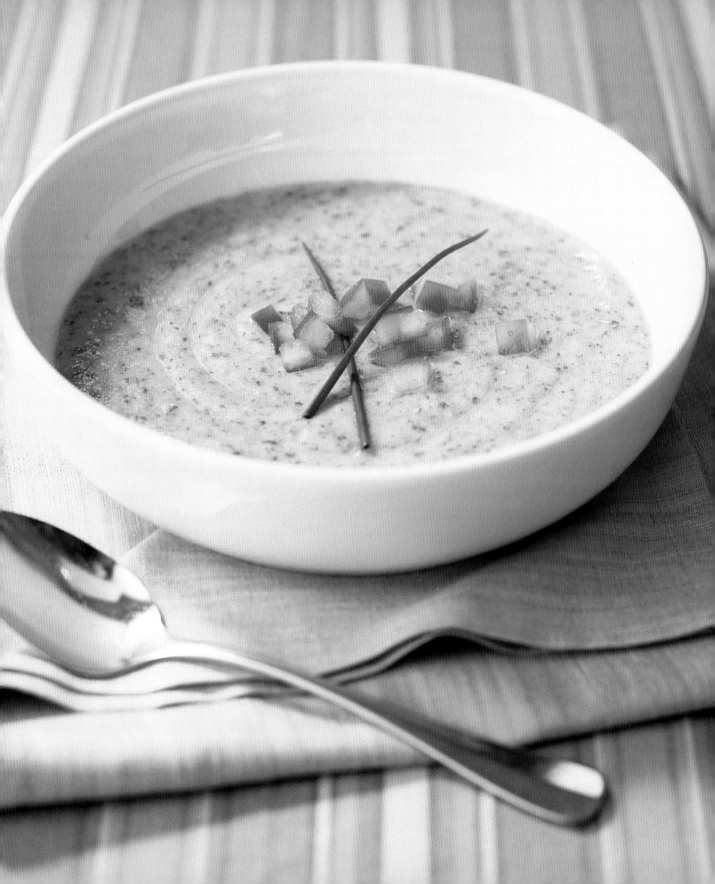

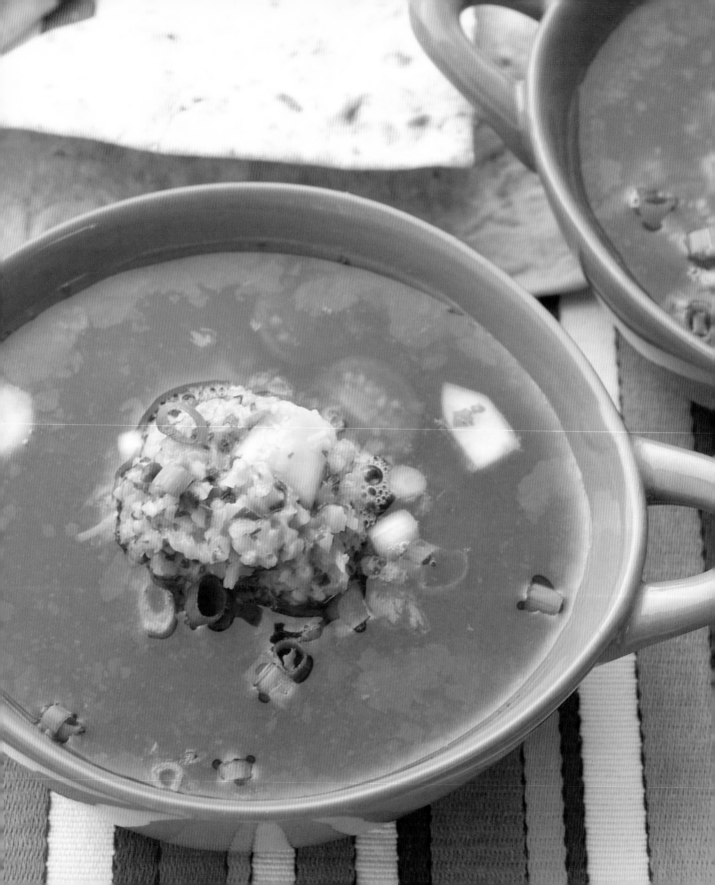

Tabbouleh with Parsley Broth

PREP TIME: 25 minutes
COOK TIME: 25 minutes plus chilling

Makes 4 to 6 servings

Inspired by the Middle Eastern dish of bulgur wheat with the same name, this soup is a refreshing start to a meal. Serve it with store-bought or homemade Lavash (page 36).

2 big bunches fresh parsley (about 4 ounces total), rinsed well, stemmed
4 cups Vegetable Stock (page 15) or water
4 teaspoons extravirgin olive oil
1 teaspoon minced garlic
½ teaspoon sea salt or more to taste
¼ teaspoon freshly ground pepper or more to taste
½ cup bulgur
2 scallions, thinly sliced crosswise
2 Kirby cucumbers, quartered lengthwise, and cut crosswise into ¼-inch wide pieces
1 cup halved mixed red and yellow cherry or grape tomatoes
¼ cup fresh lemon juice
1 tablespoon shredded fresh mint

1. Reserve a few parsley leaves for garnish and place the remaining leaves in a blender. Add 2 cups stock and pulse to combine. Blend only until the parsley is finely chopped but not pureed. Pour the liquid through a sieve into a 2-quart saucepan, pressing on the parsley to extract all the liquid. Place the parsley from the sieve in a large bowl and set aside. Add the remaining 2 cups stock, 2 teaspoons oil, ½ teaspoon garlic, and the salt and pepper to the parsley liquid. Heat to a full boil over medium-high heat and stir in the bulgur. Remove the pan from the heat and cover. Let stand until the bulgur is tender, 25 minutes or according to package directions.

2. While the bulgur stands, add the remaining 2 teaspoons oil and remaining ½ teaspoon garlic, the scallions, cucumbers, tomatoes, and lemon juice to the parsley. Mix well. Cover and let stand at room temperature.

3. When the bulgur is tender, drain the broth through a sieve into a glass measure, pressing lightly on the bulgur to drain it well. Spread out the bulgur on a plate and let it cool. Cover the broth and refrigerate until chilled.

4. Add the cooled bulgur to the parsley mixture and toss with a fork to mix. Add the mint and toss to mix. Cover and refrigerate until chilled.

5. To serve: Taste the parsley broth and the tabbouleh and season if necessary. Ladle the broth into shallow soup bowls and top with an ice-cream scoopful of the tabbouleh. Garnish with reserved parsley leaves.

Each of 4 servings: About 151 calories, 4 g protein, 24 g carbohydrate, 5 g total fat (1 g saturated), 0 mg cholesterol, 316 mg sodium.

Creamy Chilled Watercress Soup

PREP TIME: 15 minutes
COOK TIME: 40 minutes plus chilling

Makes 6 servings

Hot-pepper sauce is used here to enhance the peppery flavor of the watercress. You could also add a dash of curry powder with the leeks, or try a cream cheese flavored with chives, smoked salmon, or sundried tomatoes—whatever strikes your fancy at the deli or bagel shop.

2 English cucumbers
2 tablespoons unsalted butter
2 leeks, split lengthwise, rinsed well and chopped
1 quart Chicken or Vegetable Stock (Chapter 1)
1 big bunch watercress, leaves only, rinsed and drained
1 package (8 ounces) cream cheese, at room temperature
1 tablespoon fresh lemon juice
salt and freshly ground pepper to taste
Tabasco sauce to taste

1. Peel the cucumbers and slice in half lengthwise. Remove and discard any seeds with a teaspoon. Chop the remaining cucumber.

2. Melt the butter in a 2-quart saucepan over medium-high heat; add the leeks and sauté until softened, about 5 minutes. Add the cucumbers and sauté 1 minute. Add the stock and heat to boiling. Reduce the heat to medium and simmer soup, partially covered, 30 minutes.

3. Reserve some watercress leaves for garnish. Cut the cream cheese into 8 chunks and place half in a food processor. Drain the hot stock through a colander placed over a 2-quart heat-safe glass measure or bowl. Place the colander with the hot solids over the saucepan off the heat. Add half the solids and half the watercress to the food processor and pulse to blend. Puree, adding enough stock to puree the vegetables easily. Repeat with the remaining cream cheese, solids, and watercress. Add the puree to the hot stock.

4. Stir the lemon juice into the soup and season with salt and pepper. Cool, cover, and refrigerate until thoroughly chilled. Just before serving, taste the soup and season with Tabasco and more salt and pepper if needed.

Each serving: About 223 calories, 7 g protein, 8 g carbohydrate, 18 g total fat (11 g saturated), 52 mg cholesterol, 319 mg sodium.

STORING WATERCRESS
- The best way to store watercress is to keep it as it was grown, in water. Cut or twist off the ends of the stems and place the bouquet in a deep bowl or glass measure. Add about an inch of water, cover loosely with a plastic food storage bag, and store in the refrigerator until ready to use.

Polish Vegetable and Yogurt Soup

PREP TIME: 15 minutes
COOK TIME: 1 hour to chill

Makes 4 to 6 servings

This classic summer soup is called *chlodnik* in Polish. It is traditionally made with sour milk, but buttermilk or yogurt, or even milk and sour cream, can be used with tasty results.

1 quart plain yogurt
3 medium beets, cooked and peeled
1 English cucumber
1 bunch radishes (about 10), trimmed
1 bunch scallions (about 5), very finely chopped
1 garlic clove, crushed through a press
1 tablespoon snipped fresh dill or more to taste
salt and freshly ground pepper to taste
1 tablespoon dill pickle juice or more to taste
1 tablespoon sweet pickle juice or more to taste
3 hard-cooked eggs, chilled, for serving

1. Place the yogurt in a 2-quart bowl and whisk until blended and smooth. Finely grate the beets into the bowl (use a microplane). Peel the cucumber and cut in half lengthwise. Remove and discard any seeds with a teaspoon. Grate the cucumber and radishes into the yogurt mixture. Stir in the scallions, garlic, and dill, and season to taste with salt, pepper, and pickle juices. Cover with plastic wrap and refrigerate overnight or at least 1 hour.

2. **To serve:** Shell the eggs and quarter them lengthwise. Taste the soup and adjust seasoning if necessary. Ladle the soup into chilled soup dishes and garnish with egg wedges.

Each of 4 servings: About 307 calories, 5 g protein, 31 g carbohydrate, 8 g total fat (1 g saturated), 0 mg cholesterol, 658 mg sodium.

Chilled Roasted Beet Soup with Vegetable Polka Dots

PREP TIME: 45 minutes
COOK TIME: 45 minutes plus chilling

Makes 4 to 6 servings

You can use canned or jarred beets instead of roasting the beets, but the concentrated flavor of oven-roasted beets is, quite simply, sublime. The pea-size melon-ball scoop will have you creating dots from other vegetables as well as melons, apples and other tree fruits, cheeses, and flavored butters.

    1 very large carrot, peeled
    1 medium purple potato, peeled
    1 medium turnip, peeled
    4 small red beets, scrubbed and trimmed
    4 small golden beets, scrubbed and trimmed
    1 large red onion, cut into 6 wedges through
        the root
    2 large garlic cloves, unpeeled
    1 to 2 tablespoons olive oil
    salt and freshly ground pepper to taste
    2 cups plus 1 to 2 tablespoons water
    ½ cup fresh peas
    4 cups Vegetable Stock (page 15)
    2 Kirby cucumbers
    2 tablespoons snipped fresh dill

1. Preheat the oven to 400 degrees. Cut the carrot, potato, and turnip into balls with a pea-size melon baller; place in a bowl, cover, and refrigerate. Reserve the scraps of vegetables. Place the red beets on a piece of heavy-duty foil large enough to fold and seal around the beets. Repeat with the golden beets. On a third foil sheet, repeat with the scraps of carrot, potato, and turnip and the onion and garlic. Drizzle the vegetables with the oil, season with salt and pepper, and sprinkle with 1 to 2 tablespoons water. Seal the foil tightly around the vegetables to make 3 packets; place on a baking sheet. Bake 45 minutes or until vegetables are tender.

2. While the vegetables bake, place ice in a small bowl of water to make an ice bath. Heat 2 cups water to boiling in a small saucepan and add the peas. Cook until the peas are tender, 5 to 10 minutes. Drain the peas and immediately plunge them into the ice bath. (Chilling the peas quickly will help keep their bright green color.) When chilled, drain the peas and add them to the bowl of vegetable balls in the refrigerator.

3. When the vegetables are tender and cool enough to handle, peel the beets. Cut the flesh of 2 red beets and 2 golden beets into balls with a pea-size melon baller. Place the balls in separate bowls and refrigerate; reserve the scraps. Quarter the whole red beets and place in a blender with the scraps of red beets. Add half the roasted potato, turnip, and onion, and half the vegetable stock. Squeeze out one of the roasted garlic cloves from the root end into the mixture. Puree until smooth; taste and season with salt

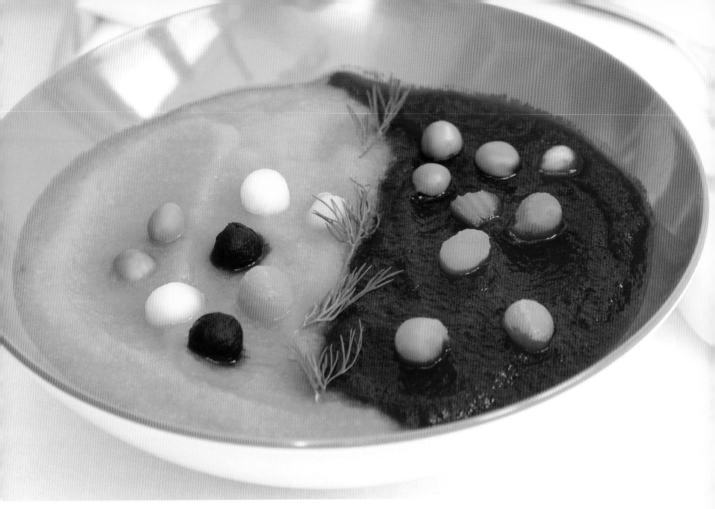

and pepper. Pour into a glass measure. Rinse out the blender and repeat with the golden beets and scraps, and remaining roasted vegetables and stock. Chill the mixtures thoroughly.

4. To serve: Peel the cucumbers and cut just the outer flesh into balls with a pea-size melon baller (do not dig deep enough to get to the seeds). Place in the bowl with the other vegetable balls. Working with one chilled shallow soup bowl at a time, pour about ¾ cup of each beet mixture into 2 separate small glass measures. Pour both mixtures at the same time into a bowl, pouring one at "3 o'clock" and the other at "9 o'clock". Gently but firmly rotate the dish clockwise and then quickly counterclockwise to create a yin-yang design with the two mixtures. Repeat with the remaining beet mixtures. Sprinkle the

cooked golden beet balls onto the red beet side and the red beet balls on the golden beet side. Sprinkle the carrot, potato, turnip, and cucumber balls and then the dill over both sides, dividing evenly among the soup bowls.

Each of 4 servings: About 156 calories, 5 g protein, 28 g carbohydrate, 4 g total fat (1 g saturated), 0 mg cholesterol, 400 mg sodium.

Vegetable-Quinoa Soup

PREP TIME: 20 minutes plus chilling
COOK TIME: 20 minutes plus chilling

Makes 6 servings

Containing more protein and fewer carbs than any other grain, quinoa (pronounced keen-wa) is an ancient staple of the Incas. When it cooks, a small spiral appears from each grain and curls around it.

1 cup quinoa, rinsed in a sieve until the water runs clear
2 cups water
2 garlic cloves, minced
½ teaspoon salt plus more if needed
2 ears yellow corn, husked
6 large, very ripe tomatoes
1 English cucumber
2 canned chipotle chiles in adobo sauce plus 2 teaspoons adobo sauce
1 small green bell pepper, seeded and cut into ¼-inch dice
1 small red bell pepper, seeded and cut into ¼-inch dice
1 small yellow bell pepper, seeded and cut into ¼-inch dice
1 small purple bell pepper, seeded and cut into ¼-inch dice
¼ cup chopped fresh cilantro leaves
¼ cup fresh lime juice plus more if needed
ground black pepper to taste

1. Combine the quinoa, water, garlic, and salt in a medium saucepan and heat to boiling over medium-high heat. Reduce the heat to medium-low, cover, and simmer until the quinoa is tender, about 15 minutes. Drain in a fine sieve and place in a large bowl. When cooled, cover and refrigerate to chill.

2. Meanwhile, over a grill, gas stovetop, or under a broiler, cook the corn until charred on all sides. When the corn is cool enough to handle, place on a cutting board and cut off the kernels, scraping the cobs to extract the juice. Place the corn and juice in a large bowl.

3. Blanch the tomatoes in a pan of boiling water. Rinse under cold water and peel. Quarter the tomatoes and discard the seeds. Chop 1 tomato and set aside. Peel the cucumber and cut in half lengthwise. Remove and discard any seeds with a teaspoon. Cut one half of the cucumber crosswise into ½-inch pieces and cut the remainder into ¼-inch dice.

4. Puree the remaining tomatoes with the ½-inch pieces of cucumber and the chipotle chiles and adobo sauce in a food mill placed over the bowl with the corn (or puree in a food processor and then add the puree to the corn). Add the chopped tomato and diced cucumber, the bell peppers, cilantro, and lime juice. Mix well and taste. Season with black pepper and more salt and lime juice if needed. Cover and refrigerate until thoroughly chilled.

5. To serve: Add the quinoa to the soup and mix well. Taste and adjust seasonings again if needed.

Each serving: About 224 calories, 8 g protein, 46 g carbohydrate, 3 g total fat (trace saturated), 0 mg cholesterol, 227 mg sodium.

Chilled Red Wine and Black Olive Soup

PREP TIME: 10 minutes
COOK TIME: 30 minutes plus chilling

Makes 4 to 6 servings

This is a delicious and interesting soup served either hot or cold. Either variation is enhanced with Brittle Bread (page 35).

   1 tablespoon olive oil
   ½ cup finely chopped shallots
   1 large garlic clove, crushed through a press
   2 tablespoons tomato paste
   1 tablespoon soy sauce
   1 tablespoon honey
   3 pounds ripe tomatoes, diced
   3 cups full-bodied red wine such a Zinfandel,
      Syrah, or Malbec
   freshly ground pepper to taste
   1 cup pitted and sliced Kalamata olives for garnish
   2 tablespoons snipped fresh dill for garnish

1. Heat the oil in a 3-quart saucepan over medium-high heat and sauté the shallots and garlic until softened and fragrant, about 3 minutes. Add the tomato paste and sauté until rust colored, about 1 minute. Stir in the soy sauce and honey until blended, and add the tomatoes and wine. Heat to boiling and reduce the heat to medium. Cover and simmer, stirring occasionally, until the tomatoes are falling apart, about 25 minutes.

2. Puree the soup in a food mill into a heat-safe bowl. Season with pepper, cover, cool, and refrigerate several hours or overnight.

3. To serve: Ladle the soup into chilled shallow soup bowls and sprinkle with the olives and dill.

Each of 4 servings: About 307 calories, 5 g protein, 31 g carbohydrate, 8 g total fat (1 g saturated), 0 mg cholesterol, 658 mg sodium.

Chilled Pea Pod Soup

PREP TIME: 15 minutes
COOK TIME: 40 minutes, plus 4 hours to chill

Makes 6 to 8 servings

As vegetables go, the pea pod is considered sweet; be very careful when you add the sugar to this savory soup or it will be too cloying.

2 pounds fresh green pea pods
½ cup margarine
8 green onions, sliced
2 quarts Vegetable Stock (page 15)
2 tablespoons fresh tarragon leaves
16 leaves romaine lettuce
½ cup crème fraîche
salt and pepper to taste
granulated sugar to taste
chopped fresh pea pods for garnish

1. Under running water, snap the ends off the pea pods and remove the strings.

2. Melt the margarine in a 6-quart pot, and sauté the pods and onions together, stirring frequently, until the onions are tender. Stir in the stock and tarragon, bring to a boil, then reduce to a simmer. Cover lightly, and cook, stirring occasionally, for about 15 minutes. Add the lettuce and continue to cook for about 5 minutes or until the lettuce is completely wilted. Remove from heat.

3. In a blender or food processor, puree the soup in batches until smooth. Strain through a fine sieve into a large bowl (discard the solids), stir in the crème fraîche, cover, and chill in the refrigerator for at least 4 hours.

4. When ready to serve, vigorously whisk the soup before adding salt and pepper to taste. Stir in the sugar. Ladle into chilled bowls and garnish with chopped pea pods.

Each of 6 servings: About 307 calories, 9 g protein, 30 g carbohydrate, 20 g total fat (5 g saturated), 13 mg cholesterol, 1,036 mg sodium.

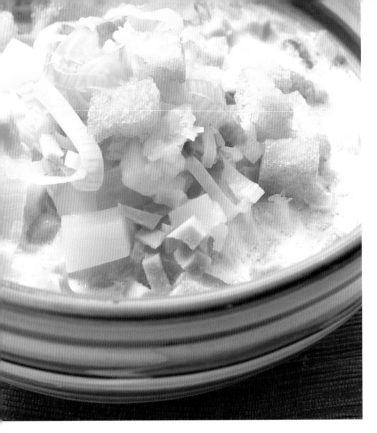

4

HOT
VEGETABLE
SOUPS

Confetti Soup

PREP TIME: 5 minutes
COOK TIME: 40 minutes

Makes 12 servings

1 tablespoon canola oil
2 medium yellow onions, minced
4 large carrots, peeled and diced
2 large fennel bulbs, cored and diced
10 cups Vegetable Stock (page 15) or water
1 teaspoon crushed dried tarragon
1 teaspoon crushed dried thyme
1 large red bell pepper, seeded and diced
2 medium zucchini, peeled and diced
12 large fresh mushrooms, quartered
salt and pepper to taste
grated Parmesan cheese for serving

1. Heat the oil in 6-quart pot and sauté the onions until soft. Add the carrots, fennel, stock, tarragon, and thyme. Bring to a boil, then reduce to a simmer, partially cover, and cook, stirring occasionally, for about 20 minutes, or until the vegetables are tender.

2. Add the red bell pepper, zucchini, and mushrooms. Cover lightly and cook for about 10 minutes.

3. Remove from the heat and add salt and pepper to taste. Serve immediately with Parmesan cheese on top.

Each serving: About 53 calories, 2 g protein, 10 g carbohydrate, 1 g total fat (trace saturated), 0 mg cholesterol, 42 mg sodium.

Minestrone (AND RIBOLLITA)

PREP TIME: 20 minutes plus chilling
COOK TIME: 1 hour 25 minutes to 2 hours

Makes 10 servings

Minestrone (or "big soup"), the traditional Italian bean and vegetable soup is cold-weather comfort food at its best. Every kitchen has its own recipe—some with pasta and/or bread, some with peas instead of beans, some sprinkled with Parmigiano-Reggiano cheese—so your house version can evolve after you've tried this one. Ribollita means "reboiled" in Italian, and in the soup world, refers to leftover minestrone that is cooked again. In this version, stale slices of Tuscan bread soak up the flavorful broth for an easy, hearty meal.

8 sprigs fresh thyme
6 sprigs fresh Italian parsley
2 sprigs fresh rosemary
¼ cup extravirgin olive oil plus your best Tuscan olive oil for serving
1 large onion, chopped
1 cup chopped carrots
1 cup chopped celery
4 garlic cloves, crushed through a press
2 tablespoons tomato paste
1 large Yukon gold potato, peeled and diced
8 cups Chicken or Vegetable Stock (Chapter 1) or water
4 cups cooked Great Northern beans from dried beans or rinsed canned beans
1 small head Savoy cabbage, large veins cut out and discarded, cut into 1-inch-thick wedges, and then cut crosswise into 1-inch pieces

1 head *cavolo nero* (Tuscan black-leaf kale) or 1
   bunch Swiss chard, large veins cut out and
   discarded, leaves cut into 1-inch squares
1 medium zucchini, quartered lengthwise, seeded
   and cut crosswise into ½-inch rounds
1 (10-ounce) package Italian green beans or
   1½ cups fresh Italian green beans or other cut
   green beans
¾ cup freshly grated Parmigiano-Reggiano
   cheese plus more for serving
salt and freshly ground pepper to taste
8 to 12 thick slices (about 8 ounces) Tuscan Bread
   (page 29), dried until stale and rubbed with
   garlic, for the Ribollita

1. Tie together the thyme, parsley, and rosemary sprigs
   with about 12 inches of cotton kitchen string and set
   aside. Heat the oil in a heavy 5-quart stockpot or
   Dutch oven over medium-high heat. Add the onion
   and sauté until softened, about 5 minutes. Add the
   carrots and celery and sauté 3 minutes. Add the garlic and sauté 1 minute. Stir in the tomato paste and
   sauté until rust colored. Add the potato. Stir in 2
   cups stock until blended with the tomato paste. Mash
   1 cup cooked Great Northern beans to a puree with a
   fork and stir into the soup. Add the herb bundle and
   the remaining stock, the cabbage, calvo nero, zucchini, and green beans and stir to mix well. Heat to
   boiling, reduce the heat to low, and simmer, partially

covered and stirring occasionally, 1 hour. Stir in the
remaining 3 cups cooked Great Northern beans and
heat through. Remove the pot from the heat.

2. To serve as minestrone: Discard the herb bunch. Stir
   in the cheese and let the soup set for 5 minutes.
   Season to taste with salt and pepper. Ladle into
   warmed soup bowls, drizzle with Tuscan olive oil,
   and sprinkle with Parmigiano-Reggiano.

3. For the ribollita: Depending how much soup is left
   over (you can turn it all into ribollita if you want),
   arrange several slices of stale Tuscan bread in a
   deep casserole and ladle enough soup on top to
   soak the bread. Repeat with as much of the remaining bread you need to soak with soup but still be
   soupy. Cover and refrigerate overnight. Remove the
   casserole from the refrigerator about 1 hour before
   serving to take the chill off. Cover and bake in the
   center of a 350-degree oven until boiling (timing will
   depend on how much soup there is). Ladle or spoon
   the soup into warmed soup bowls, drizzle with
   Tuscan olive oil, and sprinkle with Parmigiano-
   Reggiano.

Each serving: About 339 calories, 20 g protein, 43 g carbohydrate, 11 g total fat (3 g saturated), 8 mg cholesterol, 604 mg
sodium.

Quick Minestrone with Elbow Macaroni

PREP TIME: 5 minutes
COOK TIME: 35 minutes

Makes 4 servings

This easy minestrone version lives up to its namesake. Planning to double
this recipe and serve half another time? Add the macaroni to half the soup
at a time; pasta tends to oversoften when stored in a stock.

1¾ cups Vegetable Stock (page 15)
1 carrot, peeled and thinly sliced
1 celery stalk, sliced
1 cup cut green beans
⅔ cup sliced scallions
1 can (16 ounces) stewed tomatoes
1 tablespoon red wine vinegar
1 teaspoon Italian herb seasoning
pinch cayenne pepper
½ cup elbow macaroni
salt and pepper to taste
½ cup chopped fresh parsley for garnish
freshly grated parmesan cheese for garnish (optional)

Combine the stock, carrot, celery, beans, scallions, tomatoes, vinegar,
herb seasoning, and pepper in a 6-quart pot. Cover and bring to a boil.
Reduce the heat and simmer 25 minutes. Stir in the macaroni and cook
7 minutes more. Taste and season with salt and pepper if needed. Serve
the soup topped with parsley and Parmesan, if desired.

Each serving: About 136 calories, 6 g protein, 27 g carbohydrate, 1 g total fat
(trace saturated), 0 mg cholesterol, 812 mg sodium.

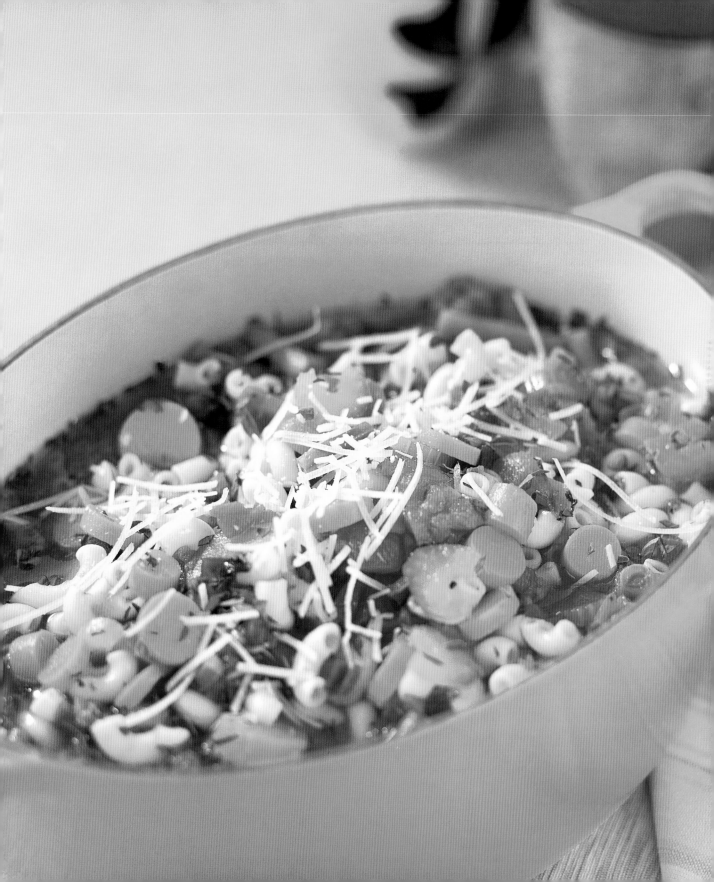

Ginger Vegetable Soup

PREP TIME: 10 minutes
COOK TIME: 15 minutes

Makes 4 servings

1 medium yellow onion, sliced
1 celery stalk, thinly sliced
1 green bell pepper, seeded and sliced
2 teaspoons minced fresh gingerroot
¼ teaspoon crushed garlic
½ cup water
4 cups Vegetable Stock (page 15)
1 can (8 ounces) tomato sauce
2 white potatoes, peeled and diced
1 small zucchini, halved lengthwise and sliced
2 cups frozen whole corn kernels
1 teaspoon crushed dried basil
1 teaspoon paprika
½ teaspoon ground black pepper
salt and pepper to taste

1. In a 6-quart pot, combine the onion, celery, green pepper, ginger, garlic, and water. Bring to a boil, and cook until the celery is tender, about 5 minutes.

2. Add the stock, tomato sauce, potatoes, zucchini, corn, basil, paprika, and pepper. Return to a boil, cover lightly, and cook, stirring occasionally, until the potatoes are tender. Remove from heat, add salt and black pepper to taste, and serve.

Each serving: About 240 calories, 9 g protein, 54 g carbohydrate, 1 g total fat (trace saturated), 0 mg cholesterol, 660 mg sodium.

Fresh Tomato-Corn Soup

PREP TIME: 5 minutes
COOK TIME: 15 minutes

Makes 4 servings

2 teaspoons olive oil
1 cup chopped red onion
4 garlic cloves, minced
1¾ cups Vegetable Stock (page 15)
2 cups diced zucchini
1 pound fresh tomatoes, chopped
1½ cups frozen corn
½ teaspoon crushed red pepper flakes
¼ cup chopped fresh basil leaves
salt and pepper to taste
2 tablespoons bacon bits for serving

1. Heat the oil in a 6-quart pot over medium-high heat for 1 minute. Add the onion and garlic and sauté until the onion is translucent, about 3 minutes.

2. Stir in the stock, zucchini, tomatoes, corn, and red pepper flakes. Cover and bring to a boil. Reduce the heat and simmer until the zucchini is tender, about 10 minutes.

3. Stir in the basil. Taste and season with salt and pepper if needed. Top each serving with bacon bits.

Each serving: About 170 calories, 7 g protein, 34 g carbohydrate, 3 g total fat (trace saturated), 0 mg cholesterol, 704 mg sodium.

Victoria's Brazilian Vegetable Soup

PREP TIME: 10 minutes
COOK TIME: 40 minutes

Makes 4 servings

You can substitute acorn, butternut, or any other winter squash for the sweet potato.

2 tablespoons vegetable oil
1 medium yellow onion, quartered
3 garlic cloves, chopped
1 serrano chile, stemmed, seeded, and diced (use rubber gloves when handling hot peppers)
2 large ripe tomatoes, quartered
1 medium carrot, peeled and diced; plus 2 carrots, peeled and thinly sliced, for garnish
1 medium sweet potato, peeled and diced
½ teaspoon black pepper
10 cups Vegetable Stock (page 15) or water
1 can (16 ounces) black beans, rinsed
1 cup finely shredded kale
salt and pepper to taste
¼ cup finely chopped fresh Italian parsley for garnish

1. Heat the oil in a 6-quart pot and sauté the onion until lightly colored. Add the garlic and chile pepper and sauté 5 minutes. Add tomatoes, diced carrot, sweet potato, pepper, and stock. Bring to a boil, then reduce to a simmer, partly cover, and cook, stirring occasionally, for about 20 minutes.

2. Add the black beans and kale, partly cover, and continue to simmer for about 15 minutes. Remove from heat and add salt and pepper to taste. Garnish with carrot slices and parsley. Serve immediately.

Each serving: About 213 calories, 9 g protein, 38 g carbohydrate, 8 g total fat (1 g saturated), 0 mg cholesterol, 583 mg sodium.

Chunky Cream of Tomato Soup with Tarragon

PREP TIME: 10 minutes
COOK TIME: 20 minutes

Makes 4 servings

3 pounds ripe tomatoes
1 teaspoon olive oil
1 large onion, chopped
1¾ cups Beef Stock (page 15)
1 tablespoon no-salt-added tomato paste
1 tablespoon brown sugar
¼ teaspoon freshly ground black pepper
1 cup 2% milk
1 teaspoon chopped fresh tarragon leaves
salt to taste
½ cup chopped fresh basil leaves for garnish

1. Peel and seed the tomatoes, reserving the juice. Cut the tomatoes into small chunks.

2. Heat the oil in a 6-quart pot over medium-high heat for 1 minute. Add the onion and sauté until golden (do not brown), about 5 minutes. Add the reserved tomato juice, tomatoes, stock, tomato paste, sugar, and black pepper. Cover and bring to a boil. Reduce the heat and simmer 10 minutes.

3. Stir in the milk and tarragon and heat through (do not boil), about 3 minutes. Taste and season with salt if needed. Top each serving with basil.

Each serving: About 159 calories, 8 g protein, 28 g carbohydrate, 3 g total fat (1 g saturated), 5 mg cholesterol, 546 mg sodium.

PEELING AND SEEDING TOMATOES

To peel and seed tomatoes easily, follow these steps:

1. Blanch tomatoes in boiling water for 1 minute and immediately plunge them into icy cold water. Slip off the skins.

2. Cut the tomatoes in half horizontally.

3. Squeeze the halves over a sieve, and discard the seeds.

Cheddar-Tomato Bisque

PREP TIME: 5 minutes
COOK TIME: 25 minutes

Makes 6 servings

This vegetable bisque has a beautiful burnt orange color, the special flavors of tomato and cheddar, and all the usual richness that comes with a bisque.

    1 teaspoon olive oil
    1 large onion, chopped
    3½ cups Beef Stock (page 15)
    2 large potatoes, peeled and cut into ½-inch cubes
    4 plum tomatoes, chopped
    1 carrot, shredded
    2 garlic cloves, crushed through a press
    ¼ teaspoon freshly ground black pepper
    ½ teaspoon ground dried savory
    1 cup 2% milk
    ¾ cup shredded reduced-fat cheddar cheese
    salt to taste
    ¼ cup chopped fresh parsley for garnish

1. Heat the oil in a 6-quart pot over medium-high heat for 1 minute. Add the onion and sauté until translucent. Stir in the stock, potatoes, tomatoes, carrot, garlic, pepper, and savory. Cover and bring to a boil. Reduce the heat and simmer until the vegetables are tender, about 15 minutes.

2. Remove from the heat and, using a handheld immersion blender, puree the mixture. Stir in the milk and cheddar and heat through (do not let it boil). Taste and season with salt if needed. Serve garnished with parsley.

Each serving: About 217 calories, 10 g protein, 27 g carbohydrate, 7 g total fat (3 g saturated), 11 mg cholesterol, 1,225 mg sodium.

Fresh Tomato and Tuscan Bread Soup

PREP TIME: 15 minutes
COOK TIME: 45 minutes

Makes 4 servings

Use only "real" seasonally ripe tomatoes (not the ones that come from a hothouse) and hearty bread with body for this soup. It just may become your September house specialty.

2 pounds any variety garden-ripe tomatoes
¼ cup extravirgin Tuscan olive oil plus more
    for serving
2 large garlic cloves, minced
3 cups 1-inch cubes Tuscan Bread (page 29), stale
    or toasted in the oven until dried and hard
6 cups Chicken or Vegetable Stock (Chapter 1)
sea salt and freshly ground pepper to taste
8 fresh basil leaves, stacked, rolled up lengthwise
    and shredded, for garnish

1. Blanch the tomatoes in a large pot of boiling water; boil 1 minute. Transfer to a bowl of ice and water. When the tomatoes are cool enough to handle, peel off and discard the skins. Cut the tomatoes crosswise in half. Remove the seeds with your thumb and place in a sieve set over a bowl. Scrape the tomato seeds against the sieve to extract the juice; discard the seeds. Dice the tomatoes and place in the bowl with the tomato juice.

2. Heat the oil in a 3-quart saucepan over medium heat. Add the garlic and sauté until fragrant, about 1 minute. Add the tomatoes and their juices and the bread and sauté until the bread is softened, about 3 minutes. Add the stock, heat to boiling, and season with salt and pepper. Reduce the heat to medium-low and simmer until the soup is thick, stirring often to break up the bread, about 30 minutes. Taste and adjust the seasoning if necessary.

3. To serve: Stir half the basil into the soup and ladle into warmed soup bowls. Sprinkle with the remaining basil and drizzle generously with olive oil.

Each serving: About 320 calories, 12 g protein, 29 g carbohydrate, 18 g total fat (3 g saturated), 0 mg cholesterol, 309 mg sodium.

Bell Pepper and Tomato Soup

PREP TIME: 10 minutes
COOK TIME: 1 hour 15 minutes

Makes 4 to 6 servings

Lightly browning the flour diminishes its thickening power a bit but adds a rich toasty flavor.

  4 tablespoons unsalted butter
  2 small green bell peppers, seeded and finely chopped
  1 small onion, finely chopped
  ¼ cup all-purpose flour
  1 pound ripe tomatoes, skinned, seeded, and chopped
  1 quart Vegetable Stock (page 15)
  2 teaspoon freshly grated horseradish or prepared horseradish
  salt and freshly ground black pepper to taste
  cayenne pepper to taste
  dash red-wine vinegar

1. Melt the butter in a 2-quart saucepan over medium heat. Add the bell peppers and onion and sauté until softened but not browned, about 7 minutes. Stir in the flour and cook, stirring, until golden, about 4 minutes. Add the tomatoes and stir to blend their juice with the flour. Gradually stir in the stock. Heat to boiling over medium-high heat; cover, and simmer over medium-low heat 1 hour.

2. Stir the horseradish into the soup and season to taste with salt, black pepper, and cayenne. Stir in the vinegar.

Each of 4 servings: About 182 calories, 3 g protein, 18 g carbohydrate, 12 g total fat (7 g saturated), 31 mg cholesterol, 311 mg sodium.

Classic Potato Leek Soup

PREP TIME: 5 minutes
COOK TIME: 20 minutes

Makes 4 servings

Seasoned with ham and celery, this popular soup makes a perfect addition to a special dinner or a speedy supper. It's light. It's easy. It's splendid.

  1 teaspoon olive oil
  3 leeks, white part only, sliced, rinsed well
  4 ounces finely diced lean deli ham
  3 cups diced potatoes
  2 cups Chicken Stock (page 14)
  ½ teaspoon ground celery seeds
  1 cup 1% milk
  ¼ teaspoon freshly ground black pepper
  salt to taste

1. Heat the oil in a 6-quart pot over medium-high heat for 1 minute. Add the leeks and ham; cook until the leeks are wilted, 3 to 5 minutes.

2. Stir in the potatoes, stock, and celery seeds. Cover and bring to a boil. Reduce the heat and simmer 10 minutes. Stir in the milk and pepper. Cook (do not boil) until the potatoes are tender, 5 to 10 minutes. Taste and season with salt if needed.

Each serving: About 158 calories, 13 g protein, 20 g carbohydrate, 3 g total fat (1 g saturated), 21 mg cholesterol, 424 mg sodium.

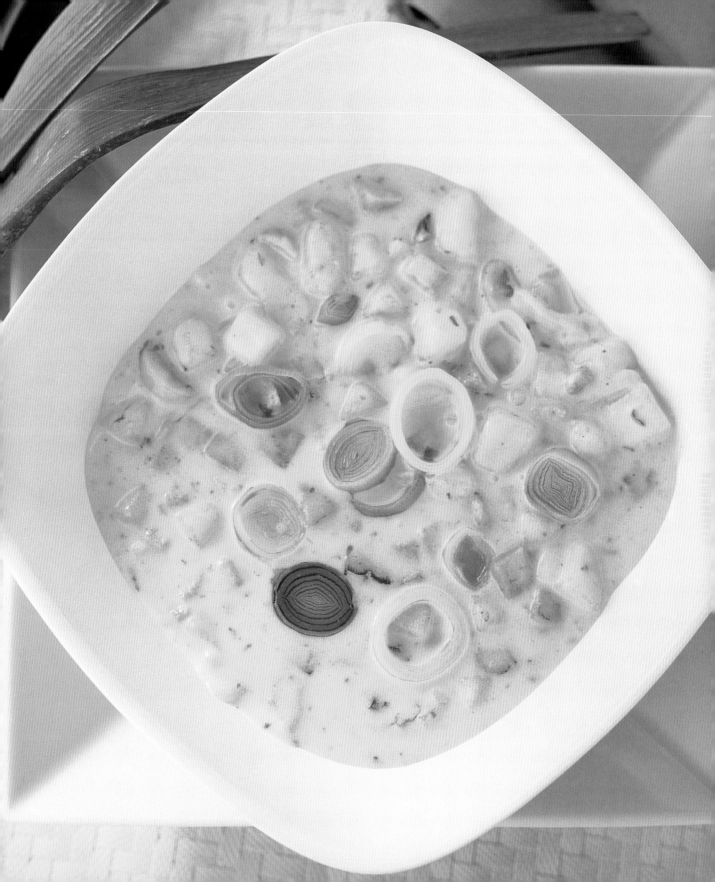

Jalapeño Jack Potato Soup

PREP TIME: 5 minutes
COOK TIME: 25 minutes

Makes 4 servings

For crunch, serve this soup with crudités, croutons, or crusty French bread.

  6 large or 10 medium potatoes, peeled and cut into
    ½-inch cubes
  1¾ cups Chicken Stock (page 14)
  1 medium onion, finely chopped
  ½ teaspoon celery seeds
  1 cup skim milk
  1 cup shredded jalapeño Monterey Jack cheese
  salt and pepper to taste
  caraway seeds for garnish

1. Combine the potatoes, stock, onion, and celery seeds in a 6-quart pot. Cover and bring to a boil. Reduce the heat and simmer until the potatoes are tender, 15 to 20 minutes.

2. Using a potato masher or handheld immersion blender, mash the potatoes, stirring in the milk a little at a time. Mix in the cheese and cook until it has melted, about 5 minutes. Taste and season with salt and pepper if needed. Garnish each serving with the caraway seeds.

Each serving: About 473 calories, 19 g protein, 80 g carbohydrate, 10 g total fat (5 g saturated), 31 mg cholesterol, 318 mg sodium.

Chipotle–Sweet Potato Soup

PREP TIME: 5 minutes
COOK TIME: 20 minutes

Makes 4 servings

Chipotles are smoked, dried jalapeño peppers. If you have trouble finding them, substitute a dried cayenne pepper and ⅛ teaspoon mesquite smoke flavoring.

  3½ cups Beef Stock (page 15)
  1 large sweet potato, peeled and shredded
  1 carrot, peeled and shredded
  1 medium onion, chopped
  1 small chipotle pepper, seeded and chopped
  ½ teaspoon cumin seed
  ¼ teaspoon allspice
  ¼ teaspoon white pepper
  ½ cup reduced-fat Monterey Jack cheese
  salt to taste

1. Combine the stock, sweet potato, carrot, onion, chipotle pepper, cumin, allspice, and white pepper in a 6-quart pot. Cover and bring to a boil. Reduce the heat and simmer 15 minutes.

2. Remove the pot from the heat; using a handheld immersion blender, partially puree the mixture. Stir in the cheese until it melts. Taste and season with salt if needed.

Each serving: About 109 calories, 8 g protein, 14 g carbohydrate, 3 g total fat (2 g saturated), 8 mg cholesterol, 1,522 mg sodium.

Asparagus Soup

PREP TIME: 10 minutes
COOK TIME: 30 minutes

Makes 6 servings

Can a soup be light, creamy, elegant, easy, and brimming with asparagus, the harbinger of spring, all at once? Absolutely.

1 pound asparagus
2 teaspoons canola oil
1 medium Spanish onion, chopped
1 medium potato, cut into ½-inch cubes
3 cups Vegetable Stock (page 15)
¼ teaspoon white pepper
1 cup 2% milk
½ teaspoon ground savory
salt to taste
¼ cup chopped fresh parsley for garnish

1. Cut off the asparagus tips. Cut the stalks into ½-inch slices, discarding the woody bases. Separately blanch the tips and stalks for 3 minutes, and then plunge them into cold water and drain. Reserve the tips for garnish.

2. Heat the oil in a 6-quart pot over medium-high heat for 1 minute. Add the onion and sauté until translucent. Stir in the asparagus stalks, potato, stock, and pepper. Cover and bring to a boil. Reduce the heat and simmer until potatoes and asparagus are tender, about 12 minutes. Using a handheld immersion blender, puree the mixture.

3. Stir in the milk and savory and heat through (do not boil), about 3 minutes. Taste and season with salt if needed. Top each serving with parsley and asparagus tips.

Each serving: About 108 calories, 5 g protein, 17 g carbohydrate, 3 g total fat (1 g saturated), 3 mg cholesterol, 557 mg sodium.

TIP
- The easiest way to remove an asparagus's woody base is to snap it off. If the stalk is tough, remove the outer layer with a vegetable peeler.

Cream of Fennel Soup

PREP TIME: 15 minutes
COOK TIME: 45 minutes

Makes 4 servings

This soup is also delicious and refreshing served cold. Hot or chilled, Quick
Pepper-Parmesan Crisps (page 37) make a perfect accompaniment.

    2 tablespoons Italian extravirgin olive oil
    1 large bulb fennel, fresh fronds coarsely chopped and reserved, bulb
      cored and finely chopped
    1 quart Chicken or Vegetable Stock (Chapter 1)
    ½ cup heavy cream
    1 teaspoon anisette or other anise-flavored liqueur such as Pernod
    pinch cayenne pepper
    salt and freshly ground black pepper to taste

1. Heat the oil in a 2-quart saucepan over medium heat. Add the chopped
   fennel bulb and sauté slowly and gently for 10 minutes. Add the stock
   and heat to boiling. Reduce the heat and simmer gently until the fennel
   is tender, about 20 minutes.

2. Pour the soup through a strainer set over a heat-safe glass measure.
   Spoon about two-thirds of the solids into a blender or food processor.
   Add enough cooking liquid to move the ingredients around easily and
   process into a puree. Pour the puree and the cooking liquid back into the
   saucepan, along with the remaining solids in the strainer, and heat
   through. Stir in the cream, anisette, and cayenne and cook until heated
   through but not boiling or simmering. Season with salt and pepper and
   ladle into warmed soup bowls. Garnish each serving with reserved
   chopped fennel fronds.

Each serving: About 161 calories, 7 g protein, 7 g carbohydrate, 12 g total fat
(4 g saturated), 11 mg cholesterol, 332 mg sodium.

Cream of Turnip Soup

PREP TIME: 15 minutes
COOK TIME: 55 minutes

Makes 4 to 6 servings

You may hear cries of "Yikes!" when you announce this soup of the day, but what a pleasant surprise it will be to taste the subtly sweet results. Small turnips are the secret: They are more delicately flavored than older ones and have a less coarse texture.

2 tablespoons unsalted butter

2 shallots, chopped

1 pound small turnips, peeled and diced

¼ cup dry white wine

2 cups Turkey or Beef Stock (Chapter 1) or more if needed

2 cups water or more if needed

2 dried bay leaves

½ teaspoon sea salt or more to taste

½ cup crème fraîche or heavy cream

¼ teaspoon freshly ground white pepper or more to taste

½ cup chopped skinned, toasted hazelnuts, for serving

1. Melt the butter in a 3-quart saucepan over medium heat. Add the shallots and sauté until softened, about 5 minutes. Add the turnips and sauté until crisp-tender, about 5 minutes. Add the wine and heat to boiling. Boil until almost evaporated, about 2 minutes. Add the stock and the water, stir, and add the bay leaves and salt. Increase the heat to medium high and bring to a boil. Reduce the heat to medium-low and simmer, covered, until the turnips are very tender, about 25 minutes.

2. Discard the bay leaves. In batches, carefully puree the soup in a blender, holding down the lid with a folded kitchen towel. Pour the soup into a clean saucepan and reheat to simmering. Whisk in a little more stock or water if the soup is too thick. Whisk in the crème fraîche and pepper. Taste and adjust the seasonings if necessary. To serve, ladle into warmed soup bowls and sprinkle with hazelnuts.

Each of 4 servings: About 244 calories, 6 g protein, 14 g carbohydrate, 18 g total fat (3 g saturated), 0 mg cholesterol, 309 mg sodium.

Cream of Cauliflower and Parsnip Soup

PREP TIME: 5 minutes
COOK TIME: 20 minutes

Makes 4 servings

Thick, satisfying, subtly nutty-tasting, and oh so good. What more could you want from a simple soup that's ready to eat in no time flat? When pureeing the potatoes and other vegetables, take care not to overwhip them as they may become gummy.

  1 teaspoon olive oil
  4 ounces mushrooms, cubed
  2 shallots, sliced
  2 large potatoes, peeled and cut into
     ½-inch cubes
  2 cups cauliflower florets
  1 cup thinly sliced parsnips
  2 cups Vegetable Stock (page 15)
  ½ cup skim milk
  ½ teaspoon sage
  ⅛ teaspoon white pepper
  salt to taste
  paprika for garnish
  fresh parsley sprigs for garnish

1. Heat the oil in a 6-quart pot over medium-high heat for 1 minute. Add the mushrooms and shallots and sauté for 3 minutes.

2. Stir in the potatoes, cauliflower, parsnips, and stock. Cover and bring to a boil. Reduce the heat and simmer until the vegetables are tender, about 10 minutes. Using a handheld immersion blender, puree the mixture.

3. Stir in the milk, sage, and pepper. Warm the soup until it is hot throughout, about 5 minutes; do not boil. Taste and season with salt if needed. Garnish each serving with the paprika and parsley.

Each serving: About 158 calories, 6 g protein, 31 g carbohydrate, 2 g total fat (trace saturated), trace cholesterol, 471 mg sodium.

Broccoli Soup

PREP TIME: 15 minutes
COOK TIME: 20 minutes

Makes 4 servings

  1 small carrot, peeled and thinly sliced
  1 celery stalk with leaves, sliced
  1 small white onion, chopped
  1 medium garlic clove, minced
  ½ teaspoon crushed dried marjoram
  ¼ teaspoon crushed dried basil
  ½ cup Vegetable Stock (page 15)
  2 cups skim milk
  2 cups coarsely chopped broccoli
  ½ cup vegetable-flavored pasta, cooked al dente
    and drained
  salt and pepper to taste
  1 cup unflavored yogurt or whipped sour cream
  ground nutmeg for garnish

1. In a 6-quart pot, combine the carrot, celery, onion, garlic, marjoram, basil, and stock and bring to a boil. Reduce to a simmer, cover lightly, and cook for about 10 minutes.

2. Add the milk and broccoli and bring to a boil. Reduce the heat, cover lightly, and simmer for about 5 minutes, until the broccoli is tender. Remove from the heat. In batches, puree the soup in a blender or food processor until smooth. Return to the pot, add the pasta, and heat through.

3. Remove from heat; add salt and pepper to taste. Top each serving with yogurt and nutmeg.

Each serving: About 179 calories, 10 g protein, 14 g carbohydrate, 1 g total fat (trace saturated), 2 mg cholesterol, 181 mg sodium.

Simple Garlic Soup

PREP TIME: 5 minutes
COOK TIME: 25 minutes

Makes 4 servings

Don't be intimidated by the amount of garlic in this recipe. Gentle cooking tames garlic's flavor and makes it mild, almost sweet.

  1 teaspoon olive oil
  1 head garlic, cloves peeled and sliced
  3½ cups Chicken Stock (page 14)
  1 tablespoon snipped fresh fennel fronds
  1 tablespoon dry sherry
  salt and pepper to taste
  ½ recipe Herb Croutons (page 22) for serving
  ¼ cup chopped fresh parsley for garnish

Heat the oil in a 6-quart pot over medium-high heat for 1 minute. Add the garlic, and sauté until golden (do not brown), 3 to 5 minutes, stirring constantly. Add the stock and fennel; simmer 15 minutes. Stir in the sherry. Taste and season with salt and pepper if needed. Top each serving with croutons and parsley.

Each serving without croutons: About 101 calories, 2 g protein, 9 g carbohydrate, 6 g total fat (1 g saturated), 1 mg cholesterol, 442 mg sodium.

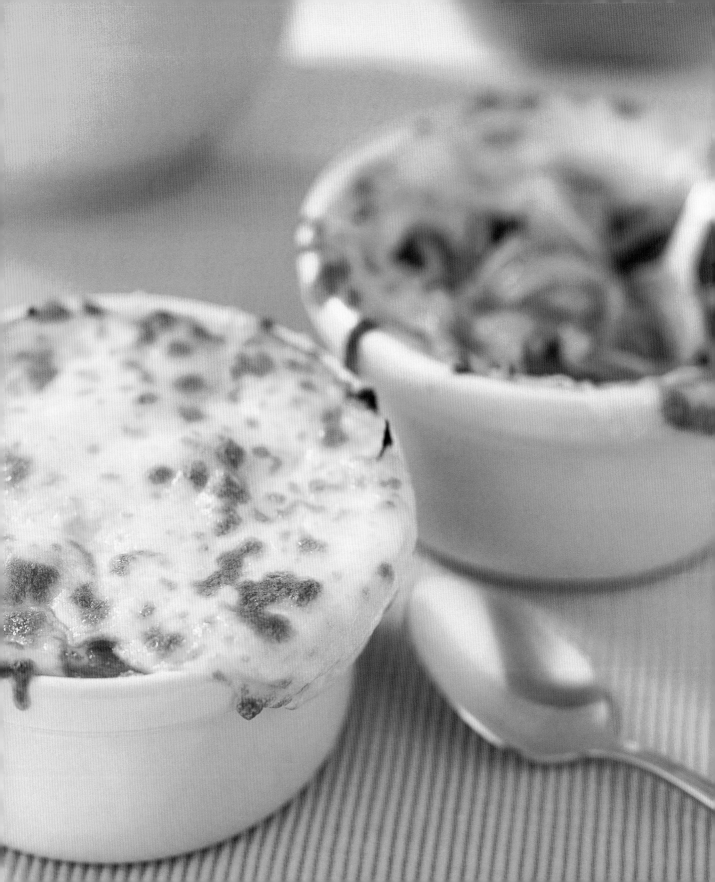

Quick French Onion Soup

PREP TIME: 5 minutes
COOK TIME: 30 minutes

Makes 4 servings

In this easy version of the French classic, Madeira wine and Gruyère cheese impart wonderful mellow and nutty flavors. Crisp croutons soak up the tasty broth.

  1 teaspoon olive oil
  4 medium onions, cut into thin wedges
  7 cups Beef Stock (page 15)
  1 tablespoon Madeira wine
  3 cups Plain Croutons (page 22)
  ½ cup shredded Gruyère cheese
  salt and pepper to taste
  chopped fresh parsley for garnish

1. Heat the oil in a 6-quart pot over medium-high heat for 1 minute. Add the onions and sauté until golden, about 8 minutes. Add the stock. Cover and bring to a boil. Reduce the heat and simmer 15 minutes. Stir in the Madeira.

2. Preheat the broiler. Divide the croutons among 4 soup bowls. Ladle in the soup and top each serving with cheese. Place the soup bowls under the broiler and broil until the cheese is melted, for 3 to 4 minutes, or until bubbling. Taste and season with salt and pepper if needed. Garnish with parsley.

Each serving without croutons: About 246 calories, 17 g protein, 27 g carbohydrate, 7 g total fat (3 g saturated), 15 mg cholesterol, 475 mg sodium.

Roasted Eggplant Soup

PREP TIME: 25 minutes
COOK TIME: 50 minutes

Makes 6 to 8 servings

The toasty flavor of Sesame Seed Crackers (page 33) goes perfectly with this soup.

2 (1-pound) eggplants
2 tablespoons extravirgin olive oil plus more for brushing
2 large red bell peppers
1 large Spanish onion, chopped
1 teaspoon ground cumin
¼ teaspoon crushed red pepper flakes
salt and freshly ground black pepper to taste
6 cups Chicken or Vegetable Stock (Chapter 1)
1 cup plain yogurt
1 medium garlic clove, crushed through a press
2 teaspoons fresh lemon juice or more to taste
2 tablespoons minced fresh mint leaves plus sprigs for garnish

1. Preheat the oven to 450 degrees. Cut the eggplants in half and brush the flesh with some olive oil. Place cut sides down on a foil-lined baking sheet. Bake until tender, about 20 minutes; let cool. Working with one half at a time, place the eggplant on a cutting board and cut lengthwise into thirds. Slide a thin-bladed knife between the skin and flesh at one end and, pressing the skin onto the cutting board, slide the knife along the skin to remove it in one piece. Discard the skins and very seedy portions; cut the eggplant flesh into ½-inch chunks. Place the eggplant in a bowl and set aside.

2. Preheat the broiler and place the bell peppers on a baking sheet. Broil the peppers 4 inches from the heat source, turning with tongs to char on all sides. Remove and cover with a dry kitchen towel. When cool enough to handle, remove the skin, stems, and seeds. Cut the flesh into ¼-inch dice and add to the bowl with the eggplant.

3. Heat 2 tablespoons olive oil in a 3-quart saucepan over medium heat. Add the onion and sauté until soft, about 7 minutes. Add the cumin and pepper flakes and sauté 1 minute. Gently stir in the eggplant and peppers and season with salt and black pepper. Add the stock and heat to simmering over medium heat. Simmer 10 minutes to blend the flavors.

4. To serve: Mix the yogurt, garlic, lemon juice, and minced mint in a bowl. Taste and season with salt and pepper and more lemon juice if needed. Ladle the soup into warmed shallow bowls and add a dollop of yogurt sauce to each. Garnish with mint leaves.

Each of 6 servings: About 176 calories, 9 g protein, 20 g carbohydrate, 8 g total fat (2 g saturated), 5 mg cholesterol, 218 mg sodium.

Portobello Mushroom Soup

PREP TIME: 5 minutes
COOK TIME: 25 minutes

Makes 4 servings

For mushroom aficionados, here's a splendid soup that's thick and dark, with loads of substantial portobello mushrooms.

2 teaspoons unsalted butter
6 ounces small portobello mushrooms, sliced, plus 4 attractive
    mushroom slices for a garnish
1 large onion, chopped
2 cups Chicken Stock (page 14)
1 large potato, peeled and shredded
2 bay leaves
¼ teaspoon white pepper
1 cup 2% milk
1 tablespoon dry sherry
salt and pepper to taste
¼ cup snipped fresh chives for garnish

1. Melt the butter in a 6-quart pot over medium-high heat. Add the mushrooms and onion and sauté until the onion is translucent. Stir in the stock, potato, and bay leaves. Cover and bring to a boil. Reduce the heat and simmer 15 minutes. Discard the bay leaves. Stir in the pepper.

2. Using a handheld immersion blender, puree the soup. Stir in the milk and sherry and heat through (do not boil), about 5 minutes. Taste and season with salt and pepper if needed. Top each serving with chives and a mushroom slice.

Each serving: About 164 calories, 9 g protein, 26 g carbohydrate, 3 g total fat (2 g saturated), 8 mg cholesterol, 143 mg sodium.

Belgian Endive Soup

PREP TIME: 10 minutes
COOK TIME: about 25 minutes

Makes 6 servings

The elongated heads (with slightly bitter leaves) of endive are white because they are grown without exposure to light.

4 tablespoons unsalted butter
4 large Belgian endives, cored and chopped
2 medium leeks, white and pale green part only, cut crosswise into thin rounds and rinsed well
1 medium baking potato, peeled and finely chopped
1 teaspoon salt
¼ teaspoon freshly ground white pepper
⅛ teaspoon freshly grated nutmeg
6 cups milk
1 cup Plain Croutons (page 22) for serving
1 cup shredded Gouda cheese for serving
2 ounces smoked ham, cut into slivers, for serving

1. Melt the butter in a 3-quart saucepan over medium heat. When the foam subsides, add the endives and leeks and stir until coated with butter. Cover and reduce the heat to low. Cook until the vegetables are soft but not browned, about 10 minutes. Stir in the potato, salt, pepper, and nutmeg and then add the milk. Heat to simmering over medium heat, stirring occasionally. Reduce the heat and cook, uncovered and without boiling, until the potato falls apart (it will thicken the soup slightly).

2. Taste the soup and adjust the seasonings if necessary. Ladle into bowls and add croutons, cheese, and ham.

Each serving: About 358 calories, 16 g protein, 24 g carbohydrate, 23 g total fat (14 g saturated), 82 mg cholesterol, 827 mg sodium.

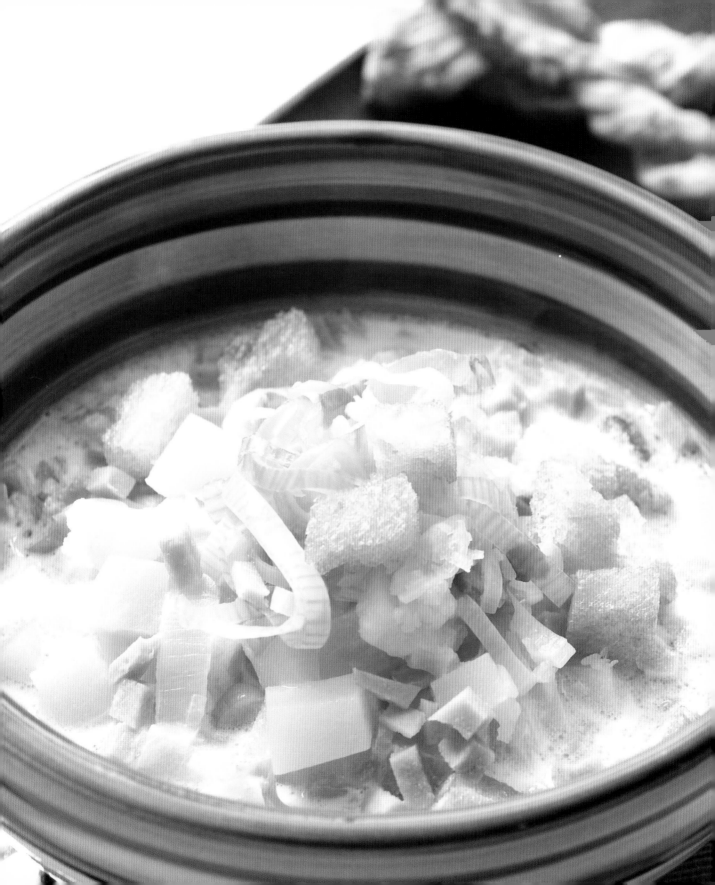

Four-Celery Soup

PREP TIME: 15 minutes
COOK TIME: 25 minutes

Makes 4 servings

For an interesting variation, omit the bacon (use butter to sauté the vegetables) and garnish the finished soup with crumbled blue cheese or shavings of Parmigiano-Reggiano cheese.

  4 slices bacon
  1 large celery root (about 1 pound)
  3 celery stalks, coarsely chopped
  1 small onion, chopped
  5 cups water or Chicken Stock (page 14)
  1 medium potato, peeled and diced
  1 teaspoon celery seeds
  1 bay leaf
  ½ teaspoon salt and more to taste
  ¾ cup cream
  freshly ground white pepper to taste
  finely chopped celery leaves for garnish
  finely chopped fresh parsley for garnish

1. Fry the bacon in a 2-quart saucepan until crisp; transfer to a paper towel–lined plate to drain. Crumble and set aside.

2. Discard all but 2 tablespoons of the bacon drippings from the pan. Heat the pan over medium-high heat. Add the celery root, celery, and onion and sauté until softened, about 10 minutes. Add the water, potato, celery seeds, bay leaf, and salt. Heat to boiling; reduce the heat to low, and simmer, partially covered, until the vegetables are very soft, about 45 minutes.

3. Pour the soup through a sieve placed over a large heat-safe glass measure; discard the bay leaf. Wash and dry the saucepan. Puree the solids through a food mill and return to the cleaned pan. (Or, puree the vegetables in a food processor and pass through a sieve.) Whisk in the cooking liquid and cream. Season to taste with salt and pepper. Heat until hot, but do not boil or the soup will curdle. Ladle into warmed bowls and sprinkle with the crumbled bacon, celery leaves, and parsley.

Each serving: About 178 calories, 5 g protein, 18 g carbohydrate, 10 g total fat (4 g saturated), 12 mg cholesterol, 532 mg sodium.

Cabbage and Beet Soup

PREP TIME: 5 minutes
COOK TIME: 30 minutes

Makes 8 servings

2 cans (16 ounces each) diced tomatoes
1 tablespoon instant vegetable bouillon granules
2½ cups fresh beets, sliced
3 medium carrots, peeled and diced
1 large yellow onion, sliced
2 celery stalks with tops, coarsely chopped
water
1 medium head cabbage, sliced or cut in wedges
3 medium garlic cloves, minced
granulated sugar to taste
salt and pepper to taste
2 tablespoons fresh lemon juice

1. In a 6-quart pot, combine the tomatoes, bouillon granules, beets, carrots, onion, celery, and enough water to cover them by at least 1 inch. Bring to a boil, then reduce to a simmer, cover lightly, and cook for about 20 minutes, or until the vegetables are tender. Add the cabbage, garlic, and sugar. Cook 10 minutes.

2. Turn off the heat, add salt and pepper to taste, and stir in the lemon juice. Serve immediately.

Each serving: About 100 calories, 4 g protein, 23 g carbohydrate, 1 g total fat (trace saturated), trace cholesterol, 594 mg sodium.

English Borscht

PREP TIME: 5 minutes
COOK TIME: 1 hour 20 minutes

Makes 4 servings

1½ cups fresh beets, peeled and grated
1½ cups red cabbage, finely shredded
3 tablespoons tomato paste
2 tablespoons red wine vinegar
3 tablespoons unsalted butter
4 cups Vegetable or Chicken Stock (Chapter 1)
1 large red onion, minced
1 large carrot, peeled and grated
salt and pepper to taste
1 tablespoon molasses
whipped sour cream or unflavored yogurt for serving

1. In a large saucepan or soup kettle, combine the beets, cabbage, tomato paste, vinegar, 1½ table-spoons butter, and the stock. Bring to a boil. Reduce to a simmer, cover, and cook, stirring occasionally, 55 to 60 minutes, or until the beets are very tender.

2. Melt the remaining 1½ tablespoons butter in a skillet and sauté the onion and carrot until the onion is browned. Transfer to the saucepan and continue to cook 10 to 12 minutes. Add salt and pepper to taste, stir in the molasses, and serve with a dollop of sour cream.

Each serving: About 201 calories, 5 g protein, 28 g carbohydrate, 9 g total fat (5 g saturated), 23 mg cholesterol, 753 mg sodium.

Spiced Chestnut Soup

PREP TIME: 15 minutes
COOK TIME: 40 minutes

Makes 4 servings

Serve this wintry soup with Herbed Garlic Bread Loaf
(page 26).

> 4 tablespoons unsalted butter
> 1 pound chestnuts, cooked and peeled
> 6 celery stalks, sliced into ¼-inch-thick pieces
> 1 medium onion, chopped
> 1 quart water or Chicken Stock (page 14)
> 1¼ teaspoons chopped fresh thyme leaves (no
>   stems) or ½ teaspoon dried thyme leaves
> ¼ teaspoon salt or more to taste
> ¼ teaspoon ground white pepper
> 1 cup loosely packed fresh parsley leaves
> 1 apple, unpeeled, cored, and diced
> ½ teaspoon curry powder
> 3 tablespoons fresh lemon juice
> ½ cup pomegranate juice for serving
> ½ cup pomegranate seeds for serving

1. Melt 3 tablespoons butter in a 2-quart saucepan over
   medium-high heat and add the chestnuts, celery, and
   onion. Cover and cook until the vegetables are softened and juicy, about 5 minutes. Add the water or
   stock, thyme, salt, and pepper; cover and heat to
   boiling. Reduce the heat to low and simmer 15 minutes. Add the parsley and cook until the chestnuts
   are soft and falling apart, about 10 minutes longer.

2. Pour the chestnut mixture through a sieve placed
   over a heat-safe glass measure. Wash and dry the
   saucepan. In batches, puree the solids in a food
   processor, adding enough cooking liquid to keep the
   mixture moving. Scrape each batch of puree into the
   saucepan. Whisk the remaining liquid into the puree
   in the pan and set aside.

3. Melt the remaining 1 tablespoon butter in a small
   skillet over medium heat. Add the apple and curry
   powder and sauté until the apple starts to soften,
   about 2 minutes. Add the lemon juice, cover, and
   simmer until apple is tender when pierced with the
   tip of a paring knife, about 3 minutes longer. Stir the
   apple mixture into the soup and heat to boiling. To
   serve: Ladle the soup into warmed bowls, drizzle
   with pomegranate juice and sprinkle with pomegranate seeds.

Each serving: About 322 calories, 4 g protein, 56 g carbohydrate, 14 g total fat (8 g saturated), 31 mg cholesterol,
359 mg sodium.

Thai Coconut Curry Soup

PREP TIME: 10 minutes
COOK TIME: 25 minutes

Makes 4 servings

Soba noodles and Chinese chili sauce can be found in Asian food stores or large supermarkets.

2 teaspoons coconut milk
2 cups unsweetened apple juice or Vegetable Stock (page 15)
1 stalk lemongrass, cut into 1-inch lengths
4-inch piece fresh gingerroot, peeled and thinly sliced
1 tablespoon curry powder
½ teaspoon turmeric
2 teaspoons grated lime zest
2 tablespoons fresh lime juice
2 teaspoons Chinese-style chili sauce
1 tablespoon sesame oil
8 white button mushrooms, trimmed
¼ pound soba noodles or thin spaghetti, cooked al dente
salt and pepper to taste
cilantro sprigs for garnish

1. In a 6-quart pot, combine the coconut milk, apple juice, lemongrass, ginger, curry powder, turmeric, lime zest and juice, and chili sauce. Bring to a boil. Reduce to a simmer, cover lightly, and cook, stirring occasionally, about 20 minutes.

2. Add the oil, mushrooms, and noodles to the hot soup.

3. Turn off the heat, and add salt and pepper to taste. Serve, garnished with cilantro sprigs.

Each serving: About 199 calories, 7 g protein, 35 g carbohydrate, 5 g total fat (trace saturated), 0 mg cholesterol, 399 mg sodium.

Sorrel Soup

PREP TIME: 5 minutes
COOK TIME: 15 minutes

Makes 4 servings

This pretty, delicate recipe calls for French sorrel, which has less acid content than wild sorrel.

3½ tablespoons unsalted butter
3 tablespoons all-purpose flour
1½ quarts Vegetable Stock (page 15)
1 bunch fresh French sorrel, tough stems removed, coarsely chopped
1 bunch fresh chervil, tough stems removed, coarsely chopped
1 egg yolk
½ teaspoon granulated sugar
salt and pepper to taste
4 to 5 tablespoons sour cream or unflavored yogurt
finely minced garlic for garnish

1. Melt the butter in a 6-quart pot over medium-high heat. Sprinkle in the flour and cook, stirring, to make a roux. Gradually stir in the stock, then add the sorrel and chervil and bring to a boil.

2. In a bowl, whisk the egg yolk until foamy. Beat in ¼ cup of hot soup, and then stir it back into the soup. Cook, stirring constantly, until thickened. Do not boil or the egg will curdle.

3. Turn off the heat, stir in the sugar, add the salt and pepper to taste, and stir in the sour cream. Serve immediately, with a sprinkling of minced garlic on top.

Each serving: About 185 calories, 5 g protein, 11 g carbohydrate, 16 g total fat (2 g saturated), 84 mg cholesterol, 1,507 mg sodium.

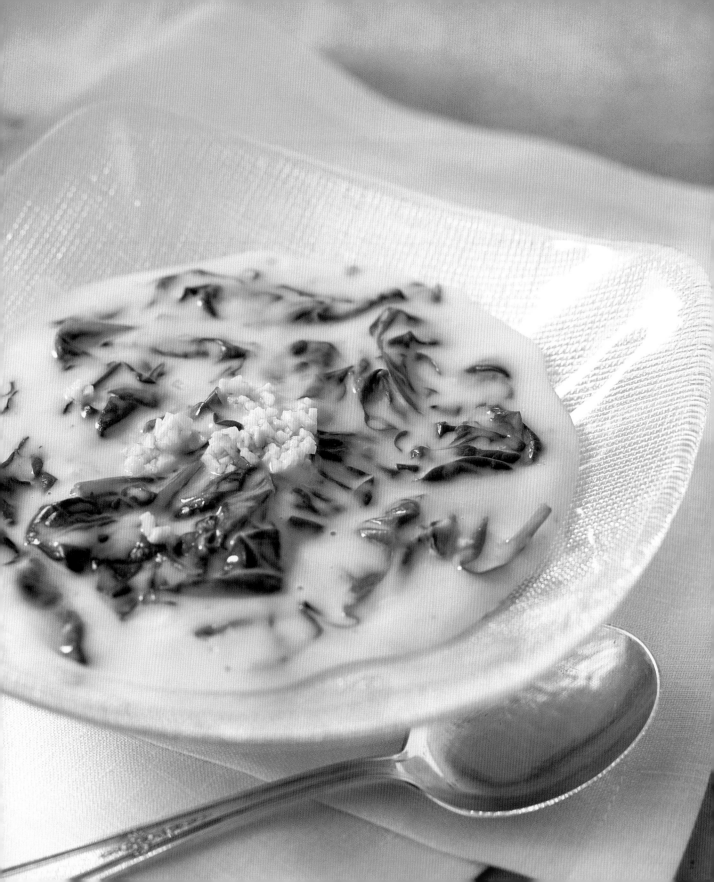

Spinach-Barley Soup

PREP TIME: 5 minutes
COOK TIME: 15 minutes

Makes 2 to 3 servings

2½ cups Vegetable Stock (page 15) or water
1 package (10 ounces) creamed spinach, drained
¼ cup quick-cooking barley
⅛ teaspoon ground nutmeg
salt and pepper to taste

1. In a 6-quart pot combine the stock and spinach. Bring to a boil, stir in the barley and nutmeg, and reduce to a simmer. Cover lightly and cook, stirring frequently, until the barley is tender.

2. Turn off the heat, add the salt and pepper to taste, and set aside for about 5 minutes. Serve immediately.

Each serving: About 185 calories, 8 g protein, 30 g carbohydrate, 4 g total fat (2 g saturated), 0 mg cholesterol, 679 mg sodium.

Green Pea Soup with Brown Rice

PREP TIME: 10 minutes
COOK TIME: 15 minutes

Makes 6 servings

You can use cut green beans instead of the peas and just about any grating
cheese for endless variety.

> 2 tablespoons unsalted butter
> 2 large shallots, minced
> 2 large garlic cloves, minced
> 5 cups Vegetable or Chicken Stock (Chapter 1)
> 2 cups fresh peas or 2 (10-ounce) packages frozen baby peas
> 1 cup cooked long-grain brown rice
> salt and freshly ground pepper to taste
> 2 tablespoons finely chopped fresh Italian parsley leaves
> 2 tablespoons toasted sesame seeds for serving
> 1 cup freshly grated Parmigiano-Reggiano cheese for serving

Melt the butter in a 3-quart saucepan over medium heat. Add the
shallots and garlic and sauté until softened, about 5 minutes. Add the
stock and heat to boiling over medium-high heat. Add the peas and rice
and simmer just until the peas are cooked through but still pop in your
mouth, about 3 minutes. Taste and season with salt and pepper. Stir in
the parsley. Ladle into warmed soup bowls and sprinkle with sesame
seeds. Pass the cheese at the table.

Each serving: About 218 calories, 12 g protein, 19 g carbohydrate, 11 g total fat
(6 g saturated), 24 mg cholesterol, 549 mg sodium.

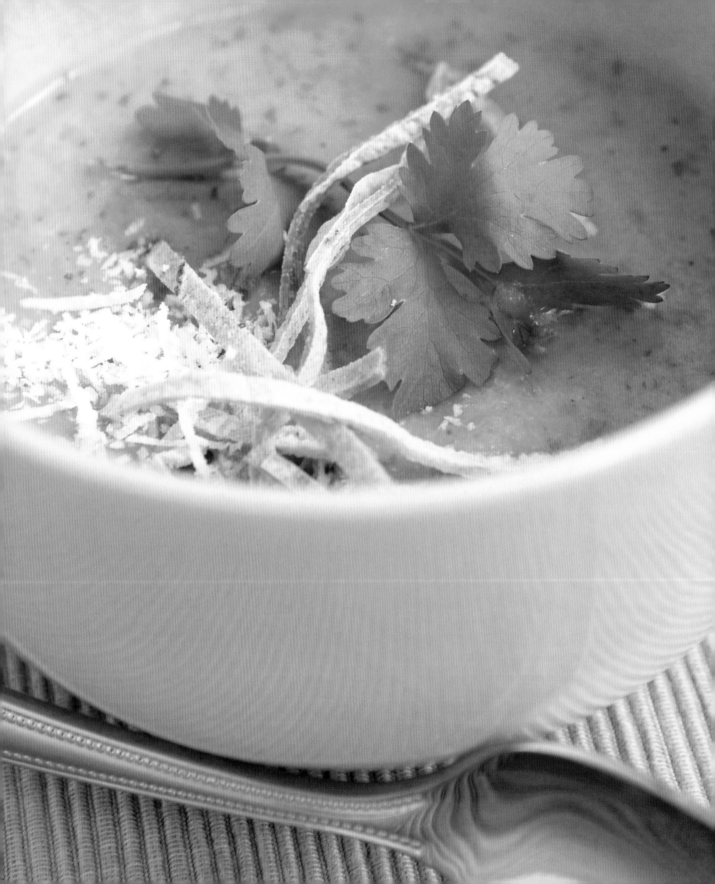

Creamy Cilantro-Chile Soup

PREP TIME: 20 minutes
COOK TIME: 35 minutes

Makes 6 servings

6 poblano chile peppers
2 bunches cilantro, rinsed well and stemmed
1 tablespoon vegetable oil
1 large onion, chopped
2 garlic cloves, minced
4½ cups Chicken or Vegetable Stock (Chapter 1)
½ cup heavy cream
½ teaspoon dried Mexican oregano
¼ teaspoon dried thyme leaves
½ cup masa harina
4 to 6 fresh corn tortillas, slivered, for serving
salt and freshly ground black pepper to taste
4 ounces coarsely grated queso fresco or
   Pecorino-Romano cheese for serving

1. Preheat the broiler or grill. Place the poblanos on a baking sheet or grill rack and broil or grill 4 inches from heat source until charred on all sides. Remove from the heat and cover loosely with a kitchen towel. Let stand 5 minutes. Wearing rubber gloves, scrape off most of the charred skin and pull out the stems and seed pods. You can rinse the poblanos to make the job easier but do it quickly or the flavorful juices will be lost. Cut into ½-inch strips.

2. Reserve a few cilantro leaves for garnish. Heat the oil in a 2-quart saucepan over medium-high heat. Add the onion and sauté until softened, about 5 minutes. Add the garlic and sauté 1 minute. Add the cilantro and poblanos and sauté until cilantro is wilted, about

1 minute. Scrape the mixture into a food processor and puree, adding 1 cup stock to get the puree moving easily; return to the saucepan. (Or pass the mixture through a food mill back into the saucepan.) Add 3 cups of the remaining stock, the cream, oregano, and thyme. Heat to simmering over medium heat.

3. Preheat the oven to 400 degrees. Mix the remaining ½ cup stock with the masa harina in a small bowl, then strain the mixture into the simmering soup, whisking constantly as it thickens. Simmer, partially covered, 10 minutes.

4. Spread the slivered tortillas on a nonstick baking sheet. Bake until lightly toasted, about 3 minutes. Transfer to a plate to cool.

5. Taste the soup and season with salt and pepper. Ladle the soup into bowls and sprinkle with the tortillas, cheese, and reserved cilantro leaves.

Each serving: About 252 calories, 10 g protein, 29 g carbohydrate, 11 g total fat (5 g saturated), 31 mg cholesterol, 275 mg sodium.

MASA HARINA
• Masa harina is a flour made from hominy that is used to make tortillas. You can find it in larger Hispanic markets and larger supermarkets.

Soup of Spring Greens

PREP TIME: 10 minutes
COOK TIME: 15 minutes

Makes 4 servings

The seasonal combination of fresh spinach and sorrel was considered to be an Old World tonic, enjoyed after a winter of root-cellar vegetables.

1 quart Vegetable Stock (page 15) or water
1 bunch fresh spinach, rinsed well, drained, and stemmed
2 bunches fresh sorrel, rinsed well, drained, and stemmed
1 small bunch watercress, rinsed well, drained, and stemmed
1 cup chopped fresh Italian parsley leaves
3 tablespoons unsalted butter
3 tablespoons all-purpose flour
salt and freshly ground pepper to taste
½ cup heavy cream, softly whipped until thick but not stiff, for serving
2 hard-cooked eggs, shelled and pressed through a fine wire sieve, for serving

1. Heat the stock to boiling in a 2-quart saucepan over medium-high heat. Add the spinach, sorrel, watercress, and parsley and simmer over medium heat until tender, about 5 minutes. Pour through a sieve placed over a heat-safe glass measure or bowl. Puree the solids in a food processor or blender, adding enough of the cooking liquid to make it easy to puree. Reserve the cooking liquid and the puree.

2. Clean the pan, add the butter, and melt it over medium heat. Remove the pan from the heat and stir in the flour until blended. Gradually whisk in 2 cups hot cooking liquid until blended. Heat to boiling, whisking constantly, over medium-high heat. Whisk until thickened, about 1 minute. Stir in the puree until smooth. Stir in the remaining cooking liquid, season with salt and pepper, and heat through.

3. To serve: Ladle the soup into warmed shallow soup bowls, dollop with the whipped cream, and sprinkle with the egg.

Each serving: About 236 calories, 13 g protein, 16 g carbohydrate, 16 g total fat (9 g saturated), 141 mg cholesterol, 545 mg sodium.

Chinese Mushroom and Wheat Berry Soup

PREP TIME: 30 minutes
COOK TIME: 1 hour

Makes 6 servings

Delightfully chewy wheat berries are whole, unprocessed kernels of wheat. You can find them in health food stores.

12 Chinese black mushrooms
1 quart hot water
1 tablespoon canola or corn oil
2 large leeks, split, rinsed well, tender green and white portions julienned
2 medium carrots, peeled and julienned
2 garlic cloves, minced
½ cup rice wine or sake
2 cups Gingered Chicken Stock (page 14) or water
2 tablespoons soy sauce
⅔ cup wheat berries

1. Place the mushrooms in a medium bowl and add the hot water. Let soak until soft, about 20 minutes. Pour the mushroom soaking water through a sieve lined with a double thickness of cheesecloth placed over a bowl. Squeeze the mushrooms into the sieve to extract the liquid. Tear or cut the stems off the mushrooms and discard. Julienne the mushroom caps. Reserve the mushrooms and the soaking liquid.

2. Heat the oil in a 3-quart saucepan over medium-high heat. Add the leeks, carrots, and garlic and sauté until fragrant, about 3 minutes. Add the rice wine and heat to boiling; boil 2 minutes. Add the mushrooms, the mushroom soaking liquid, stock, and soy sauce and heat to boiling. Reduce the heat, add the wheat berries and cook, covered, until the wheat berries are tender, about 45 minutes.

Each serving: About 146 calories, 4 g protein, 25 g carbohydrate, 3 g total fat (trace saturated), 0 mg cholesterol, 368 mg sodium.

Squash Blossom Soup

PREP TIME: 10 minutes
COOK TIME: 25 minutes

Makes 4 to 6 servings

The sunrise-colored flowers from either summer or winter squash are extremely perishable, but you can prolong their freshness for a day by layering them between paper towels to keep them dry. Store them in a plastic container in the refrigerator.

16 squash blossoms
2 tablespoons unsalted butter
1 medium red onion, finely chopped
2 jalapeño peppers, seeded and finely chopped (use rubber gloves when handling hot peppers)
1 small red bell pepper, seeded and chopped
1 medium zucchini, cut into ¼-inch cubes
2 garlic cloves, minced
½ pound mushrooms, thinly sliced
3 cups Chicken or Vegetable Stock (Chapter 1)
1 cup milk
½ cup heavy cream
salt and freshly ground black pepper to taste

1. Clean the squash blossoms: Using your fingers, break off the stems and then the little green sepals that extend from the base. Break off the long pistils in the center of each blossom and discard. Slice blossoms crosswise into ¼-inch-wide pieces with a very sharp, thin-bladed knife and set aside.

2. Melt the butter in a 2-quart saucepan over medium heat. Add the onion and sauté until softened, about 5 minutes. Add the jalapeños, bell pepper, zucchini, and garlic and sauté until softened, about 3 minutes. Add the mushrooms, increase heat to medium-high, and sauté until sizzling, about 3 minutes. Reduce the heat to medium and add the squash blossoms. Sauté until wilted, about 3 minutes. Add the stock and milk and heat to boiling over medium-high heat. Reduce the heat and simmer 10 minutes.

3. Stir the cream into the soup and taste. Season with salt and pepper. Ladle soup into bowls and serve.

Each of 4 servings: About 266 calories, 9 g protein, 14 g carbohydrate, 20 g total fat (12 g saturated), 65 mg cholesterol, 337 mg sodium.

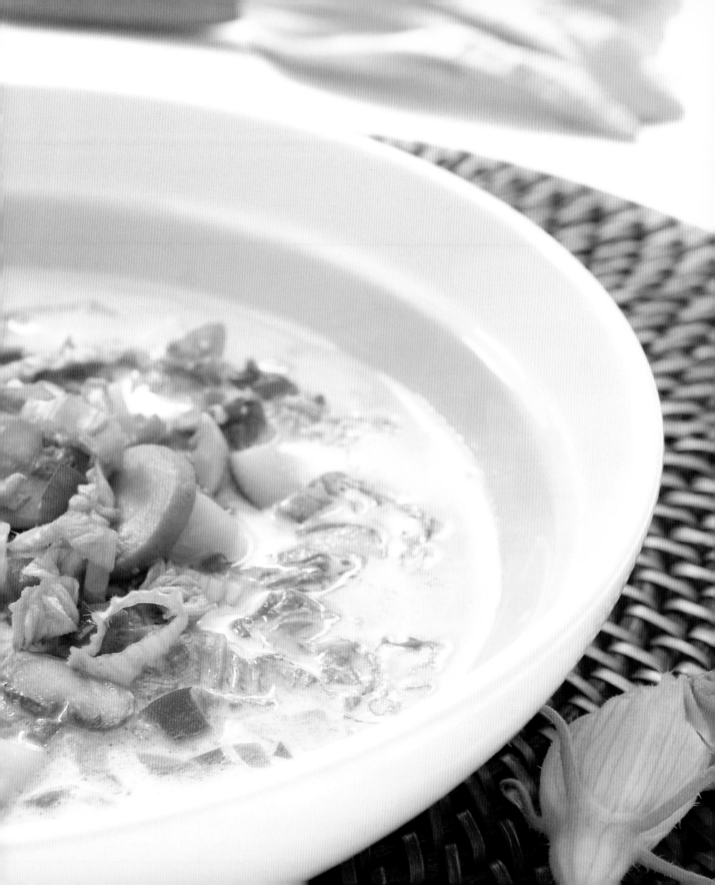

Wild Rice and Three-Mushroom Soup

PREP TIME: 30 minutes
COOK TIME: 50 minutes

Makes 6 servings

Its rice-like appearance gave wild rice its name—but it is not rice at all! The cereal grain comes from a marsh grass native to the northern Great Lakes. Wild rice should be rinsed well in a sieve before using to remove any husks or other natural debris.

1 ounce dried porcini mushrooms
1 ounce dried shiitake mushrooms
2 cups hot water
3 tablespoons unsalted butter
8 ounces fresh mushrooms, sliced
4 large shallots, chopped
2 large carrots, peeled and chopped
1 celery stalk, with some green, chopped
½ cup raw wild rice
4 cups Vegetable Stock (page 15)
¼ cup chopped fresh Italian parsley leaves
¼ cup dry sherry
salt and freshly ground pepper to taste

1. Place the dried mushrooms in a heat-safe glass measure and add the hot water. Let soak at least 20 minutes. Meanwhile, melt 1 tablespoon butter in a 3-quart saucepan over medium-high heat. Add the fresh mushrooms and sauté until golden. Transfer to a plate and set aside.

2. Melt the remaining 2 tablespoons butter in the saucepan. Add the shallots and sauté until softened but not browned, about 3 minutes. Add the carrots and celery and sauté until softened, about 4 minutes. Add the wild rice and stock and heat to boiling over medium-high heat.

3. While the soup heats, strain the mushroom soaking liquid into the soup through a sieve lined with a double thickness of cheesecloth. Place the mushrooms on a cutting board and cut off and discard any tough stems. Slice the caps into ¼-inch-wide strips and add to the soup.

4. Simmer the soup, partially covered, over medium-low heat until the rice is tender, about 30 minutes. Add the sautéed fresh mushrooms and any liquid on the plate. Stir in the parsley and sherry. Taste and season with salt and pepper.

Each serving: About 188 calories, 5 g protein, 28 g carbohydrate, 6 g total fat (4 g saturated), 16 mg cholesterol, 281 mg sodium.

Brie, Carrot, and Mushroom Bisque

PREP TIME: 10 minutes
COOK TIME: 25 minutes

Makes 8 servings

This somewhat-decadent soup gets its richness from an ample amount of Brie.

1½ pounds Brie cheese
4 tablespoons unsalted butter
8 ounces cremini or shiitake mushrooms, sliced
1 large leek, tender green and white portions only,
   cut into ¼-inch-thick rounds and rinsed well
1 package (8 ounces) peeled baby carrots, cut into
   ¼-inch thick rounds
3 tablespoons all-purpose flour
2 cups hot half-and-half
1 quart Chicken Stock (page 14)
2 tablespoons dry sherry
½ teaspoon freshly ground pepper
Garlic Croutons (page 22) for serving

1. Trim off and discard the rind from the Brie and cut into 1-inch chunks; set aside. Melt 1 tablespoon butter in a 3-quart saucepan over medium-high heat. Add the mushrooms and sauté until tender, about 5 minutes. Transfer to a bowl.

2. Wipe out the pan with a paper towel and melt the remaining 3 tablespoons butter over medium-high heat. Add the leeks and carrots and sauté until tender, about 5 minutes. Stir in the flour until blended and bubbly, then gradually whisk in the hot half-and-half until smooth. Heat to boiling, whisking; boil 1 minute.

3. Whisk in the stock, heat almost to boiling, and add the Brie. Reduce the heat to medium and stir with a wooden spoon until the cheese is melted, increasing the heat as necessary to melt the cheese. Stir in the sherry and pepper. Add the mushrooms and any liquid in the bowl; simmer over medium heat for 10 minutes. Ladle into warmed soup bowls and sprinkle with croutons.

Each serving without croutons: About 455 calories, 21 g protein, 11 g carbohydrate, 36 g total fat (23 g saturated), 123 mg cholesterol, 574 mg sodium.

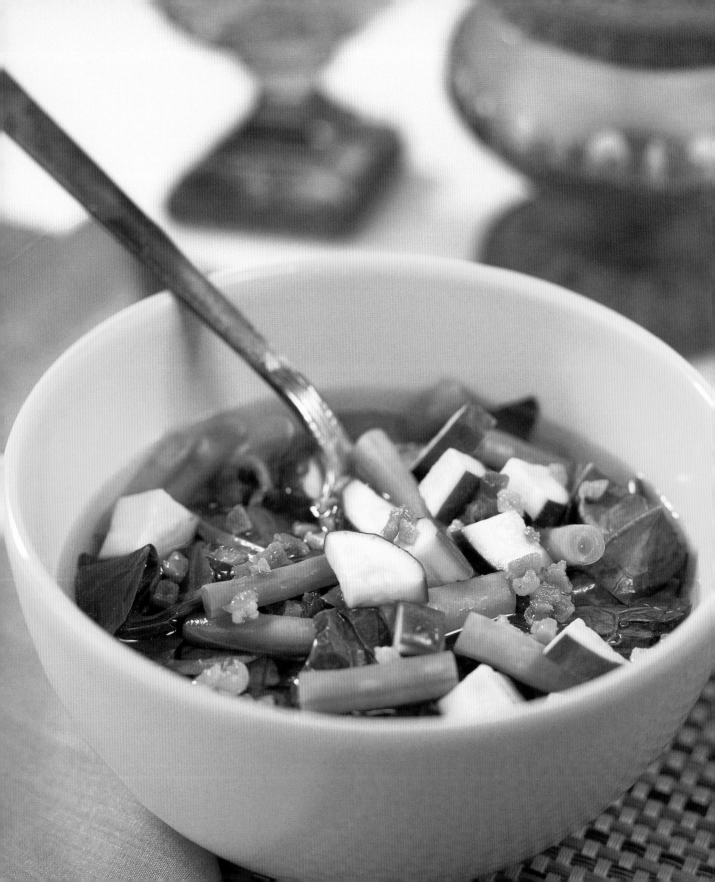

Fresh Swiss Chard and Snap Bean Soup

PREP TIME: 5 minutes
COOK TIME: 30 minutes

Makes 4 servings

Heads up, garlic lovers: This soup is brazen, bold, and assertive with the wonderful flavors of garlic and Swiss chard.

4 slices bacon
3½ cups Beef Stock (page 15)
4 large or 8 medium garlic cloves, thinly sliced
½ pound fresh green beans, cut into 1-inch lengths
1 small zucchini, quartered and sliced
4 ounces Swiss chard leaves, stems removed, torn
¼ teaspoon white pepper
1 sprig thyme
salt to taste

1. Cook the bacon in a nonstick skillet over medium-high heat until crisp. Transfer the bacon to a paper towel–lined plate to drain. Let the bacon cool; crumble it.

2. Pour the stock into a 6-quart pot. Stir in the garlic, beans, zucchini, chard, pepper, and thyme. Cover and bring to a boil. Reduce the heat and simmer until the vegetables are tender, about 20 minutes. Discard the thyme. Taste and season with salt if needed. Serve garnished with the bacon.

Each serving: About 260 calories, 10 g protein, 7 g carbohydrate, 22 g total fat (8 g saturated), 25 mg cholesterol, 475 mg sodium.

Pea, Radicchio, and Fennel Soup

PREP TIME: 10 minutes
COOK TIME: 25 minutes

Makes 4 servings

If you like, add plain toasted breadcrumbs, a favorite grated cheese,
seasoned croutons, and/or meatballs to this soup for some extra substance.

  2 tablespoons olive oil
  1 small red onion, chopped
  1 head radicchio, finely shredded
  1 small bulb fennel, bulb cored and coarsely chopped, plus the fresh
    fronds, coarsely chopped, for garnish
  1 small carrot, peeled and shredded
  1 quart Vegetable or Chicken Stock (Chapter 1)
  1 cup fresh shelled peas
  1 cup diced smoked ham (optional)
  salt and freshly ground pepper to taste

1. Heat the oil in a 2-quart saucepan over medium-high heat. Add the onion
   and sauté until softened, about 7 minutes. Add the radicchio, chopped
   fennel bulb, and carrot and sauté until wilted, about 4 minutes. Add the
   stock and heat to boiling over medium heat.

2. Add the peas and ham (if using) and cook 10 minutes or until the peas
   are tender but not mushy. Taste and season with salt and pepper. Ladle
   into warmed soup bowls and garnish with the chopped fennel fronds.

Each serving without ham: About 137 calories, 4 g protein, 16 g carbohydrate,
7 g total fat (1 g saturated), 0 mg cholesterol, 194 mg sodium.

Zucchini Soup Margherita

PREP TIME: 5 minutes
COOK TIME: 20 minutes

Makes 4 servings

Refreshing and light, this soup, which is brimming with mozzarella and basil, takes its name from Pizza Margherita. The classic Neapolitan pie was created with the colors of the Italian flag to honor Queen Margherita.

  2 teaspoons olive oil
  8 ounces small zucchini, halved lengthwise and sliced
  1 medium onion, chopped
  4 garlic cloves, chopped
  3½ cups Chicken Stock (page 14)
  8 ounces plum tomatoes, sliced
  1 teaspoon balsamic vinegar
  ¼ teaspoon freshly ground black pepper
  ½ cup shredded part-skim mozzarella cheese for serving
  salt to taste
  ½ cup chopped fresh basil for serving

1. Heat the oil in a 6-quart pot over medium-high heat for 1 minute. Add the zucchini, onion, and garlic and sauté until the vegetables start to brown, 3 to 5 minutes. Stir in the stock, tomatoes, vinegar, and pepper.

2. Cover and bring to a boil. Reduce the heat and simmer 10 minutes. Taste and season with salt if needed. Serve with the mozzarella and basil.

Each serving: About 105 calories, 7 g protein, 10 g carbohydrate, 4 g total fat (1 g saturated), 0 mg cholesterol, 373 mg sodium.

Speedy Cheese Tortellini Soup

PREP TIME: 5 minutes
COOK TIME: 10 minutes

Makes 6 servings

This easy soup takes just 10 minutes to cook and is packed with tomatoes, cheese tortellini, bell peppers, and scallions.

    2 cups coarsely chopped tomatoes
    3½ cups Chicken Stock (page 14)
    ½ cup sliced scallions
    ½ cup chopped red or green bell pepper
    1 teaspoon Italian herb seasoning
    ¼ teaspoon crushed red pepper flakes
    ⅛ teaspoon celery seeds
    1 package (about 16 ounces) frozen tricolor cheese
       tortellini
    salt and freshly ground black pepper to taste
    1 tablespoon chopped fresh basil

Combine the tomatoes, stock, scallions, bell pepper, herb seasoning, pepper flakes, and celery seeds in a 6-quart pot. Cover and bring to a boil. Stir in the tortellini and simmer the soup until the tortellini are al dente, about 10 minutes. Taste and season with salt and black pepper if needed. Stir in the basil and serve immediately.

Each serving: About 132 calories, 9 g protein, 20 g carbohydrate, 2 g total fat (1 g saturated), 7 mg cholesterol, 417 mg sodium.

VARIATIONS

• You could substitute beef stock for the chicken stock and sausage tortellini for the cheese variety. Small ravioli may be used instead of the tortellini.

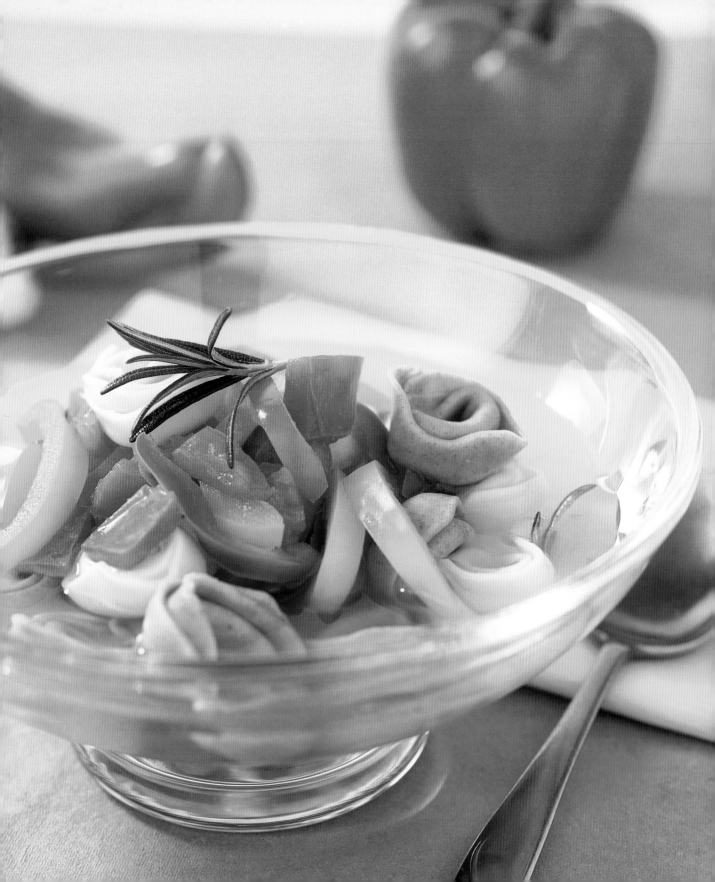

Roasted Butternut Squash and Apple Bisque

PREP TIME: 30 minutes
COOK TIME: 1 hour 40 minutes

Makes 6 servings

1 tablespoon olive oil
1½-pound butternut squash
4 tablespoons unsalted butter
3 leeks, white and tender green portions, sliced
    into thin rings and rinsed well
2 large Granny Smith apples, peeled,
    cored, and diced
3 cups Chicken Stock (page 14)
3 sprigs fresh thyme
½ teaspoon salt or more to taste
¼ teaspoon freshly ground white pepper or more
    to taste
1 cup heavy cream
2 tablespoons Calvados or other apple brandy or
    more to taste
snipped fresh chives for garnish
Plain Croutons (page 22) for serving

1. Preheat the oven to 350 degrees. Line a small baking sheet with foil and drizzle with the oil. On a cutting board, carefully cut the squash in half lengthwise; scoop out and discard the seeds. Place the halves cut side down on the foil and bake until tender, about 1 hour. When cool enough to handle, scoop out the flesh from the skins and place in a bowl.

2. Melt the butter in a 3-quart saucepan over medium-high heat. Add the leeks and apples and sauté until tender, about 7 minutes. Add the squash, stock, thyme, salt, and pepper and heat to boiling over medium-high heat. Reduce the heat to medium and simmer, partially covered, 30 minutes.

3. Pour the soup through a colander placed over a 2-quart glass measure. Wash the saucepan. Fish out the thyme stems from the solids and discard. In batches, puree the solids in a food processor until smooth, adding enough cooking liquid to each batch to move the ingredients around easily. Pour each pureed batch into the cleaned saucepan. When you have finished, add a little cooking liquid to the processor, pulse it once or twice to clean the bowl and blade, and pour the mixture into the saucepan. Whisk in the remaining cooking liquid and the cream. Taste the soup and adjust the seasoning if needed. Heat the soup to simmering. To serve: Whisk the Calvados into the soup and ladle the soup into warmed bowls. Sprinkle with chives and then croutons (if using).

Each serving without croutons: About 275 calories, 6 g protein, 29 g carbohydrate, 16 g total fat (8 g saturated), 36 mg cholesterol, 223 mg sodium.

Winter Root Vegetable Soup with Gruyère Toasts

PREP TIME: 15 minutes
COOK TIME: 40 minutes

Makes 4 servings

The earthy flavors of a mixed bag of vegetables grown underground are well matched to the toast rafts of nutty Gruyère cheese.

1 small bulb celeriac, peeled and sliced
1 small Yukon gold potato, peeled and sliced
1 small onion, sliced
1 small leek, white portion only, split, very thinly sliced, and rinsed well
6 tablespoons unsalted butter, softened
1 teaspoon salt
¼ teaspoon sugar
1 quart warm water
1¼ cups hot milk
3 slices whole-wheat bread, crusts trimmed away and toasted
½ cup grated Gruyère cheese

1. Place the celeriac, potato, onion, and leek in a 2-quart saucepan and add 4 tablespoons butter, salt, and sugar. Place a round of waxed paper that is the diameter of the saucepan over the vegetable mixture and cover. Simmer over medium-low heat until the vegetables are meltingly tender but not browned, about 20 minutes, occasionally shaking the pan gently or stirring to mix the melted butter and vegetables.

2. Add the warm water, cover, and simmer gently over medium heat for 10 minutes. Add the hot milk and simmer 5 minutes longer.

3. To serve: Spread the remaining 2 tablespoons butter over one side of the toast slices and sprinkle with the cheese. Brown in a toaster-oven or under a broiler until the cheese melts. Cut each toast into 4 thin rectangles. Ladle the soup into warmed shallow soup bowls and top each with 3 cheese toasts.

Each serving: About 347 calories, 12 g protein, 34 g carbohydrate, 20 g total fat (12 g saturated), 57 mg cholesterol, 893 mg sodium.

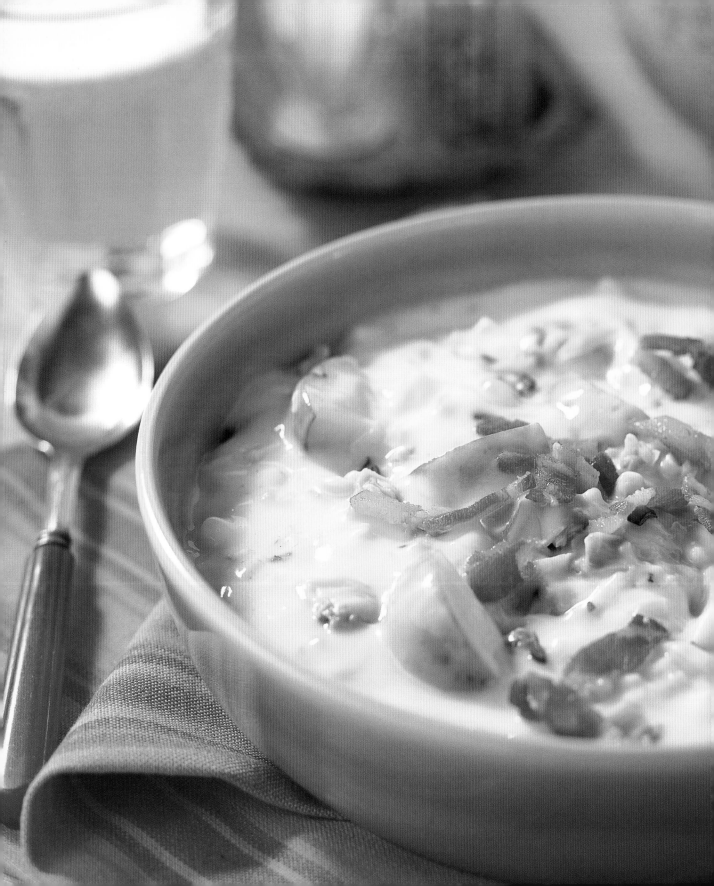

5

CHOWDERS

Cauliflower and Five-Cheese Chowder

PREP TIME: 15 minutes
COOK TIME: about 30 minutes

Makes 6 servings

Inspired by the popular side dish of cauliflower with cheese sauce, this soup takes the vegetable to new heights. A creamy fondue is lightened by stock and refreshed by juicy pear tomatoes and chives.

3 tablespoons unsalted butter
1 medium red onion, chopped
1 quart Chicken Stock (page 14)
1 cup dry white wine
2 tablespoons chopped fresh Italian parsley
3 cups bite-size cauliflower florets
1 cup heavy cream
¾ cup milk
½ cup grated Parmigiano-Reggiano cheese
½ cup grated Pecorino-Romano or other sheep's milk cheese
½ cup shredded Dutch Gouda cheese
½ cup shredded Italian Fontina cheese
¼ cup crumbled Gorgonzola or other blue cheese
1 egg yolk
¼ teaspoon freshly grated nutmeg
salt and freshly ground white pepper to taste
1 cup mixed red and yellow pear or grape tomatoes
2 tablespoons snipped fresh chives for garnish

1. Melt the butter in a 3-quart saucepan over medium-high heat. Add the onion and sauté until softened, about 7 minutes. Add the stock, wine, and parsley and heat to boiling. Add the cauliflower, reduce the heat to medium, and simmer until tender, 5 to 7 minutes.

2. Ladle about 1 cup of the cauliflower and some of the liquid into a blender and puree. Pour the puree back into the soup; add ¾ cup cream and the milk. Stir in the cheeses. Heat the soup, stirring, until the cheeses are completely melted, raising the heat a little if necessary.

3. Beat together the remaining ¼ cup cream, the egg yolk, and nutmeg in a shallow bowl; whisk in a ladleful of hot soup until blended. Whisk the mixture back into the soup, making sure the soup doesn't simmer or boil (or the egg will curdle). Taste the soup and season with salt and pepper. Stir in the tomatoes and heat through. Ladle the soup into soup bowls and sprinkle with the chives.

Each serving: About 373 calories, 21 g protein, 11 g carbohydrate, 25 g total fat (15 g saturated), 12 mg cholesterol, 646 mg sodium.

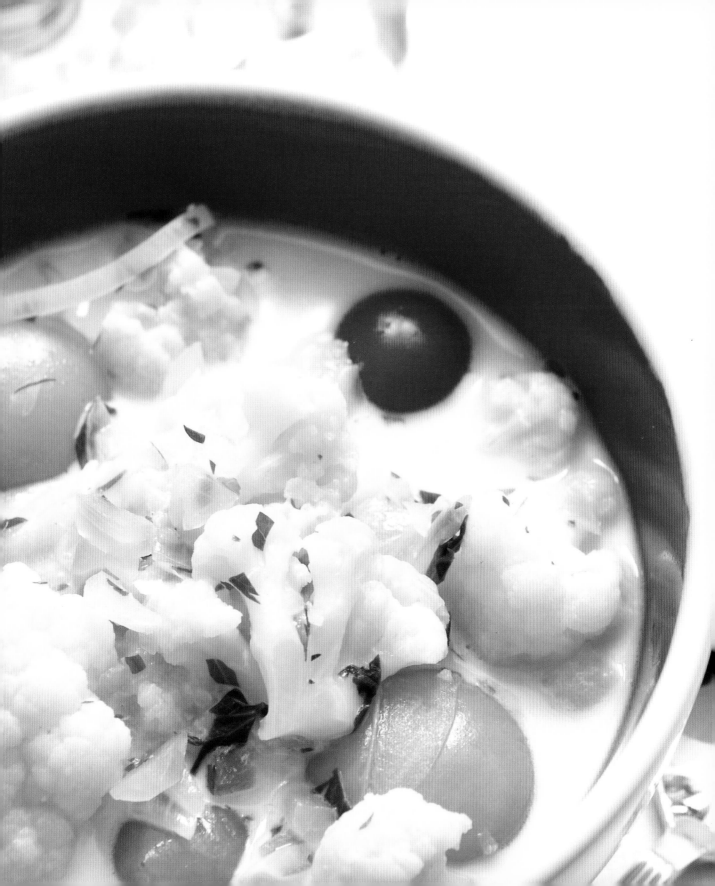

Sweet Potato Chowder

PREP TIME: 10 minutes
COOK TIME: 45 minutes

Makes 6 to 8 servings

For a vegetarian soup, substitute 2 tablespoons butter or olive oil for the pancetta.

4 ounces pancetta or bacon, cut into ¼-inch slivers
2 celery stalks, cut crosswise into ¼-inch slices
2 red onions, diced
1 Golden Delicious apple, peeled, cored, and cut into ½-inch chunks
2 tablespoons all-purpose flour
4 cups Beef, Chicken, or Vegetable Stock (Chapter 1)
3 medium sweet potatoes, peeled and cut into ½-inch chunks
2 cups half-and-half
salt and freshly ground pepper to taste
½ to 1 cup sour cream or plain yogurt
snipped fresh chives for garnish

1. Sauté the pancetta in a 3-quart saucepan over medium-high heat until crispy but not hard. Transfer to a plate with a slotted spoon. Discard all but 2 tablespoons drippings from the saucepan. Add the celery, onions, and apple to the drippings and sauté until softened, about 5 minutes. Add the flour and cook, stirring, until blended. Gradually add 2 cups stock and heat to boiling. Cook, stirring, 1 minute. Add the remaining 2 cups stock and the sweet potatoes and heat to boiling. Cover and simmer over medium-low heat until the sweet potatoes are tender but not falling apart, about 25 minutes.

2. Stir in the half-and-half and heat through. Season with salt and pepper. Ladle into warmed soup bowls and garnish each with a dollop of sour cream and a sprinkle of chives and pancetta.

Each of 6 servings: About 319 calories, 8 g protein, 29 g carbohydrate, 20 g total fat (11 g saturated), 44 mg cholesterol, 318 mg sodium.

Beautiful Bean and Vegetable Chowder for a Crowd

PREP TIME: 15 minutes plus standing
COOK TIME: 60 minutes

Makes 10 to 12 servings

You can use any type of dried beans in this soup but Great Northerns are a generous size and have a hearty texture that sops up and holds flavorful juices—just as much of a plus for baked beans as it is for soup. They also have a simply delicious "no frills" flavor that needs no other seasonings but willingly takes them if they're there.

1 pound Great Northern beans, rinsed and picked through
2 quarts water plus more for soaking the beans
2 tablespoons olive oil
8 ounces chorizo, pepperoni, or kielbasa, skinned if desired, diced
3 celery stalks, with some leaves, chopped
3 medium leeks, white and tender green portions thinly sliced crosswise and rinsed well
3 thin carrots, peeled and sliced crosswise into ½-inch-thick rounds
1 large red onion, chopped
1 large garlic clove, crushed through a press
1 can (28 ounces) crushed tomatoes in puree
1 cup diced ham (about 6 ounces)
¼ cup firmly packed brown sugar
1 teaspoon dried oregano leaves, crumbled
1 teaspoon salt
¼ teaspoon freshly ground pepper
4 ounces fresh spinach, trimmed, leaves coarsely chopped

1. Place the beans in a 3-quart saucepan and add enough cold water to cover. Heat to boiling over medium-high heat; reduce the heat, cover, and simmer 2 minutes. Remove the pan from the heat and let the beans stand, covered, 1 hour. Drain.

2. Heat the oil in a 5-quart soup pot or Dutch oven over medium heat. Add the chorizo and cook until the fat has rendered, about 4 minutes. Add the celery, leeks, carrots, onion, and garlic and sauté until tender, about 10 minutes. Add the beans and 2 quarts water. Heat the soup to boiling over medium-high heat. Reduce the heat and simmer, partially covered, until the beans are barely tender, about 30 minutes. Add the tomatoes and their liquid, the ham, brown sugar, oregano, salt, and pepper and mix well. Increase the heat to medium-high and bring to a boil. Adjust the heat and gently simmer, partially covered, until the beans are completely tender, about 15 minutes.

3. Ladle about 2 cups soup into a blender and puree, holding a folded kitchen towel firmly on the lid. Stir the puree back into the soup and add the spinach. Cook until the spinach is wilted.

Each of 10 servings: About 395 calories, 21 g protein, 49 g carbohydrate, 14 g total fat (4 g saturated), 30 mg cholesterol, 886 mg sodium.

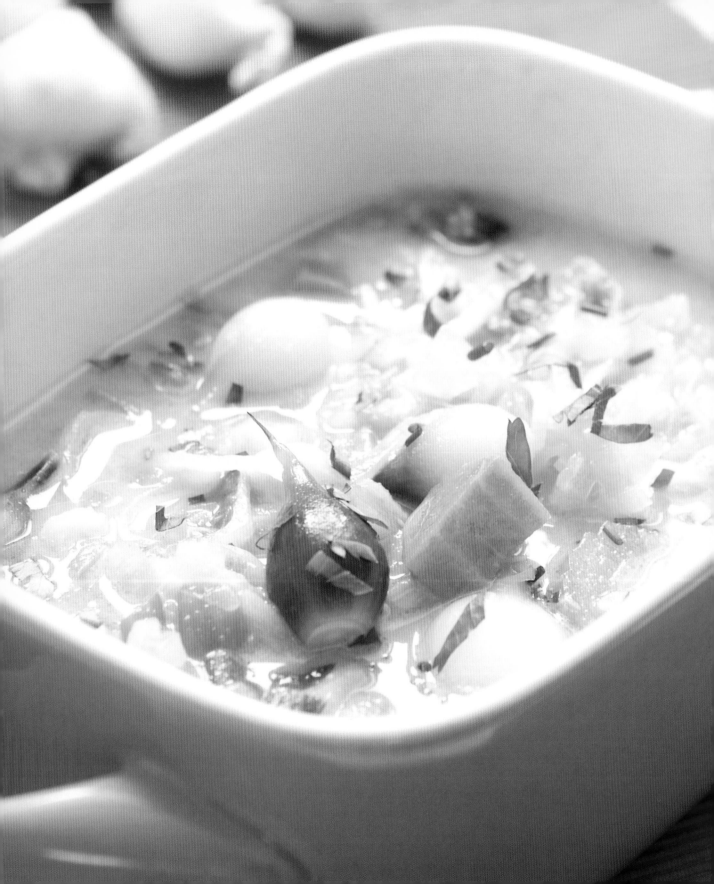

Seven-Onion Chowder

PREP TIME: 20 minutes
COOK TIME: 45 minutes

Makes 6 servings

This creamy tasting soup has no cream in it! Instead, the texture comes from thickening the liquid with a mayonnaise-like sauce. To make the soup ahead, which is not only convenient but gives the ingredients time to marry and mellow, make it through step 2, cool it completely, cover, and refrigerate up to 3 days. Then, make the sauce, heat the soup just to a boil, and add the sherry, sauce, and herbs. You can season and thicken the chowder using an Aioli sauce (page 38) instead of the egg mixture in this recipe.

4 tablespoons unsalted butter
4 shallots, thinly sliced
3 scallions, cut crosswise into ¼-inch pieces
2 large leeks, tender green and white portions cut crosswise into thin rings and rinsed well
1 large Vidalia or other sweet onion, chopped
1 medium red onion, chopped
1 cup mixed red and white pearl onions, peeled
1 large carrot, peeled and chopped into rough ½-inch chunks
1 celery stalk including some leaves, chopped into rough ½-inch chunks
1 tablespoon sugar
1 teaspoon sea salt or more to taste
¼ teaspoon freshly ground pepper or more to taste
6 cups Chicken, Beef, or Vegetable Stock (Chapter 1)
1 large egg
½ cup extravirgin olive oil

3 tablespoons fresh lemon juice
2 tablespoons dry sherry
¼ cup snipped chives
2 tablespoons chopped fresh Italian parsley

1. Melt the butter in a 3-quart saucepan over medium-high heat and add the shallots, scallions, leeks, Vidalia onion, red onion, pearl onions, carrot, and celery. Sauté until the vegetables soften, about 5 minutes. Reduce the heat to low. Cover the mixture with a sheet of waxed paper and cover the pan with the lid. "Sweat" the vegetables until soft, about 10 minutes.

2. Remove the lid and waxed paper. Stir in the sugar, salt, and pepper and sauté until the vegetables are glazed with lightly caramelized sugar, about 3 minutes. Add the stock and heat to boiling. Reduce the heat to low and simmer, partially covered, for 10 minutes.

3. Make the sauce: Place the egg in a blender and turn the machine on to blend. With the machine running, add the oil through the hole in the lid, pouring in a thin, steady stream. With the machine running, add the lemon juice and then gradually add ½ cup hot soup. Taste the sauce, and season with salt and pepper.

4. Stir the sherry into the soup and remove the pan from the heat. Stir the sauce into the soup and then the chives and parsley. Do not let boil. Taste the soup again and adjust the seasonings if necessary. Ladle the soup into warmed bowls and serve.

Each serving: About 382 calories, 9 g protein, 24 g carbohydrate, 28 g total fat (8 g saturated), 56 mg cholesterol, 426 mg sodium.

Alder-Smoked Salmon and Roasted Pumpkin Chowder

PREP TIME: 20 minutes
COOK TIME: 1 hour 45 minutes

Makes 6 servings

Because of the long summer days in Alaska, vegetables (like pumpkins) can grow to the size of small children. Harvest time is salmon-running time, which inspired this Alaskan combination of flavors.

1 tablespoon olive oil

1½-pound cooking pumpkin

4 tablespoons unsalted butter

3 leeks, white and tender green portions sliced crosswise into ½-inch wide rings and rinsed well

1 large red bell pepper, seeded and diced

2 tablespoons finely grated peeled fresh gingerroot

6 cups Chicken or Vegetable Stock (Chapter 1)

1 teaspoon chopped fresh thyme leaves (no stems)

¼ teaspoon saffron threads, crumbled (optional)

½ teaspoon salt or more to taste

¼ teaspoon freshly ground white pepper or more to taste

8 ounces alder-smoked salmon, flaked into bite-size pieces

ALDER-SMOKED SALMON

• Smoking fish and meat over alder wood is a Native American form of preserving that rivals salt-cured and sun-dried curing in flavor. Alder-smoked salmon can be found online and in many fish markets.

1. Preheat the oven to 350 degrees. Line a small baking sheet with foil and drizzle with the oil. Carefully cut the pumpkin in half lengthwise and scoop out the seeds. Place the halves cut side down on the foil and bake until tender, about 1 hour. When cool enough to handle, scoop out the flesh from the skin and chop into ½-inch pieces.

2. Melt the butter in a 3-quart saucepan over medium-high heat. Add the leeks, bell pepper, and ginger and sauté until tender, about 5 minutes. Add the pumpkin, stock, thyme, saffron (if using), salt, and pepper and heat to boiling over medium-high heat. Reduce the heat to medium and simmer, partially covered, 30 minutes. Add the salmon and simmer until cooked through, about 10 minutes. Taste and adjust the seasoning if needed.

Each serving: About 245 calories, 15 g protein, 14 g carbohydrate, 15 g total fat (6 g saturated), 44 mg cholesterol, 222 mg sodium.

Chilled Garden Chowder with Smoked Salmon and Fresh Dill

PREP TIME: 15 minutes
COOK TIME: 15 minutes

Makes 4 servings

You can use 8 ounces of cooked baby shrimp (the canned ones are nice for this soup) instead of the smoked salmon.

2 cups Vegetable Stock (page 15) or water
8 peeled baby carrots, cut crosswise into
   ¼-inch-thick rounds
4 radishes, cut into ¼-inch-thick rounds
2 new Yukon gold or other waxy potatoes, peeled
   and cut into ¼-inch dice
2 spring onions, sliced crosswise into thin rounds
¼ teaspoon sea salt
¼ teaspoon freshly ground white pepper or more
   to taste
8 asparagus stalks, tough ends snapped off,
   remaining stalk peeled
½ cup shelled peas
4 ounces fresh spinach leaves, washed well,
   stacked, and shredded
2 trays ice cubes
8 ounces smoked salmon, cut into
   ½- by-1-inch pieces
2 tablespoons snipped fresh dill fronds
sour cream or crème fraîche for serving (optional)
Scandinavian or other crisp crackers for serving

1. Combine the stock, carrots, radishes, potatoes, onions, salt, and ¼ teaspoon pepper in a 2-quart saucepan; heat to boiling over medium-high heat. Simmer until the vegetables are tender, 5 to 8 minutes. Add the asparagus, peas, and spinach and cook until tender, about 4 minutes.

2. Pour the chowder into a 2-quart heat-safe glass measure or bowl and immediately add the ice cubes. Stir until the ice cubes mostly melt and the vegetables are chilled. Let stand until the ice melts. Stir in the salmon and dill. Taste and add more pepper if needed.

3. To serve: Ladle the soup into chilled soup bowls. Add a dollop of sour cream to each bowl if you like. Serve with crackers.

Each serving (without sour cream or crackers): About 142 calories, 14 g protein, 16 g carbohydrate, 3 g total fat (1 g saturated), 13 mg cholesterol, 624 mg sodium.

Nor'easter Clam Chowder

PREP TIME: 5 minutes
COOK TIME: 50 minutes

Makes 4 servings

When cold winds blow, warm up with this robust New England–style chowder. It holds its own against the elements of hunger, and it's chockablock with flavor from clams, potatoes, corn, and bacon. For a thicker chowder, use less clam juice.

3 slices (about 2 ounces) smoked bacon
1 medium onion, chopped
2 cans (about 6 ounces each) minced clams
1 can (11 ounces) clam juice
2 medium red potatoes, diced
¾ cup frozen corn
1½ cups 2% milk
2 teaspoons Worcestershire sauce
¾ teaspoon dried savory leaves
salt and pepper to taste

1. Cook the bacon in a 3-quart saucepan until browned, about 5 minutes. Transfer the bacon to a paper towel–lined plate to drain. Add the onion to the pan, and sauté until translucent, about 3 minutes.

2. Drain the clams in a fine mesh sieve set over the saucepan. Set the clams aside. Add the canned clam juice and the potatoes to the pan. Cook until the potatoes are tender, 15 to 20 minutes.

3. Using a slotted spoon, transfer half the mixture to a bowl. Using a handheld immersion blender, puree the soup in the pan. Return the reserved vegetables to the pan and stir in the corn, milk, Worcestershire sauce, savory, and clams.

4. Heat the chowder on low (do not boil), stirring occasionally, until it is hot, 5 to 10 minutes. Taste and season with salt and pepper if needed. Crumble the bacon and sprinkle on top of each.

Each serving: About 229 calories, 29 g protein, 33 g carbohydrate, 4 g total fat (2 g saturated), 18 mg cholesterol, 1,469 mg sodium.

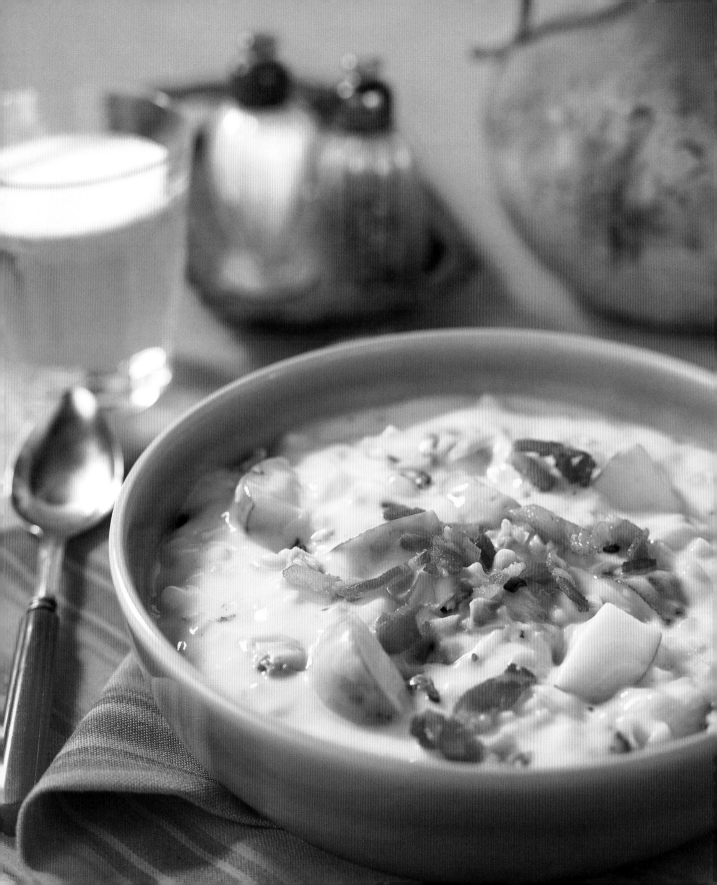

Scrod Chowder with Broccoflower

PREP TIME: 5 minutes
COOK TIME: 40 minutes

Makes 4 servings

Broccoflower, which is a cross between broccoli and cauliflower, gives this chowder a splash of bright green color and mild cauliflower flavor.

3 cups cubed peeled potatoes
1 large onion, chopped
1½ cups clam juice
2 bay leaves
2 ounces prosciutto, finely chopped
½ teaspoon freshly ground black pepper
2 cups broccoflower florets
1 pound scrod fillet, cut into ½-inch pieces
1 cup 2% milk
salt and pepper to taste

1. Combine the potatoes, onion, clam juice, and bay leaves in a 6-quart pot. Cover and bring to a boil. Reduce the heat and simmer until the potatoes are tender, about 15 minutes. Using a slotted spoon, transfer half the potatoes and onions to a bowl. Discard the bay leaves.

2. Using a potato masher, mash the vegetables in the pot. Stir in the prosciutto, pepper, and reserved vegetables. Cover and bring to a simmer. Add the broccoflower and scrod. Cook, covered, until the broccoflower is tender and the scrod is cooked through, 5 to 10 minutes.

3. Stir in the milk and heat the chowder through, 3 to 5 minutes. Taste and season with salt and pepper if needed.

Each serving: About 211 calories, 20 g protein, 23 g carbohydrate, 7 g total fat (2 g saturated), 32 mg cholesterol, 1,133 mg sodium.

Mixed Seafood Chowder

PREP TIME: 10 minutes
COOK TIME: 40 minutes

Makes 8 servings

Here's a soup in the European tradition, a "whatever got caught in the net" assortment that marries well in the pot. Be sure to stir in either of the bold finishing sauces to add color and zip.

2 tablespoons vegetable oil
3 medium potatoes, peeled and diced
3 celery stalks, chopped
1 large leek, tender green and white portions thinly sliced crosswise and rinsed well
2 medium garlic cloves, crushed through a press
1 can (16 ounces) crushed tomatoes
2 cups Basic Fish Stock (page 16) or 1 cup bottled clam juice and 1 cup water
½ cup dry white vermouth
¾ teaspoon dried oregano leaves
1 yellow zucchini or summer squash, halved lengthwise, seeded, and cut into ½-inch chunks
1 pound skinned halibut fillets, cut into 1-inch chunks
1 pound skinned very fresh bluefish or mackerel fillets, cut into 1-inch chunks
1 pound bay scallops
1 pint shucked oysters with liquor
Romesco Sauce (page 40) or Saffron-Orange Aioli (page 38) for serving
croutons of choice (page 22) for serving

1. Heat the oil in a 4-quart saucepan over medium heat. Add the potatoes, celery, leek, and garlic and sauté 5 minutes. Add the tomatoes, stock, vermouth, and oregano and heat to boiling. Reduce the heat to medium-low and simmer, covered, 20 minutes.

2. Add the zucchini, halibut, and bluefish to the soup. Cover and simmer until the fish starts to flake apart when prodded with a fork and is almost cooked through, about 7 minutes. Add the scallops and cook 1 minute. Add the oysters and their liquor and simmer just until the oysters are cooked, about 2 minutes.

3. To serve: Ladle the chowder into warmed soup bowls. Pass the Romesco sauce or Aioli and croutons at the table.

Each serving without sauce or croutons: About 336 calories, 38 g protein, 21 g carbohydrate, 9 g total fat (1 g saturated), 85 mg cholesterol, 352 mg sodium.

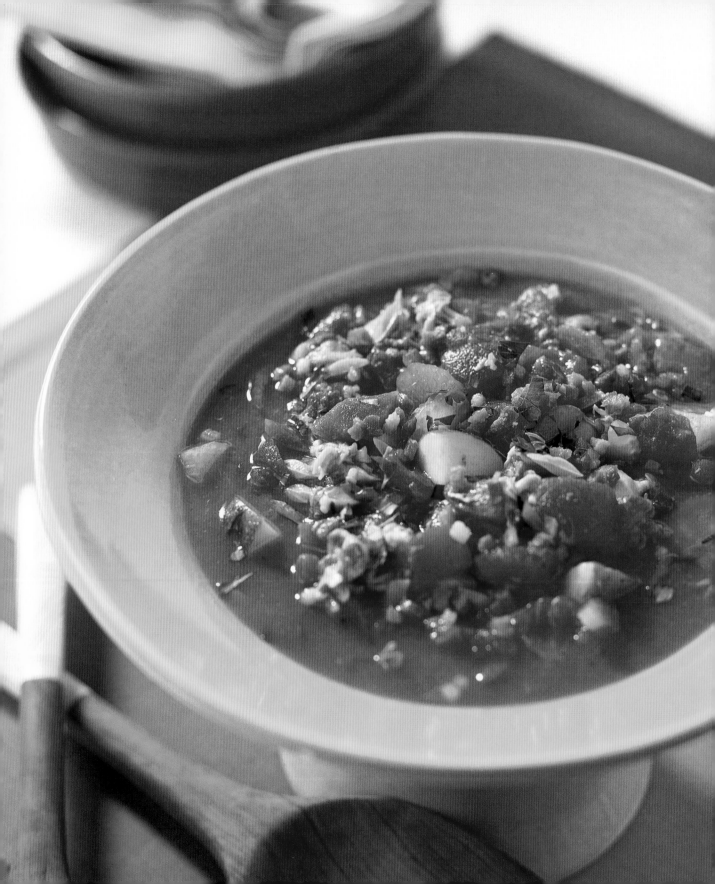

Easy Manhattan-Style Clam Chowder

PREP TIME: 5 minutes
COOK TIME: 20 minutes

Makes 4 servings

Tomato-based clam chowder aficionados: This chunky version is brimming with clams, tomatoes, potatoes, and bacon, and is ready to serve in less than 30 minutes.

    4 ounces Canadian bacon, diced
    1 large Spanish onion, chopped
    1 stalk celery, thinly sliced
    1 can (10 ounces) clam juice
    1 can (15 ounces) whole tomatoes, chopped
    2 medium red potatoes, chopped
    2 bay leaves
    ¼ teaspoon lemon pepper
    1 can (6 ounces) minced clams with juice
    salt and pepper to taste
    ¼ cup chopped fresh parsley for garnish

1. Sauté the bacon in a 6-quart pot until lightly browned. Add the onion and celery and sauté until the onion is transparent, about 3 minutes.

2. Stir in the clam juice, tomatoes, potatoes, bay leaves, and lemon pepper. Cover the pot and bring the mixture to a boil. Reduce the heat and simmer until the potatoes are tender, 12 to 15 minutes.

3. Stir in the clams and simmer the soup for 5 minutes more. Taste and season with salt and pepper if needed. Discard the bay leaves. Top each serving with the parsley.

Each serving: About 166 calories, 18 g protein, 27 g carbohydrate, 2 g total fat (1 g saturated), 23 mg cholesterol, 1,219 mg sodium.

Smoked Haddock Chowder

PREP TIME: 15 minutes
COOK TIME: 55 minutes

Makes 8 servings

8 ounces pancetta, cut into ½-inch dice
1 large red onion, chopped
1 small inner celery stalk with leaves, chopped
2 garlic cloves, minced
1 teaspoon chopped fresh thyme leaves (no stems)
2 medium Yukon gold or Yellow Finn potatoes, peeled and cut into ½-inch cubes
2 small carrots, peeled and sliced crosswise into thin rounds
1 cup dry white wine
5 cups Basic Fish Stock (page 16) or water
1¼ pounds smoked haddock (finnan haddie)
2 cups whole milk
1 cup heavy cream
sea salt and freshly ground pepper to taste
2 egg yolks
2 tablespoons chopped fresh Italian parsley
paprika for garnish

1. Sauté the pancetta in a 3-quart saucepan over medium heat until it is crisp but not hard and the fat is rendered, about 7 minutes. With a slotted spoon, transfer the pancetta to a paper towel–lined plate to drain. Discard all but 3 tablespoons of the rendered fat.

2. Heat the fat in the pot over medium-high heat until hot. Add the onion and celery and sauté 3 minutes. Add the garlic and thyme and sauté 1 minute. Add the potatoes and carrots and sauté 1 minute. Add the wine and heat to boiling, stirring; boil 1 minute. Add the stock, cover, and heat to boiling. Reduce the heat to medium-low and simmer until the potatoes and carrots are tender, about 25 minutes.

3. Meanwhile, place the haddock in a skillet large enough to hold the fish in a single layer and add the milk. Heat to boiling over medium-high heat. Reduce the heat to medium-low and simmer, covered, until the fish flakes with a fork, about 15 minutes. With a slotted spatula, transfer the fish to a shallow bowl and flake it into 1-inch chunks with a fork. Reserve the cooking liquid.

4. With a slotted spoon, transfer half of the vegetables in the saucepan to a food processor or blender and puree, adding enough cooking liquid to allow the vegetables to process easily. Stir the puree back into the saucepan. Add the fish and its cooking liquid and ½ cup cream. Simmer over medium heat 10 minutes. Taste the soup and season with salt and pepper.

5. Beat the egg yolks and remaining ½ cup cream in a medium bowl until blended; whisk in a ladleful of hot soup. Stir the mixture back into the soup and cook, stirring gently and making sure the soup does not simmer or boil (or the egg yolks will curdle). Cook until the soup thickens, about 2 minutes, removing the pan from the stove if necessary to keep the soup from simmering.

6. To serve: Ladle the soup into soup bowls and sprinkle each with pancetta, parsley, and paprika.

Each serving: About 345 calories, 29 g protein, 16 g carbohydrate, 16 g total fat (7 g saturated), 149 mg cholesterol, 971 mg sodium.

Flounder-Jack Chowder

PREP TIME: 10 minutes
COOK TIME: 25 minutes

Makes 4 servings

2 teaspoons unsalted butter
1 large onion, chopped
2 celery stalks, chopped
2 garlic cloves
2 large potatoes, peeled and cut into ½-inch cubes
1¾ cups Chicken Stock (page 14)
1 pound flounder fillets, cut into bite-size pieces
½ cup skim milk
½ cup shredded reduced-sodium Monterey Jack cheese
1 teaspoon Louisiana-style hot-pepper sauce
salt and pepper to taste
2 tablespoons snipped fresh chives for garnish

FLOUNDER
- Flounder is a delicate fish. To keep it from falling apart, simmer and stir the soup gently.

1. Melt the butter in a 6-quart pot over medium-high heat. Add the onion, celery, and garlic and cook until the onion is golden, about 3 minutes. Add the potatoes and stock. Cover the pot and bring the mixture to a boil. Reduce the heat and simmer until the potatoes and celery are tender, about 12 minutes. Using a slotted spoon, transfer 2 cups of the vegetables to a bowl.

2. Using a handheld immersion blender, puree the vegetables remaining in the pot. Add the flounder. Cover the pot and gently simmer until the fish is tender, 3 to 5 minutes. Gently stir in the milk, Monterey Jack cheese, hot-pepper sauce, and reserved vegetables. Heat the soup throughout; do not boil. Taste and season with salt and pepper if needed. Top each serving with chives.

Each serving: About 281 calories, 30 g protein, 21 g carbohydrate, 8 g total fat (4 g saturated), 75 mg cholesterol, 296 mg sodium.

Pea and Cabbage Chowder with Seafood Dumplings

PREP TIME: 15 minutes
COOK TIME: 15 minutes

Makes 4 to 6 servings

The dumpling mixture makes a delicious filling for wontons, too.

Seafood Dumplings
8 ounces bay scallops
8 ounces shelled, deveined shrimp
2 scallions, finely sliced crosswise
1 large egg white
1 tablespoon low-sodium soy sauce
2 teaspoons grated peeled fresh gingerroot
2 teaspoons vegetable oil
1½ teaspoons dark sesame oil
1 teaspoon cornstarch
½ teaspoon fine sea salt
pinch cayenne pepper

1 quart Gingered Chicken Stock (page 14) or
   1 quart regular Chicken Stock (page 14) with
   2 tablespoons grated peeled fresh gingerroot
   and 1 tablespoon roasted garlic teriyaki sauce
16 Chinese pea pods, stripped of stems and
   strings
3 cups slivered Napa Cabbage or Savoy cabbage
2 tablespoons cilantro leaves
1 tablespoon minced scallions
1 teaspoon dark sesame oil

1. Make the dumplings: Combine the scallops, shrimp, scallions, egg white, soy sauce, ginger, vegetable oil, sesame oil, cornstarch, salt, and pepper in a food processor; pulse until blended and chunky. Scrape down the sides of the bowl and pulse to combine, still keeping the mixture chunky. Scrape into a bowl, cover, and refrigerate until ready to cook.

2. Make the chowder: Place the stock in a 3-quart saucepan and heat to boiling over medium-high heat. Add the pea pod strips and cabbage strips and heat to simmering.

3. Drop scant teaspoonfuls of the dumpling mixture into the pea-pod broth. Cover and simmer over low heat until the dumplings are barely cooked through, about 2 minutes. Add the cilantro, scallions, and sesame oil and ladle into warmed soup bowls.

Each of 4 servings: About 138 calories, 22 g protein, 4 g carbohydrate, 3 g total fat (1 g saturated), 105 mg cholesterol, 630 mg sodium.

Chili Chicken Chowder

PREP TIME: 5 minutes
COOK TIME: 20 minutes

Makes 6 servings

Here's an easy-to-make knockout chowder with signature Southwest flavors.

½ pound cooked chicken breast, cubed
1¾ cups Chicken Stock (page 14)
1 can (14 ounces) diced tomatoes
1 can (15 ounces) black beans, rinsed and drained
1 red potato, diced
1 large carrot, thinly sliced
2 garlic cloves, minced
2 teaspoons chili powder
½ teaspoon cumin seeds
salt and pepper to taste

Combine the chicken, stock, tomatoes, beans, potato, carrot, garlic, chili powder, and cumin seeds in a 6-quart pot. Cover and bring to a boil. Reduce the heat, and simmer until the potato and carrot are tender, 15 to 20 minutes. Taste and season with salt and pepper if needed.

Each serving: About 137 calories, 16 g protein, 14 g carbohydrate, 1 g total fat (trace saturated), 33 mg cholesterol, 518 mg sodium.

CUMIN
- Use ground cumin if you can't find cumin seeds.

VARIATION
- Variation: Substitute turkey for the chicken, and pinto beans for the black beans.

Chicken-Corn Chowder with Stuffed Olives

PREP TIME: 5 minutes
COOK TIME: 35 minutes

Makes 4 servings

A tasty combination—chicken and corn—makes for a family-favorite chowder. Mashed potatoes thicken the stock; garlic and hot-pepper sauce impart zing.

1 teaspoon olive oil
¾ pound skinless boneless chicken breast, cut into ½-inch cubes
1½ cups Chicken Stock (page 14)
1 large potato, peeled and cut into ½-inch cubes
4 garlic cloves, crushed through a press
1 can (15 ounces) reduced-sodium cream-style corn
1½ cups frozen corn
4 scallions, sliced
½ cup 2% milk
2 to 3 drops Louisiana hot-pepper sauce
salt and pepper to taste
1 tablespoon stuffed olives, chopped

1. Warm the oil in a 6-quart pot over medium-high heat for 1 minute. Add the chicken and sauté until the pieces are cooked through and lightly browned, 5 to 10 minutes. Transfer to a bowl.

2. Pour 1 cup of the stock into the same pot. Add the potato and garlic. Cover and bring to a boil. Reduce the heat, and simmer the mixture until the potato is tender, about 12 minutes. Using a potato masher, mash the potato mixture.

3. Stir in the chicken, cream-style corn, frozen corn, scallions, milk, hot sauce, and remaining ½ cup stock. Heat thoroughly, about 6 minutes. Taste and season with salt and pepper if needed. Stir in the olives and serve immediately.

Each serving: About 367 calories, 25 g protein, 48 g carbohydrate, 11 g total fat (3 g saturated), 57 mg cholesterol, 620 mg sodium.

HOT SAUCE WARNING
- Add hot-pepper sauce with caution, tasting the soup after each drop. Why? The firepower of hot-pepper sauces varies dramatically. Some are relatively mild; others are scorching.

Turkey and Broccoli Chowder

PREP TIME: 10 minutes
COOK TIME: 35 minutes

Makes 6 servings

Utilize your Thanksgiving leftovers with this chow-der. If you have lots of different cooked vegetables left over, and even some gravy, add them all with the turkey and forget about the broccoli.

4 tablespoons unsalted butter
3 scallions, cut crosswise into ¼-inch-thick rounds
1 medium green bell pepper, seeded and diced
1 medium red bell pepper, seeded and diced
8 ounces small mushrooms, quartered lengthwise
¼ cup all-purpose flour
2 cups hot whole milk or half-and-half
3 cups Turkey Stock (page 18)
2 medium potatoes, peeled and coarsely diced
½ teaspoon salt or more to taste
¼ teaspoon freshly ground white pepper or more
   to taste
1½ pounds cooked turkey breast, cut into
   bite-size chunks
2 cups broccoli florets, split in half lengthwise
2 tablespoons fresh lemon juice

1. Melt the butter in a 3-quart saucepan over medium-high heat. Add the scallions and bell pepper and sauté until softened, about 2 minutes. Add the mushrooms and sauté 1 minute. Stir in the flour until blended with the butter. Gradually stir in the hot milk. Heat to boiling and cook 1 minute. Stir in the stock.

2. Add the potatoes, salt, and pepper and heat to boiling. Reduce the heat to medium and simmer, partially covered, until the potatoes are tender, about 20 minutes. Add the turkey and broccoli and simmer until the broccoli is crisp-tender, about 5 minutes. Stir in the lemon juice. Taste and adjust the season-ing if needed.

Each serving: About 378 calories, 43 g protein, 23 g carbohy-drate, 12 g total fat (7 g saturated), 126 mg cholesterol, 383 mg sodium.

Homespun Sausage and Hominy Chowder

PREP TIME: 15 minutes
COOK TIME: about 35 minutes

Makes 6 servings

Hominy is hulled white or yellow corn with the germ removed; it was introduced to the early colonists by Native Americans. When the dried kernels are ground, hominy is called grits.

4 scallions, trimmed
1 roll (12 or 16 ounces) refrigerated Southern-style hot breakfast sausage
1 medium green bell pepper, seeded, finely chopped
1 cup chopped Vidalia or other sweet onion
1 package (12 or 16 ounces) coleslaw mix (red and green cabbage and carrots)
2 garlic cloves, minced
1 quart Chicken or Vegetable Stock (Chapter 1)
1 can (15½ ounces) white hominy, drained and rinsed
2 cups cooked black-eyed peas from dried, or 1 can (about 15 ounces) black-eyed peas, drained and rinsed
2 ripe tomatoes, seeded and diced
¼ cup chopped fresh Italian parsley
¼ cup chopped fresh cilantro
freshly ground black pepper to taste
1 cup shredded Cheddar cheese for serving

1. Cut 3 scallions crosswise into ½-inch pieces and place in a bowl. Slice the remaining scallion crosswise into very thin rounds and set aside in another bowl.

2. Cook the sausage in a 3-quart saucepan over medium heat, breaking the sausage into bite-size pieces with a wooden spoon, until the sausage is browned and the fat is rendered. Transfer the sausage to a bowl with a slotted spoon. Discard all but 2 tablespoons drippings from the saucepan.

3. Add the ½-inch pieces of scallion, bell pepper, ½ cup onion, the coleslaw mix, and garlic, to the drippings in the pan and sauté until softened, 5 minutes. Add the sausage, stock, hominy, and black-eyed peas and stir to mix. Heat to boiling over medium heat; simmer 20 minutes. Meanwhile, mix the sliced scallion and remaining ½ cup onion with the tomatoes, parsley, and cilantro in a bowl.

4. To serve: Taste the soup and season with black pepper. Ladle the soup into soup bowls. Sprinkle with the tomato mixture and then the cheese.

Each serving: About 382 calories, 22 g protein, 32 g carbohydrate, 19 g total fat (8 g saturated), 48 mg cholesterol, 441 mg sodium.

Parsnip-Tomato Chowder with Little Meatballs

PREP TIME: 20 minutes
COOK TIME: about 15 minutes

Makes 8 servings

For a bit thinner soup, omit the tomato paste. There will still be lots of tomato presence to balance the sweet flavor of the parsnips.

   6 cups Vegetable Stock (page 15)

Meatballs
   8 ounces ground veal, pork, and/or beef
   1 tablespoon finely chopped fresh parsley
   ¼ teaspoon salt plus more to taste
   pinch freshly grated nutmeg
   pinch freshly ground black pepper
   flour for dusting your hands

   1 pound parsnips, peeled and cut into ¼-inch dice
   1 slender carrot, peeled and cut into thin rounds
   1 bulb fennel, cored and thinly sliced
   1 small zucchini, cut into ¼-inch dice
   1 can (about 14 ounces) diced tomatoes with garlic and basil
   1 scallion, grated
   ¼ cup tomato paste

1. Heat the stock to boiling in a 4-quart saucepan over medium-high heat. Meanwhile, make the meatballs: Place the meat in a bowl and add the parsley, salt, nutmeg, and pepper. Mix gently until combined. Dust your hands with flour and shape the meat into marble-size balls (about ½-inch in diameter). Gently drop the balls into the boiling stock and cook until they rise to the surface, about 2 minutes. Transfer the meatballs to a bowl with a slotted spoon and set aside.

2. Add the parsnips, carrot, fennel, zucchini, tomatoes, and scallion to the stock. Heat to a gentle boil and cook until the vegetables are tender, about 5 minutes. Transfer 1 cup of soup to a bowl; whisk in the tomato paste until smooth and then pour back into the soup. Simmer 3 minutes. Add the meatballs and heat through. Taste and season with salt and pepper. Ladle into warmed shallow soup bowls.

Each serving: About 139 calories, 8 g protein, 16 g carbohydrate, 5 g total fat (2 g saturated), 25 mg cholesterol, 257 mg sodium.

Beef and Roasted Corn Chowder

PREP TIME: 15 minutes
COOK TIME: 50 minutes

Makes 4 servings

You can make this chili-infused chowder with boneless pork or lamb instead of beef.

4 ears corn on the cob, husked
1 tablespoon vegetable oil
1 large onion, chopped
1 slender carrot, peeled and sliced crosswise into thin rounds
2 garlic cloves, minced
1 pound round steak, cut into small cubes
2 teaspoons chili powder
½ teaspoon ground cumin
½ teaspoon dried oregano leaves
1 can (about 14 ounces) diced tomatoes with zesty mild green chilies
1 quart Beef Stock (page 15)
salt and freshly ground pepper to taste
2 tablespoons chopped fresh cilantro leaves

1. Preheat the broiler, prepare an outdoor grill, or use a gas burner. Place the corn ears close to the heat source and roast, turning as the kernels brown, to cook on all sides. Transfer to a cutting board and remove the kernels with a sharp knife.

2. Heat the oil in a 3-quart saucepan over medium-high heat; sauté the onion and carrot until softened, about 5 minutes. Add the garlic and sauté 1 minute. Add the steak, chili powder, cumin, and oregano. Reduce the heat to medium-low and cook until the meat is tender, about 20 minutes. Add the tomatoes and their juices; cover and simmer 20 minutes. Add the stock and heat to boiling, covered, over medium-high heat. Stir in the corn, taste, and season with salt and pepper. Stir in the cilantro. Ladle into warm soup bowls.

Each serving: About 405 calories, 31 g protein, 32 g carbohydrate, 19 g total fat (6 g saturated), 74 mg cholesterol, 526 mg sodium.

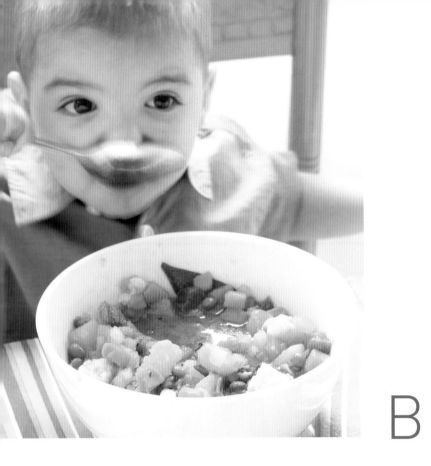

6

BEAN &
LEGUME SOUPS

Black Bean Soup

PREP TIME: 10 minutes plus overnight soak
COOK TIME: 3 hours 30 minutes

Makes 6 servings

1 pound dried black beans, soaked in water
   overnight
2 bay leaves
3 quarts Vegetable Stock (page 15) or water
1 cup olive or canola oil
3 small shallots, diced
1 small white onion, diced
1 large red bell pepper, seeded and diced
1 large green bell pepper, seeded and diced
3 garlic cloves, minced
1 tablespoon ground cumin
2 teaspoons crushed dried oregano
2 tablespoons chopped fresh parsley
2 tablespoons light brown sugar
salt and pepper to taste

1. Drain the beans and transfer to a 6-quart pot.
   Add the bay leaves and stock and bring to a boil.
   Reduce to a simmer, partially cover, and cook,
   stirring occasionally, for 2½ to 3 hours, or until
   the beans are very tender. Add more water if
   necessary during cooking.

2. Meanwhile, heat the oil in a skillet and sauté the
   shallots and onion until translucent. Add the red
   pepper, green pepper, and garlic, and continue to
   cook, stirring frequently, for about 3 minutes. Add
   the cumin, oregano, and parsley. Heat through and
   add the sugar. Remove from heat and cool slightly.

3. In a blender or food processor, puree the sautéed
   vegetables until smooth; stir into the cooking
   beans. Cover and continue to cook for an additional
   30 minutes.

4. Turn off the heat, discard the bay leaves, and add
   salt and pepper to taste. Serve immediately.

Each serving: About 445 calories, 5 g protein, 20 g carbohydrate, 38 g total fat (5 g saturated), 0 mg cholesterol, 285 mg
sodium.

Tex-Mex Black Bean Soup with Jalapeños

PREP TIME: 10 minutes, plus overnight soak
COOK TIME: 2 hours 30 minutes

Makes 6 servings

This soup is south-of-the-border hot and spicy. Dried chili powder will be hotter than fresh red chiles.

2 tablespoons vegetable oil
2 medium yellow onions, chopped
4 medium garlic cloves, minced
8 jalapeño peppers, seeded and chopped (use rubber gloves when handling hot peppers)
2 cups dried black beans, soaked in water overnight
1 cup canned diced tomatoes
1 tablespoon crushed fresh red chile (use rubber gloves when handling hot peppers) or dried red chili powder
1 tablespoon red wine vinegar
2 teaspoons ground cumin
1 teaspoon ground ezpazote (Mexican tea)
1 teaspoon ground coriander
¼ teaspoon ground cloves
6 to 8 cups water
salt and pepper to taste
3 tablespoons tequila (optional)
sour cream for serving

1. Heat the oil in a saucepan and sauté the onions and garlic until the onions are tender.

2. In a 6-quart pot, combine the onions and garlic with the jalapeños, beans, tomatoes, crushed red chile, vinegar, cumin, ezpazote, coriander, cloves, and water. Bring to a boil. Reduce to a simmer, partly cover, and cook until the beans are tender, about 2 hours.

3. In a blender or food processor, puree one half of the soup until smooth. Pour the puree back into the soup and continue to simmer until thickened to desired consistency, about 15 minutes.

4. Taste and season with salt and pepper if needed. Remove from the heat and stir in the tequila if using. Serve immediately with dollops of sour cream.

Each serving: About 154 calories, 6 g protein, 22 g carbohydrate, 6 g total fat (1 g saturated), 0 mg cholesterol, 902 mg sodium.

Barbecued Pork and Bean Soup

PREP TIME: 15 minutes
COOK TIME: 1 hour 30 minutes to 1 hour 40 minutes

Makes 8 servings

Serve hot cornbread, cornsticks, or garlic bread made from hamburger buns with this fusion-flavored soup.

- 2 strips applewood or other smoked bacon, cut into ½-inch-wide strips
- 1 large onion, chopped
- 1 large garlic clove, chopped
- 1 tablespoon Mexican chili powder
- 1 teaspoon smoked Spanish paprika (Pimentón de la Vera) or 2 teaspoons sweet paprika and ¼ teaspoon cayenne pepper)
- 2 tablespoons tomato paste
- 2 tablespoons ketchup
- 2 tablespoons Dijon mustard
- 12 ounces (1½ cups) beer (preferably lager)
- 2 quarts water
- 1½-pound fully cooked smoked boneless pork butt (shoulder)
- 1 bag (12 or 16 ounces) coleslaw mix (red and green cabbage and carrots)
- 4 cups cooked Great Northern beans or 2 cans (16 ounces each) white beans, rinsed
- 1 chipotle chile in adobo sauce, finely chopped, plus 1 teaspoon adobo sauce or more to taste (optional)

1. Sauté the bacon in a 3-quart saucepan over medium heat until the pieces are crisp but not hard and the fat has rendered. Transfer the bacon to paper towels to drain. Add the onion to the drippings and sauté over medium heat until softened, about 5 minutes. Add the garlic and sauté 1 minute. Add the chili powder and paprika and sauté until fragrant, about 30 seconds. Add the tomato paste and sauté until rust-colored, about 1 minute. Stir in the ketchup and mustard until blended. Slowly whisk in the beer until blended. Add the water and pork and heat to boiling, skimming off any foam on the surface. Reduce the heat to medium, cover, and simmer until the pork is tender, about 1 hour.

2. With tongs, transfer the pork to a bowl. Add all but 1 cup of the coleslaw mix and the beans to the soup and stir to mix. Simmer, uncovered, 10 to 20 minutes.

3. Cut the pork into bite-size chunks or strips and add to the soup with any juices in the bowl. Taste the soup and stir in the chipotle chile and adobo sauce to taste if needed. To serve: Ladle the soup into warmed bowls and sprinkle with reserved coleslaw mix and bacon.

Each serving: About 409 calories, 24 g protein, 29 g carbohydrate, 21 g total fat (7 g saturated), 64 mg cholesterol, 251 mg sodium.

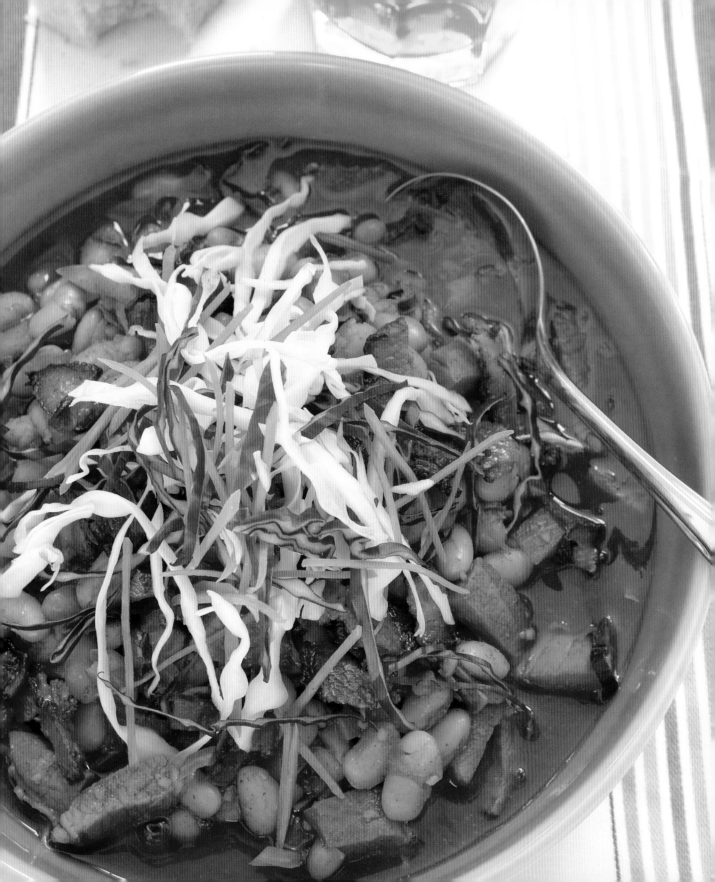

Bean and Bread Soup

PREP TIME: 15 minutes
COOK TIME: 20 minutes

Makes 8 servings

Here's a traditional Italian dish that's called a soup but actually contains very little liquid.

½ cup extravirgin olive oil
1 medium onion, finely chopped
1 celery stalk, finely chopped
1 small garlic clove, minced
6 cups rinsed, canned cannellini beans or 2 cups dried cannellini
     beans (white kidney beans), soaked and cooked as package label
     directs and drained
1 cup Beef Stock (page 15)
salt and freshly ground pepper to taste
1 loaf Italian bread, cut into thick slices and toasted
2 ripe plum tomatoes, diced and mashed with a fork, for serving
¼ cup finely chopped fresh Italian parsley leaves for garnish

1. Heat the oil in a 4-quart saucepan over medium heat. Add the onion
   and sauté until softened, about 5 minutes. Add the celery and sauté
   2 minutes. Add the garlic and sauté 1 minute. Add the beans and stock,
   season with salt and pepper, and heat until simmering. Simmer, covered,
   5 minutes.

2. To serve: Place slices of toasted bread in warmed shallow soup bowls and
   ladle beans on top. Repeat. Spoon tomatoes on top, sprinkle with parsley,
   and serve.

Each serving: About 339 calories, 13 g protein, 40 g carbohydrate, 15 g total fat
(2 g saturated), 0 mg cholesterol, 420 mg sodium.

Quick Sausage and Bean Soup

PREP TIME: 10 minutes
COOK TIME: about 40 minutes

Makes 6 servings

8 ounces sweet Italian sausage, removed
   from casings
1 small onion, chopped
1 medium garlic clove, crushed through a press
1 can (28 ounces) Italian plum tomatoes
1 quart Chicken Stock (page 14)
1 cup uncooked small bow-tie pasta
1 can (16 ounces) cannellini beans, drained
   and rinsed
Classic Pesto (page 46) for serving

1. Place the sausage in a 3-quart saucepan and sauté
   over medium-high heat, breaking the sausage into
   small pieces with a wooden spoon. Add the onion
   and garlic and sauté until the onion is softened,
   about 5 minutes. Add the tomatoes and their juice,
   squeezing the tomatoes with your hand to break into
   bite-size pieces. Add the stock and heat to boiling.
   Add the pasta and cook until al dente according to
   package directions. Stir in the beans.

2. Simmer the soup 10 minutes. Ladle into warmed
   soup bowls and add a dollop of pesto to each. Swirl
   the pesto through the soup.

Each serving without Pesto: About 332 calories, 16 g
protein, 30 g carbohydrate, 17 g total fat (6 g saturated),
26 mg cholesterol, 452 mg sodium.

Chili Bean Soup with Summer Squash

PREP TIME: 5 minutes
COOK TIME: 15 minutes

Makes 4 servings

Few dishes are faster, easier, or tastier than this
chunky bean soup: It's ready to eat in just 20 minutes.
If the summer squash doesn't look up to par, use zucchini instead.

3½ cups Beef Stock (page 15)
1 large onion, chopped
2 carrots, peeled and thinly sliced
1 medium yellow summer squash, halved and
   sliced
3 cups canned chili beans with liquid
2 cups fresh chopped tomatoes
¼ teaspoon freshly ground black pepper
1 teaspoon dried cilantro
salt and pepper to taste

1. Combine the stock, onion, carrots, and squash in a
   6-quart pot. Cover and bring to a boil. Reduce the
   heat and simmer until the carrots are almost tender,
   about 10 minutes.

2. Stir in the chili beans, tomatoes, and pepper and
   simmer 5 minutes more. Stir in the cilantro. Taste
   and season with salt and pepper if needed.

Each serving: About 289 calories, 17 g protein, 63 g carbohydrate, 2 g total fat (1 g saturated), 0 mg cholesterol,
1,385 mg sodium.

Bean Soup
with Pistou

PREP TIME: 5 minutes plus overnight soak
COOK TIME: 3 hours

Makes 4 to 6 servings

1 cup dried navy beans
1 cup dried cannellini beans
1 large yellow onion, chopped
5 cups boiling Vegetable Stock (page 15)
2 large carrots, peeled and minced
1 cup shredded cabbage
2 small red potatoes, peeled and diced
1 package (10 ounces) frozen cut green
    beans, thawed
salt and pepper
Pistou (page 47)

1. The night before, place the navy beans and cannellini beans in separate large bowls or saucepans. Cover with cold water and soak overnight.

2. Position the rack in the center of the oven and preheat to 400 degrees. Drain the soaked beans and rinse several times. Place together in a large bean pot or saucepan. Add the onion and enough water to cover the beans. Cover tightly and bake in the oven until the beans are very tender, 1½ to 2 hours.

3. Remove from the oven and drain. Using a blender or food processor, puree the soup in batches until smooth. Return to the pot and slowly add the stock, carrots, cabbage, potatoes, and green beans. Add salt and pepper to taste, cover again, and return the pot to the oven. Reduce the heat to 350 degrees and bake for 1 hour.

4. Remove the soup from the oven and stir in one half of the pistou. Ladle the soup into warmed bowls and pass the remaining pistou at the table.

Each serving: About 440 calories, 28 g protein, 82 g carbohydrate, 3 g total fat (trace saturated), 0 mg cholesterol, 1,291 mg sodium.

Red Kidney Bean Soup with Tomatoes and Cheese

PREP TIME: 10 minutes plus overnight soak
COOK TIME: 2 hours 10 minutes to 3 hours 10 minutes

Makes 8 servings

More flavorful than white kidney beans (cannellini), red beans are most often seen in chili con carne and red beans and rice. You can use 3 cups drained and rinsed canned beans if you don't want to take the time to cook dried beans.

¼ cup extravirgin olive oil plus more for serving
1 medium carrot, peeled and chopped
1 medium onion, chopped
1 tablespoon tomato paste
4 sprigs fresh thyme
4 sprigs fresh parsley
1 bay leaf
2 quarts Vegetable or Chicken Stock (Chapter 1)
1 cup dried red kidney beans, soaked overnight in
   water and drained
8 plum tomatoes, skinned, seeded, and chopped
salt and freshly ground pepper to taste
2 cups grated Asiago or Manchego cheese
   for serving

1. Heat the oil in a 3-quart saucepan over medium heat. Add the carrot and onion and sauté until softened, about 5 minutes. Add the tomato paste and sauté until rust colored. Tie the thyme, parsley, and bay leaf together with cotton kitchen string. Add the herb bundle, stock, beans, and half the tomatoes. Heat to boiling over medium-high heat. Reduce the heat, cover, and simmer until the beans are tender, 2 to 3 hours.

2. To serve: Season the soup with salt and pepper. Discard the herb bundle. Ladle the soup into warmed soup bowls, drizzle with olive oil, and sprinkle with the remaining tomatoes and plenty of cheese.

Each serving: About 260 calories, 14 g protein, 19 g carbohydrate, 15 g total fat (5 g saturated), 20 mg cholesterol, 348 mg sodium.

Cabbage Bean Soup with Rivels

PREP TIME: 10 minutes
COOK TIME: 30 minutes

Makes 6 servings

Rivels are small chunks of homemade pasta or very tiny dumplings. Flavor the rivels by sprinkling them with finely chopped fresh basil or another herb.

Rivels
1 cup all-purpose flour
2 tablespoons milk
1 egg, beaten

4 cups water or Vegetable Stock (page 15)
5 cups shredded green cabbage
1⅓ cups shredded carrots
2 tablespoons bacon bits
1 tablespoon vegetable bouillon granules
1 tablespoon cider vinegar
1 teaspoon caraway seeds
1 large onion, chopped
1 medium apple, cored and coarsely chopped
1 can (about 15 ounces) Great Northern beans, rinsed
salt and pepper to taste

1. To make the rivels, in a bowl, using a fork or pastry blender, combine the flour, milk, and egg until coarse crumbs (about the size of raisins) form. Set aside.

2. In a 6-quart pot, combine the water, cabbage, carrots, bacon bits, bouillon granules, vinegar, caraway seeds, onion, apple, and beans. Bring to a boil, then reduce to a simmer, partly cover, and cook for about 5 minutes.

3. Sprinkle in the rivels, stirring to separate them, and cover the pot again. Continue to simmer for about 20 minutes or until the vegetables are tender.

4. Turn off the heat, and add salt and pepper to taste. Serve immediately.

Each serving: About 226 calories, 10 g protein, 42 g carbohydrate, 2 g total fat (trace saturated), 31 mg cholesterol, 397 mg sodium.

Bean, Escarole, and Ravioli Soup

PREP TIME: 10 minutes
COOK TIME: about 20 minutes

Makes 8 servings

To make ahead, prepare the soup without the ravioli, cover, and refrigerate. When ready to serve, reheat the soup while cooking the ravioli in a separate saucepan of boiling water. Drain the ravioli and add it to the soup.

  4 ounces pancetta, diced
  2 medium garlic cloves, thinly sliced
  ¼ teaspoon crushed red-pepper flakes
  4 cups Chicken Stock (page 14)
  1 package (7 ounces) refrigerated small ravioli
    (any filling)
  4 cups washed and coarsely chopped escarole
    or chicory
  1 can (16 ounces) white beans (Great Northern or
    navy), rinsed and drained
  1 medium yellow bell pepper, seeded and diced
  1 can (28 ounces) Italian plum tomatoes
  grated Parmigiano-Reggiano cheese for serving

1. Sauté the pancetta in a 3-quart saucepan over medium heat until the fat has rendered and the pancetta is crisp but not dry, about 3 minutes. Transfer the pancetta to a plate with a slotted spoon. Add the garlic and pepper flakes to the drippings and sauté 1 minute. Add the stock and heat to boiling.

2. Stir the ravioli into the stock and cook according to package directions until not quite al dente. Add the escarole, beans, and bell pepper. Add the tomatoes and their liquid, squeezing the tomatoes with your hand to break into bite-size chunks. Heat soup until simmering. Ladle into warmed soup bowls and sprinkle each serving with the cooked pancetta and cheese.

Each serving: About 265 calories, 14 g protein, 28 g carbohydrate, 18 g total fat (5 g saturated), 17 mg cholesterol, 519 mg sodium.

Pigeon Pea Soup with Cornmeal Dumplings

PREP TIME: 15 minutes
COOK TIME: 2 hours 10 minutes

Makes 8 to 10 servings

Native to Africa, pigeon peas are a flavorful legume popular in the Caribbean and the American South.

1 pound dried pigeon peas, soaked in water overnight
1 smoked ham hock
2 cups peeled, ½-inch cubes pumpkin or other winter squash
2 quarts water
2 tablespoons unsalted butter
2 celery stalks, finely chopped
1 medium onion, chopped
1 garlic clove, crushed through a press
1 pound sweet potatoes or yam, peeled and cut into bite-size cubes
1 can (14 ounces) diced tomatoes
½ teaspoon dried thyme leaves
½ teaspoon salt or more to taste
¼ teaspoon freshly ground pepper or more to taste

Dumplings
1 cup all-purpose flour
¼ cup cornmeal
1 teaspoon sugar
¼ teaspoon salt
⅛ teaspoon freshly ground black pepper
1 tablespoon vegetable oil
3 tablespoons milk or water plus more if needed

1. Drain and rinse the peas and place in a 6-quart pot. Add the ham hock, pumpkin, and water and heat to boiling over medium-high heat. Simmer, partially covered, until tender, about 2 hours.

2. While the beans cook, melt the butter in a 3-quart saucepan over medium heat. Add the celery, onion, and garlic and sauté until softened, about 5 minutes. Add the sweet potatoes, tomatoes with their juice, thyme, salt, and pepper and heat to boiling. Simmer, partially covered, until the sweet potatoes are tender, about 40 minutes.

3. When the beans are tender, add the sweet-potato mixture and mix well. Heat to a gentle boil. Taste and add more salt and pepper if necessary.

4. Make the dumplings: Mix the flour, cornmeal, sugar, salt, and pepper in a small bowl. Make a well in the center and add the oil and milk. Stir and add more milk, 1 tablespoon at a time, until the dough is soft enough to form a spoonable batter.

5. To serve: Drop the batter by scant tablespoonfuls into the soup. Cook, partially covered, until firm, about 5 minutes. Ladle into warmed soup bowls.

Each of 8 servings: About 485 calories, 24 g protein, 74 g carbohydrate, 11 g total fat (4 g saturated), 31 mg cholesterol, 679 mg sodium.

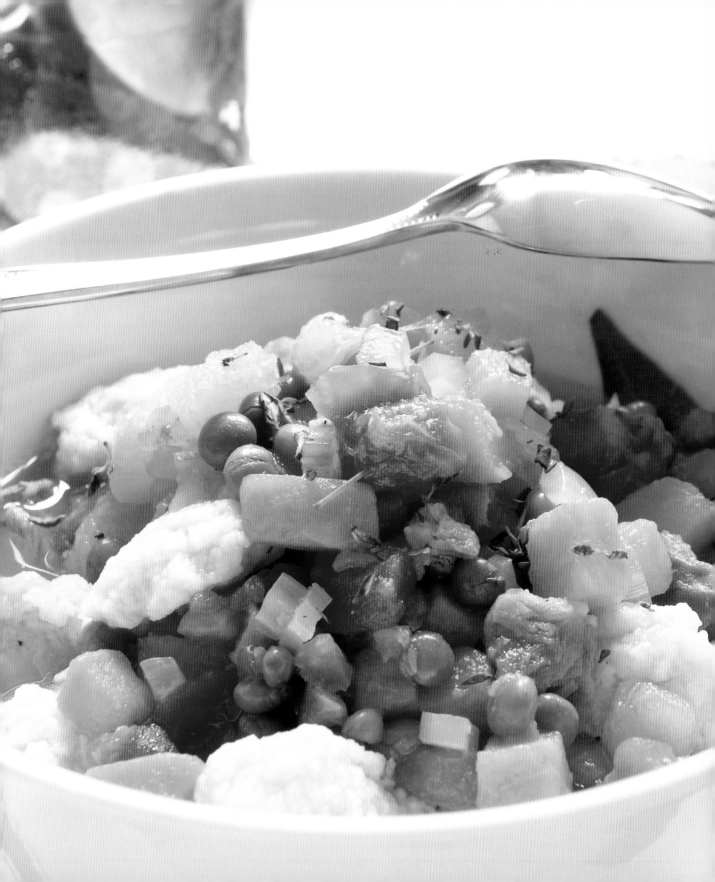

Spicy Pinto Bean Soup

PREP TIME: 15 minutes
COOK TIME: 45 minutes

Makes 6 servings

One of the more flavorful beans, pintos are pretty, too, with reddish streaks on the pale pink skin. They are aptly named pinto, which is Spanish for "painted."

1 tablespoon olive oil
1 medium onion, chopped
1 large garlic clove, crushed
1 tablespoon Mexican chili powder
1 teaspoon ground cumin
2 cans (about 16 ounces each) pinto beans, drained and rinsed, or 4 cups cooked pinto beans from soaked, dried beans
1 quart Chicken Stock (page 14)
salt to taste
½ cup sour cream
1 tablespoon fresh lime juice
1 tablespoon tequila (optional)
¼ cup toasted pine nuts, chopped, for serving
2 thin scallions, thinly sliced crosswise, for serving
2 tablespoons chopped fresh cilantro for serving
2 tablespoons diced red bell pepper for serving

1. Heat the oil in a 3-quart saucepan over medium-high heat. Add the onion and sauté until softened, about 5 minutes. Add the garlic and sauté 1 minute. Add the chili powder and cumin and stir until blended. Add the beans and stock and heat to boiling. Reduce the heat to medium and simmer, partially covered, 30 minutes.

2. Drain the soup through a colander placed over another 3-quart saucepan. In batches, puree the solids from the colander in a food processor or blender, adding enough cooking liquid to make it easier to puree. Pour the puree into the pan with the cooking liquid and whisk until smooth. Taste and season with salt. Heat until simmering.

3. To serve: Whisk the sour cream with the lime juice and tequila (if using) until smooth in a bowl. Ladle the soup into warmed soup bowls. Drizzle with the sour-cream mixture and flick a skewer through the cream to swirl it decoratively. Sprinkle each serving with pine nuts, scallions, cilantro, and red bell pepper.

Each serving: About 243 calories, 11 g protein, 34 g carbohydrate, 7 g total fat (3 g saturated), 7 mg cholesterol, 219 mg sodium.

Chickpea and Spinach Soup

PREP TIME: **5 minutes**
COOK TIME: **30 minutes**

Makes 4 servings

1 tablespoon unsalted butter
1 large yellow onion, chopped
4 small garlic cloves, minced
1 cup milk
1 can (16 ounces) chickpeas, drained and rinsed
4 to 5 cups fresh spinach, shredded
1 teaspoon curry powder
¼ teaspoon turmeric
⅛ teaspoon cardamom powder
⅛ teaspoon ground nutmeg
salt and pepper to taste

1. Melt the butter in a 4-quart pot and sauté the onion and garlic until the onion is translucent. Stir in the milk and bring to a boil. Reduce to a simmer and add the chickpeas, spinach, curry powder, turmeric, cardamom, and nutmeg. Cook, stirring occasionally, about 15 minutes.

2. Transfer about 1½ cups of the soup to a blender and puree until smooth. Return to the pot and heat through. Season to taste with salt and pepper and serve immediately.

Each serving: About 278 calories, 15 g protein, 43 g carbohydrate, 5 g total fat (2 g saturated), 10 mg cholesterol, 1,273 mg sodium.

Indian Tomato Lentil Soup

PREP TIME: 5 minutes
COOK TIME: 35 minutes

Makes 4 servings

2 tablespoons olive oil
1 medium red onion, chopped
4 cups Vegetable Stock (page 15)
1 can (16 ounces) chopped tomatoes
1 package (12 ounces) dried red lentils, rinsed and drained
1 teaspoon ground coriander
¾ teaspoon turmeric
¾ teaspoon ground cumin
light pinch curry powder
pinch ground cloves
salt and pepper to taste

1. Heat the oil in a saucepan or soup kettle and sauté the onion until translucent. Add the stock, tomatoes, lentils, coriander, turmeric, cumin, curry powder, and cloves. Bring to a boil. Reduce to a simmer, cover lightly, and cook, stirring, 20 to 30 minutes, or until the lentils are very tender.

2. Remove from the heat and puree in batches in a blender or food processor. Return to the saucepan and heat through. Taste and season with salt and pepper if needed.

Each serving: About 427 calories, 25 g protein, 62 g carbohydrate, 9 g total fat (1 g saturated), 0 mg cholesterol, 995 mg sodium.

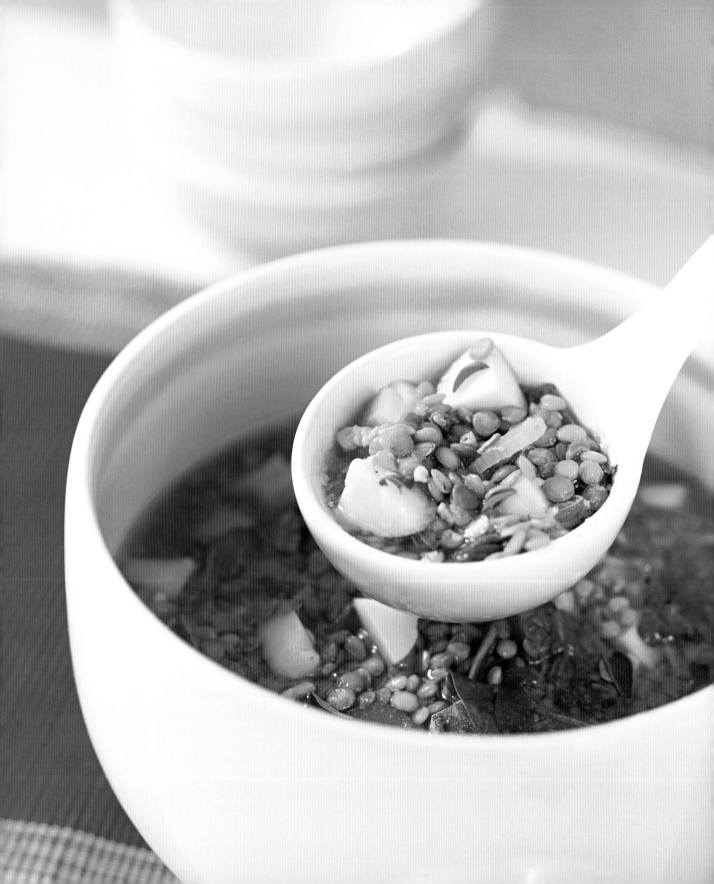

Lentil Soup with Prosciutto

PREP TIME: 5 minutes
COOK TIME: 10 minutes plus standing

Makes 4 servings

Prosciutto and Provolone cheese provide the pizzazz that sets this singular soup apart. Lentils don't have to be soaked before they're cooked. If you skip that step, simply increase the cooking time by 30 to 45 minutes.

1 cup dried lentils
3½ cups Beef Stock (page 15)
1 medium red potato, diced
1 medium onion, chopped
2 stalks celery, sliced
2 garlic cloves, crushed through a press
2 ounces thinly sliced prosciutto, chopped
¼ teaspoon freshly ground black pepper
1 cup packed torn fresh spinach
⅓ cup reduced-sodium Provolone cheese, shredded
salt and pepper to taste
2 tablespoons fresh oregano leaves for garnish

1. Fill a 6-quart pot with water. Add the lentils. Cover and bring to a boil. Reduce the heat and simmer 3 minutes. Remove from the heat and let sit for 30 to 60 minutes.

2. Drain the lentils, and return them to the pot. Stir in the stock, potato, onion, celery, garlic, prosciutto, and pepper. Cover and bring to a boil. Reduce the heat, and simmer until the lentils and potatoes are tender, 12 to 15 minutes.

3. Stir in the spinach and cheese. Taste and season with salt and pepper if needed. Top each serving with oregano.

Each serving: About 337 calories, 27 g protein, 43 g carbohydrate, 7 g total fat (1 g saturated), 21 mg cholesterol, 1,575 mg sodium.

Lentil and Chickpea Soup

PREP TIME: 10 minutes
COOK TIME: 50 minutes to 1 hour

Makes 6 servings

You can buy pappadoms, the wafer-thin breads made from lentil flour, in East Indian grocery stores. When they are fried in hot oil, they puff to disks twice their original size.

3 tablespoons olive oil
3 medium onions, chopped
2 celery stalks, thinly sliced
1 bag (8 ounces) peeled baby carrots, cut into thirds
1 small garlic clove, minced
1 teaspoon ground coriander
1 teaspoon ground cumin
½ teaspoon hot Madras curry powder
¼ teaspoon ground cardamom
3-inch cinnamon stick
1 cup dried lentils, washed and picked over
4 cups Vegetable Stock (page 15) or water
2 cups cooked chickpeas from soaked, dried chickpeas or 1 can (about 16 ounces) chickpeas, rinsed
salt to taste
⅓ cup toasted chopped cashews for serving
fried pappadoms or Indian bread such as naan for serving

1. Heat the oil in a 3-quart saucepan over medium-high heat. Add the onions and sauté until soft but not browned, about 7 minutes. Add the celery and carrots and sauté until softened, about 3 minutes. Add the garlic and sauté 1 minute. Add the coriander, cumin, curry powder, and cardamom and sauté until fragrant, about 2 minutes. Add the cinnamon stick, lentils, and stock and heat to boiling. Reduce the heat to medium-low, cover, and simmer until the lentils are tender but not mushy, 35 to 45 minutes. (Taste the lentils at 35 minutes.)

2. Stir the chickpeas into the soup and heat through. Taste and season with salt as needed. Ladle the soup into warmed soup bowls and sprinkle with cashews. Serve with pappadoms.

Each serving without pappadoms or bread: About 343 calories, 16 g protein, 45 g carbohydrate, 12 g total fat (2 g saturated), 0 mg cholesterol, 275 mg sodium.

Red Lentils in Coconut-Curry Broth

PREP TIME: 10 minutes
COOK TIME: 20 minutes

Makes 6 servings

Curry pastes (found in Asian grocery stores) have more "life" to them than
curry powder. They'll keep indefinitely in the refrigerator.

1 tablespoon red curry paste
2 teaspoons vegetable oil
1 quart Chicken or Vegetable Stock (Chapter 1)
1 can (about 14 ounces) unsweetened coconut milk
1 cup red lentils
1 cup peeled baby carrots, quartered lengthwise
4 kaffir lime leaves, shredded
1 cup snow peas, stings removed
1 can (about 14 ounces) baby corn, drained and rinsed
1 teaspoon sugar or more to taste
¼ teaspoon salt or more to taste

1. Heat the curry paste and oil in a 2-quart saucepan over medium-low
   heat until sizzling, about 2 minutes. Whisk in a little of the stock until
   blended. Add the remaining stock, the coconut milk, lentils, carrots, and
   lime leaves and heat to boiling over medium heat. Simmer, partially covered and stirring occasionally, until the lentils and carrots are softened,
   about 10 minutes.

2. Add the snow peas, corn, sugar, and salt and simmer until the snow
   peas are tender, about 5 minutes. Taste and adjust the seasonings if
   necessary.

Each serving: About 357 calories, 15 g protein, 38 g carbohydrate, 18 g total fat
(13 g saturated), 0 mg cholesterol, 137 mg sodium.

Black-Eyed Pea and Corn Soup

PREP TIME: 5 minutes
COOK TIME: 30 minutes

Makes 4 servings

Here's a hearty, homey soup that's high in flavor and low in fat.

   4 slices smoked bacon
   2 cups Chicken Stock (page 14)
   1 can (15 ounces) black-eyed peas, rinsed and drained
   1 can (14 ounces) cream-style corn
   1 cup chopped red onions
   4 garlic cloves
   1 teaspoon dried thyme
   ¼ teaspoon white pepper
   1 cup roasted red peppers
   salt to taste
   ¼ cup chopped fresh parsley for garnish

1. Cook the bacon in a 3-quart saucepan over medium-high heat until browned. Transfer to a paper towel–lined plate to drain.

2. Add the stock, black-eyed peas, corn, onion, garlic, thyme, and white pepper to the saucepan. Cover and bring to a boil. Reduce the heat and simmer 15 minutes to blend the flavors.

3. Stir in the roasted peppers and heat the soup for 1 minute more. Taste and season with salt if needed. Crumble the bacon. Top each serving of soup with bacon and parsley.

Each serving: About 245 calories, 19 g protein, 39 g carbohydrate, 2 g total fat (1 g saturated), 25 mg cholesterol, 1,326 mg sodium.

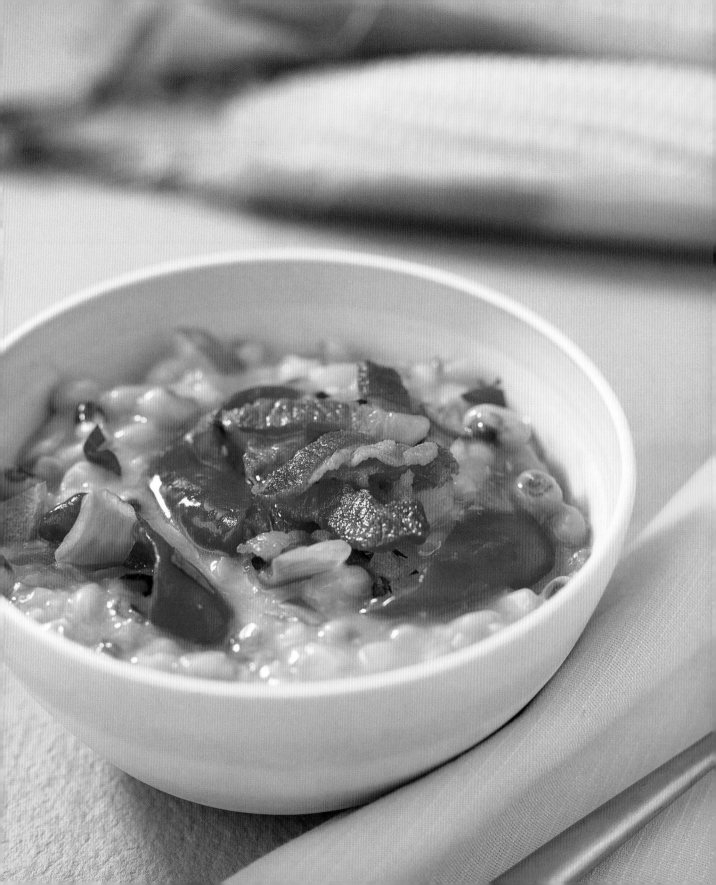

Yellow Split-Pea Soup with Canadian Bacon and Whiskey

PREP TIME: 15 minutes
COOK TIME: 1 hour 15 minutes

Makes 6 servings

Here's a salute to our northern neighbors, using ingredients from or in the style of Canada. It's a bowl of instant warmth. You can, of course, use green split peas instead of yellow.

1 pound dried yellow split peas
2 quarts cold water
4 tablespoons unsalted butter
2 slender carrots, peeled and cut into thin rounds
2 small turnips, peeled and diced
1 medium red onion, finely chopped
8 ounces Canadian bacon, trimmed and diced
2 tablespoons chopped fresh Italian parsley
2 tablespoons fresh lemon juice
2 tablespoons Canadian whiskey or more to taste
salt and freshly ground pepper to taste

1. Rinse the split peas and pick through for any stones. Place the peas and water in a 4-quart saucepan and heat to boiling over medium-high heat. Reduce the heat to low and simmer, partially covered and stirring occasionally, for 40 minutes.

2. While the peas cook, melt the butter in a 10-inch skillet over medium heat. Add the carrots, turnips, and onion and sauté until softened, about 10 minutes. Add the bacon and sauté until sizzling, about 2 minutes.

3. When the peas have cooked for 40 minutes, stir in the bacon mixture. Cook, partially covered, until the peas are soft, about 30 minutes longer. To serve, stir the parsley, lemon juice, and whiskey into the soup and season with salt and pepper. Ladle into warmed soup bowls.

Each serving: About 407 calories, 26 g protein, 52 g carbohydrate, 11 g total fat (6 g saturated), 39 mg cholesterol, 611 mg sodium.

Quick Fava Bean Soup

PREP TIME: 5 minutes
COOK TIME: 20 minutes

Makes 4 servings

Buttery-tasting fava beans and fresh tomatoes steal the show in this robust
shortcut soup.

   1 teaspoon olive oil
   1 medium onion, chopped
   4 garlic cloves
   1 can (14 ounces) fava beans, rinsed and drained
   1 medium yellow summer squash, chopped
   2¾ cups Beef Stock (page 15)
   2 cups diced plum tomatoes
   4 ounces Canadian bacon, chopped
   1 teaspoon Italian herb seasoning
   1 teaspoon red wine vinegar
   salt and pepper to taste

Heat the oil in a 6-quart pot over medium-high heat. Add the onion and
garlic and sauté until the onion is golden. Add the beans, squash, stock,
tomatoes, bacon, herb seasoning, and vinegar. Cover and bring to a
boil. Reduce the heat and simmer until the squash is tender, about
15 minutes. Taste and season with salt and pepper if needed.

Each serving: About 240 calories, 19 g protein, 32 g carbohydrate, 6 g total fat
(2 g saturated), 15 mg cholesterol, 970 mg sodium.

Bean Lover's Soup

PREP TIME: 10 minutes plus standing
COOK TIME: 1 hour 20 minutes

Makes 8 servings

16 ounces bean soup mix (mixed beans)
3½ cups Beef Stock (page 15)
2 cups water
2 carrots, peeled and sliced
2 cups torn fresh spinach
2 ounces deli baked ham, cut into ¼-inch cubes
1 teaspoon chopped fresh tarragon leaves
½ teaspoon lemon pepper
salt to taste
paprika for garnish
fresh parsley sprigs for garnish

> ### OVERNIGHT SOAK
> - If you can plan ahead, soak the beans in cold water in the refrigerator overnight; then you won't need the soak in hot water in step 1.

1. Rinse the beans and sort through them to remove any debris. Place the beans in an 8-quart pot and add 6 cups water. Cover the pot and bring the water to a boil. Simmer for 3 minutes and remove the pot from the heat. Let sit for 1 hour. Drain the beans and return them to the pot.

2. Add the stock, 2 cups water, carrots, spinach, ham, tarragon, and lemon pepper. Cover and bring to a boil. Reduce the heat and simmer until the beans are tender, about 1¼ hours.

3. Transfer half the soup to a bowl. Using a handheld immersion blender, puree the soup in the pot. Return the reserved soup to the pot. Heat the soup throughout, about 5 minutes; do not boil. Taste and season with salt if needed. Top each serving with the paprika and parsley.

Each serving: About 233 calories, 16 g protein, 40 g carbohydrate, trace total fat (trace saturated), 3 mg cholesterol, 698 mg sodium.

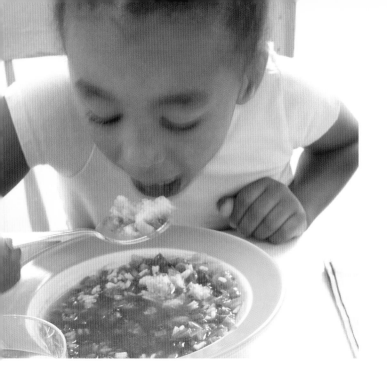

7

SEAFOOD SOUPS

Orange Roughy and Carrot Soup

PREP TIME: 5 minutes
COOK TIME: 40 minutes

Makes 6 servings

In this enticing soup, a hint of orange makes for a perfect complement to orange roughy. Pureed carrots and diced red pepper complete the flavor balance while giving the dish its eye-catching color. If you can't find orange roughy, substitute another white-fleshed flatfish, such as flounder.

2 slices turkey bacon
1 large onion, chopped
3 cups clam juice
2 carrots, peeled and chopped
2 large potatoes, cut into ½-inch cubes
1 red bell pepper, seeded and chopped
2 teaspoons grated orange zest
½ teaspoon lemon pepper
1 pound orange roughy fillets, cut into
   bite-size pieces
1 cup 2% milk
salt to taste

1. Cook the bacon in a 6-quart pot over medium-high heat until browned and crisp. Transfer to a paper towel–lined plate to drain.

2. Add the onion to the pot and sauté until translucent, about 5 minutes. Stir in the clam juice, carrots, and potatoes. Cover and bring to a boil. Reduce the heat and simmer until the potatoes are tender, about 12 minutes.

3. Using a potato masher, mash the mixture. Bring to a simmer and stir in the bell pepper, orange zest, and lemon pepper. Add the orange roughy, and cook, covered, until it is cooked through, 3 to 5 minutes.

4. Stir in the milk and heat the soup through, about 2 minutes. Taste and season with salt if needed. Crumble the bacon and top each serving with it.

Each serving: About 222 calories, 18 g protein, 32 g carbohydrate, 3 g total fat (1 g saturated), 22 mg cholesterol, 307 mg sodium.

Salmon Wonton Soup

PREP TIME: 25 minutes
COOK TIME: about 20 minutes

Makes 4 servings

When cooking the wontons, a little cold water is added to the boiling water to "shock" the wontons. This trick cooks the wontons quickly without hard boiling, which might break them apart.

Wontons

8 ounces diced skinless salmon fillet
1 small onion, finely chopped
1 tablespoon grated peeled fresh gingerroot
1 tablespoon minced fresh cilantro
1 tablespoon soy sauce
36 to 48 wonton wrappers (more or less, depending on how stuffed you make them)

3 cups Asian Shrimp Stock (page 21) or Basic Fish Stock (page 16) made with salmon bones
1 cup baby spinach or arugula
2 teaspoons minced scallions
2 teaspoons dark sesame oil
2 teaspoons soy sauce
¼ teaspoon ground white pepper

1. Make the wontons: Combine the salmon, onion, ginger, cilantro, and soy sauce in a bowl and mix well. For each wonton, place a wrapper with the points arranged like a compass (north, south, east, and west) on the work surface and brush lightly with water. Spoon about a teaspoon of filling in the middle, just below the center. Fold the south corner up and over the filling (not onto the wrapper) and roll towards the center, leaving about 1 inch of the north corner of the wrapper unrolled. Press lightly around the sides of the filling to seal but be sure to get the air out first. Brush the east corner with water and fold it over the west corner to seal like a tortellini. As you work, set the finished wontons aside on a baking sheet and cover with a dry kitchen towel.

2. Heat 2 quarts water to boiling in a 4-quart saucepan over high heat. Add the wontons and return to the boil. Add ½ cup cold water and heat to boiling. Add another ½ cup cold water. Continue to cook wontons until they float to the surface. Drain and keep warm.

3. To serve: Heat the stock to boiling in a 1-quart saucepan, add the spinach and cook until wilted, about 1 minute. Divide the stock, wontons, scallions, sesame oil, soy sauce, and pepper among four warmed soup bowls.

Each serving based on 36 wrappers: About 338 calories, 20 g protein, 45 g carbohydrate, 8 g total fat (1 g saturated), 42 mg cholesterol, 874 mg sodium.

Catfish and Tomato Gumbo

PREP TIME: 10 minutes
COOK TIME: 35 to 45 minutes

Makes 8 servings

For a shrimp gumbo, use 2 pounds peeled deveined shrimp instead of catfish and Shrimp Stock (page 20) for part or all of the fish stock.

½ cup vegetable oil
1 cup all-purpose flour
1 pound okra, cut crosswise into ½-inch-wide rounds
1 large yellow onion, finely chopped
1 green bell pepper, seeded and finely chopped
1 stalk celery with leaves, finely chopped
3 large garlic cloves, finely chopped
2 tablespoons unsalted butter
1 can (35 ounces) crushed Italian tomatoes
½ cup coarsely chopped fresh Italian parsley
3 bay leaves
1 tablespoon chopped fresh thyme leaves (no stems)
4 fresh basil leaves, slivered
8 cups Basic Fish Stock (page 16) or water, heated to boiling
1 cup dry white wine
juice of 1 lemon
2 pounds skinless catfish fillets, cut into 1-inch pieces
½ cup finely chopped scallions
cayenne pepper to taste
salt to taste
4 cups cooked long-grain white rice for serving

1. Heat the oil in a heavy-bottomed 5-quart saucepan or enamel-lined Dutch oven until smoking. Add the flour and stir until blended. Cook, stirring constantly, until the mixture is smooth and straw colored, about 3 minutes. Stir in the okra, onion, bell pepper, celery, and garlic. Reduce the heat to medium and stir in the butter. Cook, stirring constantly, until the vegetables begin to soften, about 5 minutes.

2. Stir in the tomatoes with their liquid, the parsley, bay leaves, thyme, and basil. Stir in the stock, wine, and lemon juice and simmer until the gumbo has thickened, 20 to 30 minutes. Add the fish, scallions, and cayenne and stir gently until mixed well. Cook until the fish layers separate when gently prodded with a fork, 2 minutes. Taste and season with salt. Discard the bay leaves. To serve: Ladle the gumbo into large bowls and pass the rice at the table.

Each serving: About 501 calories, 26 g protein, 50 g carbohydrate, 21 g total fat (4 g saturated), 74 mg cholesterol, 179 mg sodium.

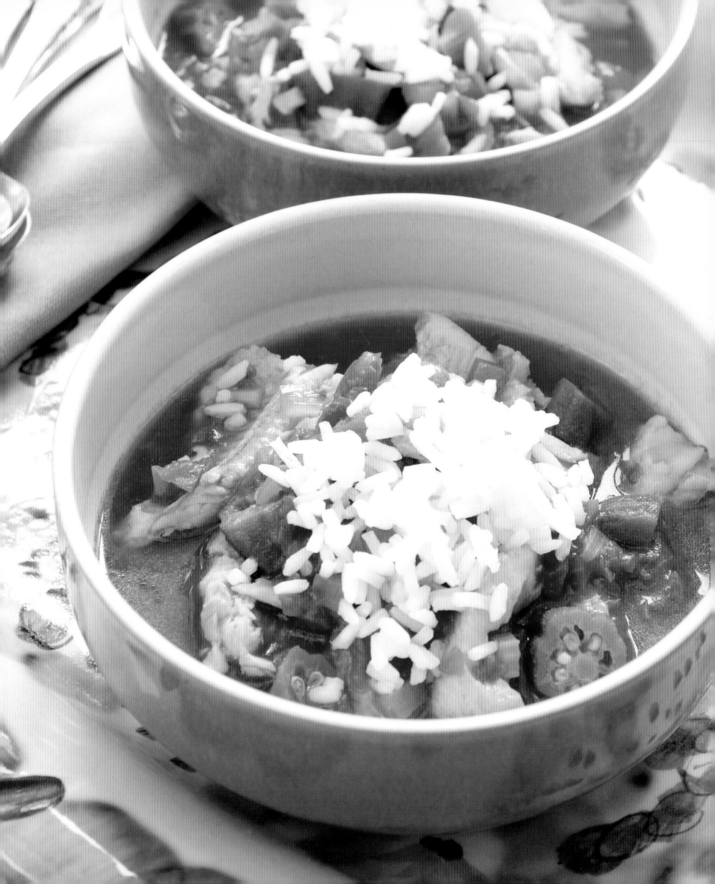

Shrimp Gumbolaya

PREP TIME: 15 minutes
COOK TIME: 1 hour 25 minutes

Makes 8 servings

This is a soup version of a marriage of jambalaya, the classic Creole ham-seafood-rice casserole, and gumbo, another Louisiana dish of shellfish (or meat), okra, and tomatoes.

2 tablespoons vegetable oil
8 ounces spicy smoked sausage (preferably andouille or kielbasa), skinned, cut into ½-inch cubes
8 ounces smoked ham, cut into ½-inch cubes
1 large red onion, finely chopped
6 large scallions, including fresh, tender green portion, chopped
2 large celery stalks, chopped
1 red bell pepper, seeded and chopped
1 green bell pepper, seeded and chopped
1 yellow bell pepper, seeded and chopped
3 cloves garlic, minced
½ cup all-purpose flour
1 can (about 15 ounces) diced tomatoes with green chiles
5 to 6 cups Spicy Shrimp Stock (page 20), or 6 cups Shrimp Stock (page 20) plus 1 tablespoon Maryland- or New Orleans–style seafood seasoning
1 pound okra, cut crosswise into ½-inch pieces
1½ pounds shrimp, shelled and deveined
4 cups cooked long-grain white rice for serving
4 basil leaves, slivered, for garnish

1. Heat the oil in a 4-quart saucepan over medium-high heat until hot. Add the sausage and ham and sauté until lightly browned, about 5 minutes. Transfer to a bowl with a slotted spoon. Add the onion, scallions, celery, and bell peppers to the fat in the pan and sauté over medium heat until softened, about 5 minutes. Add the garlic and cook 1 minute. Add the flour and cook, stirring, until the flour browns, about 10 minutes.

2. Add the tomatoes with their juice; stir until the juices are blended with the flour. Gradually stir in 1 cup stock. Add the remaining stock and the okra; heat to boiling. Reduce the heat and simmer, stirring occasionally, 45 minutes. Add the sausage, ham, and shrimp and cook just until the shrimp are pink and cooked through, about 3 minutes.

3. To serve: Ladle the gumbo into shallow bowls and add a spoonful of rice to each bowl. Sprinkle with the basil.

Each serving: About 454 calories, 32 g protein, 44 g carbohydrate, 17 g total fat (5 g saturated), 165 mg cholesterol, 980 mg sodium.

Shrimp-Rice Soup

PREP TIME: 5 minutes
COOK TIME: 45 minutes

Makes 4 servings

A generous splash of lime gives this simple soup a refreshing twist.

3½ cups Chicken Stock (page 14)
1 small onion, finely chopped
1 celery stalk, thinly sliced
¼ cup uncooked brown rice
½ pound medium shrimp, shelled, deveined, and cut into thirds
1 tablespoon grated lime zest
juice of 1 lime
⅛ teaspoon crushed red pepper flakes
salt and freshly ground black pepper to taste

1. Combine the stock, onion, celery, and rice in a 6-quart pot. Cover and bring to a boil. Reduce the heat and simmer until the rice is tender, about 40 minutes.

2. Stir in the shrimp and simmer until they are pink and cooked through, about 5 minutes. Stir in the lime zest, lime juice, and pepper flakes. Taste and season with salt and black pepper if needed.

Each serving: About 139 calories, 18 g protein, 12 g carbohydrate, 1 g total fat (trace saturated), 86 mg cholesterol, 234 mg sodium.

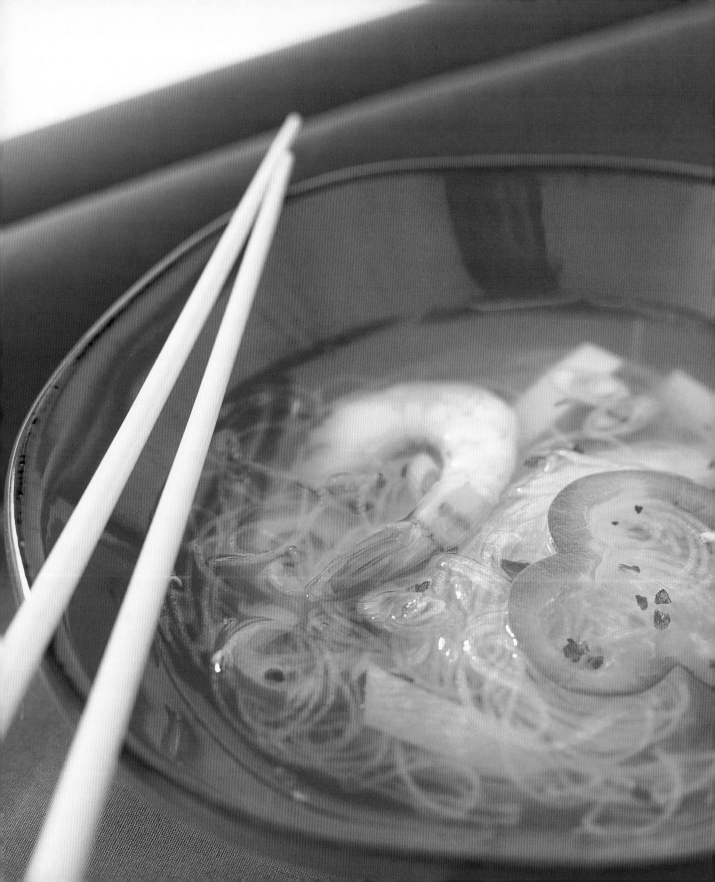

Szechuan Shrimp Soup with Cellophane Noodles

PREP TIME: 5 minutes
COOK TIME: 20 minutes

Makes 4 servings

Got a yen for something slightly spicy? Chinese chili sauce and five-spice powder give this quick soup just the right Chinese character and zest. If you can't find cellophane noodles, substitute bean threads or rice sticks.

4 ounces cellophane noodles, broken into short pieces
3½ cups Vegetable Stock (page 15)
¼ cup rice wine vinegar
2 tablespoons Chinese chili sauce with garlic
½ pound large shrimp, peeled and deveined
½ (4-ounce) can sliced bamboo shoots, drained
1 cup sliced scallions
1 red bell pepper, seeded and cut into thin rings
¼ teaspoon Chinese five-spice powder
salt and pepper to taste

1. Fill a 3-quart saucepan with water. Warm it over medium-high heat until hot but not boiling. Add the noodles. Soak for 10 minutes and drain.

2. Combine the stock, vinegar, and chili sauce in a 6-quart pot. Cover and bring to a boil. Add the shrimp, bamboo shoots, scallions, pepper, and five-spice powder. Cover and bring to a boil. Reduce the heat and simmer 2 to 3 minutes. Stir in the noodles. Simmer until the shrimp are cooked through, about 3 minutes more. Taste and season with salt and pepper if needed.

Each serving: About 305 calories, 18 g protein, 58 g carbohydrate, 2 g total fat (trace saturated), 86 mg cholesterol, 1,574 mg sodium.

Teriyaki Scallop Soup

PREP TIME: 5 minutes
COOK TIME: 25 minutes

Makes 4 servings

Here's a light and delightful Asian-style soup with an unforgettable balance of complex flavors—snow peas and scallops seasoned with gingerroot, garlic, teriyaki sauce, and Marsala. Take care not to overcook scallops or they will become tough and rubbery; they're done when they are opaque from top to bottom.

2 cups water
2 cups Vegetable Stock (page 15)
1 tablespoon grated fresh gingerroot
4 garlic cloves, crushed through a press
1 tablespoon Marsala wine
2 teaspoons teriyaki sauce
1 teaspoon peanut oil
¼ pound snow peas, strings removed
1 pound bay scallops
2 scallions, sliced
¼ teaspoon lemon pepper
salt to taste

1. Combine the water, stock, gingerroot, and garlic in a 6-quart pot. Cover and bring to a boil. Reduce the heat and simmer 15 minutes.

2. Stir in the Marsala, teriyaki sauce, and oil. Cover and return to a boil. Add the snow peas, and cook for 1 minute. Stir in the scallops, scallions, and lemon pepper and simmer until the peas are crisp and tender and the scallops are done, about 3 minutes. Taste and season with salt if needed.

Each serving: About 160 calories, 22 g protein, 14 g carbohydrate, 2 g total fat (trace saturated), 37 mg cholesterol, 544 mg sodium.

Scallop Soup St. Jacques

PREP TIME: 15 minutes
COOK TIME: 40 minutes

Makes 4 to 6 servings

This memorable starter incorporates the elements in *Coquilles St. Jacques*, the classic French appetizer of scallops poached in wine and combined with a rich cream sauce, then gratinéed in their shells. The scallop is linked to the apostle St. James (St. Jacques in French) by legend: It is said that St. James saved the life of a drowning knight, who emerged from the sea covered in scallop shells. Thereafter, crusading knights of the Order of St. James wore a scallop shell to signify their allegiance.

2 sprigs fresh thyme
1 small bay leaf
4 tablespoons unsalted butter
8 ounces sliced cremini or shiitake mushrooms
2 large leeks, split, rinsed and coarsely chopped
1 small garlic clove, minced
4 cups water
1 baking potato (8 ounces), peeled and coarsely chopped
½ teaspoon salt or more to taste
8 ounces bay scallops
2 egg yolks
½ cup heavy cream
2 tablespoons dry sherry or more to taste
freshly ground white pepper to taste
1 cup grated Gruyère cheese for serving

1. Tie the thyme and bay leaf together in a square of cheesecloth. Melt 2 tablespoons butter in a 2-quart saucepan over medium-high heat. Add the mushrooms and sauté until golden, about 5 minutes. Transfer to a bowl with a slotted spoon and set aside. Heat the remaining 2 tablespoons butter in the saucepan. Add the leeks and sauté until wilted, about 5 minutes. Add the garlic and sauté 1 minute. Add the herb packet, water, potato, and salt and heat to boiling. Cover and simmer over medium heat until the potato is falling apart, about 20 minutes.

2. Discard the herb packet. In batches, carefully puree the soup in a blender, holding down the top with a folded kitchen towel. Pour the puree into a 3-quart saucepan and heat to simmering over medium heat. Add the scallops and heat just until cooked through, about 5 minutes. Add the mushrooms to the soup.

3. Mix the egg yolks with the cream in a small bowl. Whisk a ladleful of hot soup into the yolk mixture and then whisk back into the soup. Heat the soup but do not let it boil or the egg yolks will curdle; stir until thickened. Stir in the sherry, taste, and season with additional salt if needed and pepper. Ladle into warmed bowls and sprinkle with some Gruyère.

Each of 4 servings: About 429 calories, 24 g protein, 22 g carbohydrate, 27 g total fat (15 g saturated), 197 mg cholesterol, 504 mg sodium.

Sherried Scallop Soup with Havarti

PREP TIME: 5 minutes
COOK TIME: 30 minutes

Makes 4 servings

This rich restaurant-style soup is easy enough to make at home and fast enough to prepare on weeknights.

2 cans (11 ounces each) clam juice
½ cup water
2 potatoes, peeled and cut into ½-inch cubes
1 medium onion, chopped
2 bay leaves
½ cup cream sherry
½ cup shredded creamy Havarti cheese
1 pound bay scallops
½ cup 2% milk
salt and pepper to taste
¼ cup snipped fresh chives for garnish

1. Combine the clam juice, water, potatoes, onion, and bay leaves in a 6-quart pot. Cover and bring to a boil. Reduce the heat and simmer until the potatoes are tender, 10 to 15 minutes. Discard the bay leaves.

2. Using a slotted spoon, transfer half the vegetables to a bowl. Add the sherry and Havarti to the pot. Using a handheld immersion blender, puree the mixture in the pot. Return the reserved vegetables to the pot.

3. Stir in the scallops. Cover the pot and just barely simmer until the scallops are cooked through, about 3 minutes (do not boil). Stir in the milk and heat through. Taste and season with salt and pepper if needed. Top each serving with chives.

Each serving: About 307 calories, 37 g protein, 14 g carbohydrate, 13 g total fat (trace saturated), 71 mg cholesterol, 1,619 mg sodium.

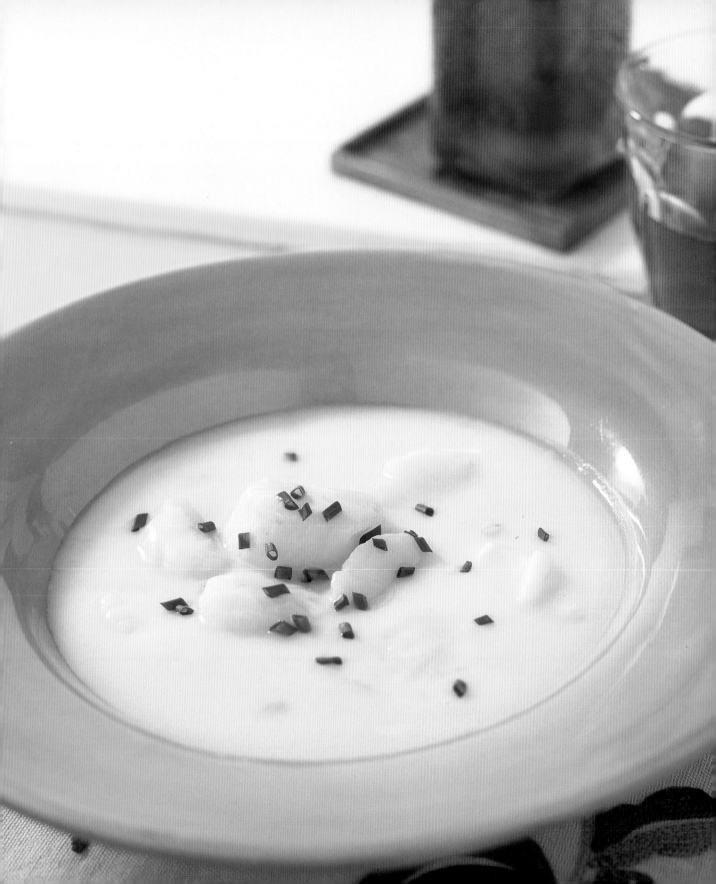

Crawfish and Fennel Soup

PREP TIME: 20 minutes
COOK TIME: about 30 minutes

Makes 6 servings

You can find many suppliers of fresh farm-raised crawfish online if your fish market doesn't carry them. Also look for frozen crawfish in your grocery store.

  4 tablespoons unsalted butter
  3 small fennel bulbs, fronds coarsely chopped, bulbs cored and thinly sliced
  1 large shallot, finely chopped
  3 cups Shrimp Stock or Basic Fish Stock (Chapter 1) or more if needed
  ½ teaspoon salt or more to taste
  freshly ground black pepper to taste
  1 pound fresh or parboiled crawfish tails (thaw if frozen)
  ½ cup heavy cream
  2 tablespoons herbsaint or other anise-flavored liqueur

1. Melt the butter in a 2-quart saucepan over medium-high heat. Add the sliced fennel bulbs and shallot and sauté until crisp-tender, about 7 minutes. Add 1 cup stock and the salt and heat to boiling. Reduce the heat to low, cover, and simmer until fennel is soft, about 10 minutes.

2. Transfer the soup to a food processor and wash the pan. Puree the soup and scrape it back into the clean pan. Add the remaining 2 cups stock and a few grindings of pepper; heat to boiling over medium-high heat. Add the crawfish with any liquid, the cream, and liqueur; stir well and thin with more stock if needed. Reduce the heat to and simmer just until the crawfish are cooked or heated through, about 2 minutes. Taste and adjust seasoning if necessary. Ladle soup into bowls and sprinkle with chopped fennel fronds.

Each serving: About 267 calories, 25 g protein, 13 g carbohydrate, 12 g total fat (7 g saturated), 190 mg cholesterol, 435 mg sodium.

Bergen Fish Soup

PREP TIME: 15 minutes
COOK TIME: about 15 minutes

Makes 6 servings

This classic Norwegian soup is usually a home-specific recipe, but cups of it are available in several variations from stands in the fish market in the harbor town of Bergen. The fish is cooked inside a cheesecloth bag so that the fish isn't smashed to smithereens.

6 cups Basic Fish Stock with Root Vegetables (page 17)
1 pound (1-inch-thick) skinless fish fillets such as haddock, halibut, or cod, or a mix, wrapped in cheesecloth and tied with cotton string
1 small carrot, peeled and finely chopped
1 small parsnip, peeled and finely chopped
1 small leek, white part only, split, rinsed, and thinly sliced
2 egg yolks
salt and freshly ground pepper to taste
2 tablespoons fresh chervil leaves or chopped Italian parsley for garnish

1. Combine the stock in a 3-quart saucepan with the fish, carrot, and parsnip. Heat to boiling; reduce the heat and simmer 6 minutes. Add the leek and simmer until tender, about 2 minutes. Remove the pan from the heat and lift the fish onto a plate. Untie and test the fish with a fork; it should separate easily into flakes. If not, tie up again and cook another 2 to 3 minutes. Transfer the fish to a plate, remove the cheesecloth, and separate into flakes.

2. Place the egg yolks in a medium bowl and pour in 1 ladle of hot soup in a thin stream, whisking until blended. Whisk the yolk mixture back into the soup. Add the fish and season with salt and pepper. Reheat the soup but do not let it boil or the egg yolks will curdle. Ladle the soup into bowls and sprinkle with chervil.

Each serving: About 122 calories, 16 g protein, 9 g carbohydrate, 3 g total fat (1 g saturated), 114 mg cholesterol, 259 mg sodium.

Ceviche Soup with Roasted Popcorn

PREP TIME: 15 minutes
COOK TIME: 5 minutes plus chilling

Makes 6 to 8 servings

Ceviche is a Latin American appetizer of fish (usually fillets) and shellfish (usually scallops and shrimp) that are marinated in a mixture of citrus juice and other seasonings. The marinade is acidic enough to "cook" the seafood, almost as if it were heated. In Ecuador and Peru, ceviche is traditionally served with fire-roasted popcorn.

¾ pound clean squid, cleaned,
2 tablespoons Spanish extravirgin olive oil (oil from arbequina olives is fruity and sweet)
¾ pound medium shrimp, shelled and deveined
¾ pound bay scallops
½ cup fresh lime juice
¼ cup fresh lemon juice
1 small Vidalia or other sweet onion, finely chopped
1 jalapeño pepper, seeded and minced (use rubber gloves when handling hot peppers)
1 garlic clove, crushed through a press
¼ cup minced fresh cilantro
2 cups canned petite-diced tomatoes, drained, or seeded, chopped, skinned fresh tomatoes
2 cups blood-orange juice
1 cup tomato juice cocktail (Clamato juice)
¼ cup sliced pitted olives (mixed or all one kind)
sea salt and freshly ground black pepper to taste
bittersweet Spanish paprika for dusting
2 cups popcorn popped in a wire basket over a wood fire or unsalted, unbuttered popcorn

1. Cut the tentacles of the squid in half if large and cut the bodies crosswise into ¼-inch-wide rings. Heat the oil in a skillet over medium-high heat. Add the shrimp and sauté 1 minute. Add the squid and sauté 1 minute. Transfer the shrimp, squid, and oil to a large nonreactive bowl. Add the scallops, lime juice, lemon juice, onion, jalapeño, garlic, and cilantro and mix well. Cover with plastic wrap and refrigerate until the scallops are "cooked," 30 minutes to 1 hour.

2. Add the tomatoes, orange juice, tomato juice cocktail, and olives to the ceviche and mix well. Season with salt and pepper. Ladle the soup into chilled large shallow soup bowls and sprinkle with paprika and popcorn.

Each serving: About 318 calories, 32 g protein, 36 g carbohydrate, 10 g total fat (2 g saturated), 237 mg cholesterol, 684 mg sodium.

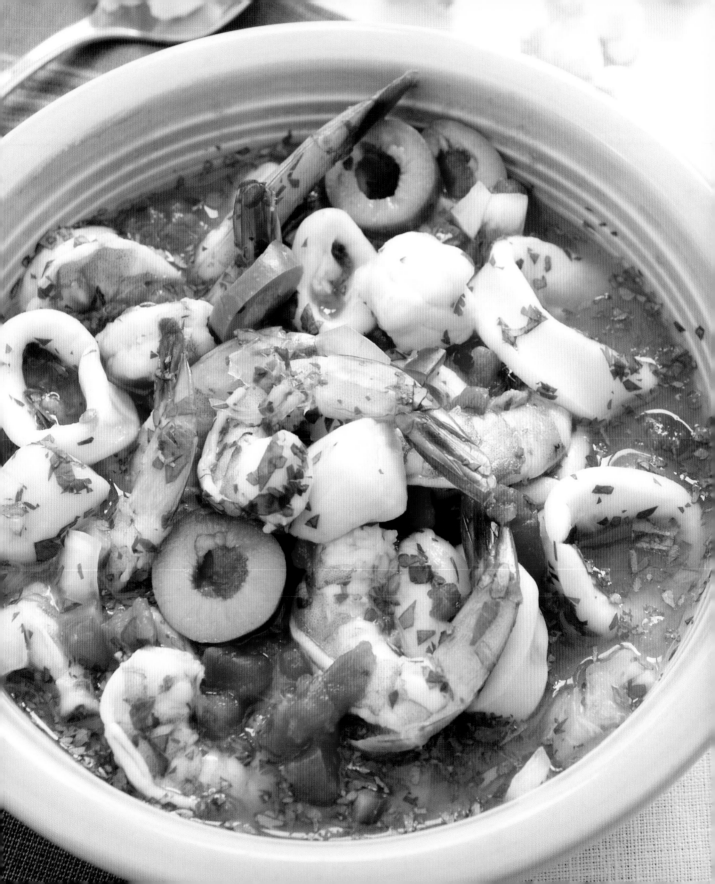

Saffron-Mussel Soup with Rouille Croûtes

PREP TIME: 15 minutes
COOK TIME: 25 minutes

Makes 4 servings

The black mussel shells are extremely glamorous when they are poking out of this fiery-orange broth, but if you think your guests would prefer to forgo the messiness of eating mussels on the shell, by all means remove the shells before serving. The rouille-topped croûtes will still be a tasty focal point and the submerged shelled mussels will be happily devoured.

2 cups Basic Fish Stock (page 16) or water
1 cup dry white wine
24 mussels, scrubbed, debearded just before cooking
½ teaspoon chopped fresh thyme leaves (no stems) or ¼ teaspoon dried thyme
½ teaspoon saffron threads, crushed
2 tablespoons unsalted butter
1 large leek, thinly sliced crosswise and rinsed well
2 large shallots, chopped
2 large egg yolks
½ cup crème fraîche
Garlic Croûtes (page 27) spread with Rouille (page 44) for serving

1. Combine the stock and wine in a 3-quart saucepan and heat to boiling over medium-high heat. Add the mussels and cover. Steam, stirring every few minutes to make sure the mussels have room to open, until the mussels open, about 8 minutes. Transfer to a bowl with a slotted spoon. Discard any unopened mussels. Remove the mussels from the shells if you like.

2. Strain the stock through a large fine sieve lined with a double thickness of cheesecloth into a heat-safe glass measure. Discard the solids. Add the thyme and saffron to the hot stock. Clean the pan and return to the stove. Melt the butter over medium-high heat. Add the leek and shallots and sauté until soft but not browned, about 7 minutes. Add the stock, scraping in the pieces of thyme and saffron, and heat to boiling.

3. Mix the egg yolks and crème fraîche in a small bowl until blended; whisk in a ladleful of hot stock. Pour the mixture back into the soup and heat until hot but do not let it boil or the egg yolks will curdle. Whisk until the soup thickens and add the mussels. Serve with the croûtes in the soup, stirring to mix the rouille into the stock.

Each serving without Croûtes: About 310 calories, 18 g protein, 14 g carbohydrate, 16 g total fat (8 g saturated), 166 mg cholesterol, 429 mg sodium.

Clam Soup with Sausage and Linguine

PREP TIME: 10 minutes
COOK TIME: about 30 minutes

Makes 6 to 8 servings

A not-too-great leap from linguine with clam sauce, this soup is a quick comfort food. Make it a pantry dish by using a 6.5-ounce can of chopped clams and their juice instead of fresh clams in the shell.

8 ounces hot Italian sausage, removed from casings
2 tablespoons olive oil
1 medium red onion, chopped
1 large red bell pepper, chopped
2 garlic cloves, crushed through a press
3 cups Chicken Stock (page 14)
1 (12-ounce) bottle clam juice
1½ cups water
2 tablespoons fresh lemon juice
8 ounces linguine
1 pound littleneck clams, scrubbed
1 tablespoon minced fresh Italian parsley for garnish

1. Cook the sausage in a 3-quart saucepan over medium heat until browned, breaking it into bite-size pieces with a wooden spoon. Add the oil and onion and sauté until the onion is softened, about 7 minutes. Add the bell pepper and garlic and sauté 1 minute. Add the stock, clam juice, water, and lemon juice and heat to boiling over medium-high heat. Add the linguine and cook, partially covered, 5 minutes.

2. Add the clams and stir to separate so they can open. Cover and reduce the heat to medium-low. Simmer, stirring occasionally, until the clams open and the linguine is al dente, about 5 minutes longer. Discard any clams that do not open. Sprinkle with parsley and serve in warmed soup bowls.

Each of 6 servings: About 403 calories, 14 g protein, 38 g carbohydrate, 21 g total fat (6 g saturated), 30 mg cholesterol, 408 mg sodium.

Herb Cheese, White Wine, and Littleneck Clam Soup

PREP TIME: 10 minutes
COOK TIME: about 20 minutes

Makes 4 servings

Purge clams of any sand by placing them in a bowl of cold water to cover and sprinkle a little cornmeal over them. Let stand in the refrigerator 2 to 24 hours before using.

2 tablespoons unsalted butter
½ cup chopped scallions
2 cups dry white wine
1 package (5 ounces) imported garlic-and-herb cheese spread
3 dozen littleneck clams, scrubbed and purged
2 cups heavy cream
¼ teaspoon salt
¼ teaspoon freshly ground black pepper
¼ cup chopped fresh Italian parsley for garnish

1. Melt the butter in a 3-quart saucepan over medium heat. Add the scallions and sauté until softened, 2 minutes. Add 1 cup wine and the cheese and whisk until the cheese is melted. Gradually whisk in the remaining 1 cup wine until the mixture is smooth. Heat to boiling, add the clams, and cover tightly. Cook until the clams start to open, 5 minutes.

2. Add the cream, salt, and pepper. Stir well so all the closed or partially opened clams are free to open fully. Cover tightly and cook until the clams open, about 5 minutes longer. Discard any unopened clams. Sprinkle the soup with parsley and ladle into warmed bowls.

Each serving: About 513 calories, 23 g protein, 12 g carbohydrate, 33 g total fat (20 g saturated), 143 mg cholesterol, 440 mg sodium.

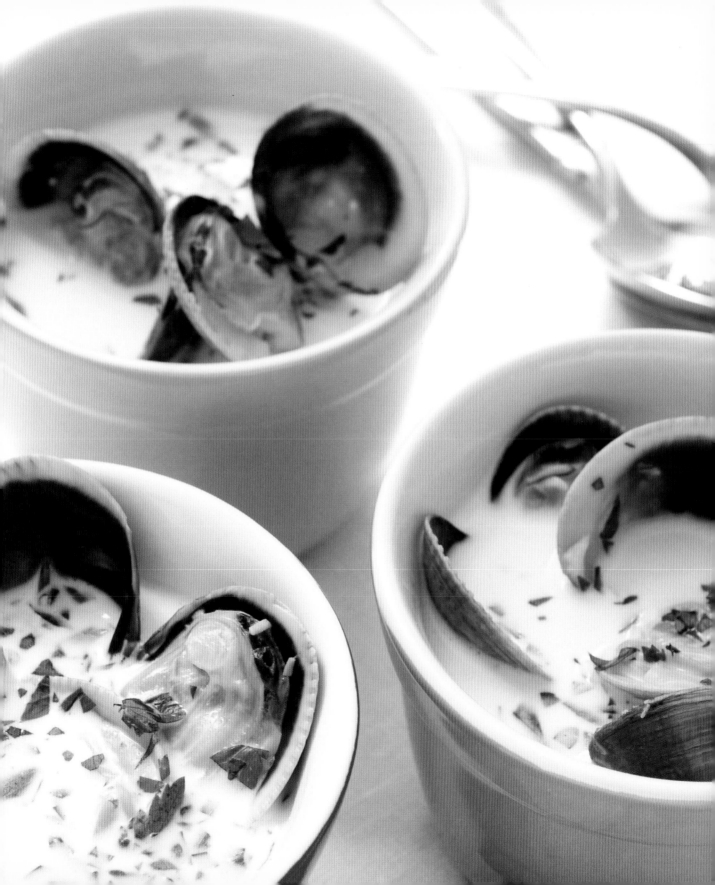

Jamaican Curried Crab Soup

PREP TIME: 20 minutes
COOK TIME: about 20 minutes

Makes 6 to 8 servings

Follow this spicy soup with an assortment of tropical fruit sorbets to cleanse and cool the palate.

1 pound crabmeat, picked over
2 tablespoons fresh lemon juice
2 tablespoons unsalted butter
3 tablespoons Madras curry powder
½ cup chopped red onion
½ cup chopped scallions, including fresh,
    tender green portion
2 teaspoons minced peeled fresh gingerroot
1 garlic clove, minced
1 quart Basic Fish Stock or Chicken Stock
    (Chapter 1)
1 cup drained canned small-diced tomatoes
    (plain or with green chiles)
1 teaspoon soy sauce
dash Jamaican hot-pepper sauce or Tabasco sauce
    or more to taste
2 cups cooked white rice
salt and freshly ground pepper to taste
salted banana chips for serving
bottled mango chutney for serving

1. Combine the crabmeat and lemon juice in a bowl and toss to mix. Let stand 10 minutes.

2. Meanwhile, melt the butter in a 3-quart saucepan over medium heat and add 2 teaspoons curry powder; stir until blended. Add the onion, scallions, ginger, and garlic and sauté until the vegetables are soft but not brown, about 7 minutes.

3. Add the remaining curry powder to the vegetables and stir until blended. Add the stock, tomatoes, soy sauce, and hot-pepper sauce; heat to boiling. Stir in the crabmeat and rice and heat through. Taste and season with salt and pepper and additional hot-pepper sauce if needed. Ladle the soup into warmed bowls, and pass around the banana chips and chutney at the table.

Each serving without banana chips or chutney: About 172 calories, 18 g protein, 21 g carbohydrate, 2 g total fat (trace saturated), 114 mg cholesterol, 259 mg sodium.

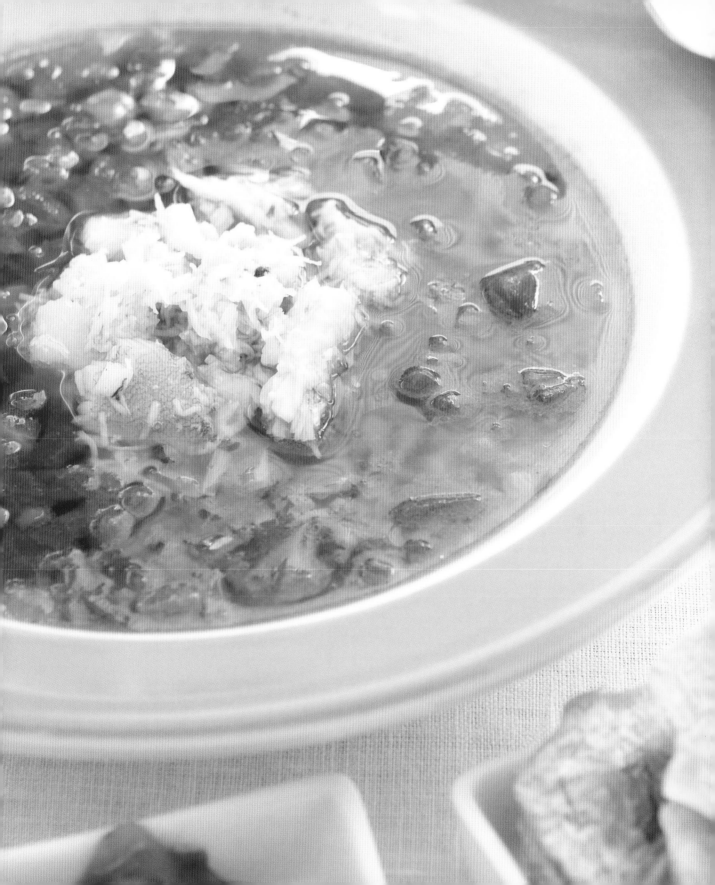

Creole Crab and Oyster Soup

PREP TIME: 15 minutes
COOK TIME: 50 minutes to 1 hour 5 minutes

Makes 6 servings

The flavor of anise goes well with seafood. Pass a bottle of herbsaint (a New Orleans specialty) or another anise-flavored liqueur at the table to splash at will into the soup.

  2 large lemons
  1 bay leaf
  1 large sprig fresh parsley
  1 sprig fresh marjoram
  1 sprig fresh thyme
  3 tablespoons unsalted butter
  1 medium yellow onion, chopped
  1 celery stalk, thinly sliced
  1 green bell pepper, seeded and chopped
  2 cloves garlic, minced
  4 cups canned peeled Italian tomatoes, seeded
    and chopped, with their juice
  4 cups Shrimp Stock, Spicy Shrimp Stock or Basic
    Fish Stock (Chapter 1)
  2 tablespoons chopped fresh mint
  1 pound lump crabmeat, picked over
  16 shucked oysters and their liquor
  salt to taste
  Tabasco sauce to taste

1. Peel the zest from 1 lemon in one long strip if possible with a vegetable peeler; set aside. Juice the peeled lemon. Thinly slice the remaining lemon; remove the seeds and set aside. Tie the bay leaf, parsley, marjoram, and thyme together with a piece of cotton string.

2. Melt the butter in a stockpot or Dutch oven over medium heat. Add the onion, celery, green pepper, and garlic and sauté over medium heat until soft, about 4 minutes. Add the tomatoes with their juice and the stock; heat to boiling over medium high heat. Add the herb bundle, the lemon zest strip, 1½ tablespoons lemon juice, and 1 tablespoon chopped mint to the soup. Reduce the heat and simmer, partially covered, 30 to 45 minutes.

3. Gently stir in the crabmeat and simmer gently until slightly thickened, about 10 minutes more. Stir in the oysters and their liquor and cook just until the oysters are plumped, about 1 minute. Taste and season with salt, Tabasco and additional lemon juice if needed. Discard the herb bundle. Ladle the soup into bowls, sprinkle with the remaining 1 tablespoon chopped mint, and top each serving with a lemon slice.

Each serving: About 201 calories, 19 g protein, 14 g carbohydrate, 8 g total fat (4 g saturated), 101 mg cholesterol, 676 mg sodium.

Cioppino (SAN FRANCISCAN SEAFOOD SOUP)

PREP TIME: 20 minutes
COOK TIME: 1 hour 10 minutes

Makes 6 to 8 servings

1 quart Basic Fish Stock (page 16) or water
1½ pounds shrimp, with shells and heads on, or
   1 pound shelled and deveined shrimp
24 mussels, scrubbed, beards removed just
   before cooking
18 littleneck clams, scrubbed
3 tablespoons olive oil
1 medium onion, chopped
1 green bell pepper, seeded and chopped
2 medium garlic cloves, crushed through a press
2 cans (about 14 ounces each) diced tomatoes
2 cups dry white wine
1 teaspoon chopped fresh thyme leaves (no stems)
   or ½ teaspoon dried thyme leaves
2 teaspoons chopped fresh oregano or marjoram
   leaves or 1 teaspoon dried
1 cup torn fresh basil leaves
2 pounds skinned haddock, cod, or sea bass fillet
   or a mixture, cut into 1-inch chunks
salt and freshly ground pepper to taste
sliced Italian or French bread for serving

1. Heat the stock in a 3-quart saucepan over medium-high heat. Add the shrimp, cover, and cook just until pink and curled, 2 to 3 minutes. Transfer the shrimp to a bowl with a slotted spoon. Set aside to cool.

2. Add the mussels to the stock and cover. Steam, stirring every few minutes to make sure the mussels have room to open, until the mussels open, about 8 minutes. Transfer the mussels to a bowl with a slotted spoon. Discard any unopened mussels. Repeat with the clams.

3. Remove the heads and shells from the shrimp; set the shrimp aside and add the shells and heads to the stock, smashing and breaking them up with the back of a large wooden spoon. Cover and simmer over medium heat 20 minutes. Strain the stock through a large fine sieve lined with a double thickness of cheesecloth into a heat-safe glass measure. Discard the solids.

4. Clean the saucepan and return to the stove. Add 2 tablespoons oil and heat over medium-high heat. Add the onion and sauté until softened, about 5 minutes. Add the bell pepper and sauté 2 minutes. Add the garlic and sauté 1 minute. Add the strained stock, the tomatoes with their juice, the wine, thyme, and oregano; simmer over medium heat, partially covered, 25 minutes.

5. While the soup simmers, remove the mussels and clams from their shells, adding any liquid to the soup. Place the basil on a cutting board, drizzle with the remaining 1 tablespoon oil, and finely chop.

6. Ten minutes before serving, stir the haddock into the soup. About 9 minutes later, stir in the shrimp, mussels, clams, and basil and heat through. Taste and season with salt and pepper. Ladle the soup into warmed shallow soup bowls and serve with the bread.

Each of 6 servings: About 509 calories, 69 g protein, 16 g carbohydrate, 12 g total fat (2 g saturated), 296 mg cholesterol, 821 mg sodium.

Provençale Bourride

PREP TIME: 5 minutes
COOK TIME: 30 minutes

Makes 4 servings

This quick version of the classic Mediterranean seafood soup nets unforgettable flavor from garlic and orange zest.

    2 tablespoons olive oil
    1 cup sliced leeks, rinsed well
    4 teaspoons minced garlic
    1 cup sliced carrots
    1 can (11 ounces) clam juice
    2 cups dry white wine
    ¼ teaspoon freshly ground black pepper
    pinch saffron threads
    ¾ pound flounder fillets, cut into bite-size pieces
    ½ teaspoon grated orange zest
    salt to taste
    4 slices French bread, toasted, for serving

1. Heat the olive oil in a 6-quart pot. Add the leeks and garlic and sauté until the leeks are wilted, 3 to 5 minutes.

2. Add the carrots, clam juice, wine, pepper, and saffron. Cover and bring to a boil. Reduce the heat and simmer until the carrots are tender, about 15 minutes.

3. Add the flounder and orange zest and simmer 10 minutes. Taste and season with salt if needed. Serve with the toasted bread.

Each serving: About 400 calories, 28 g protein, 35 g carbohydrate, 9 g total fat (1 g saturated), 41 mg cholesterol, 989 mg sodium.

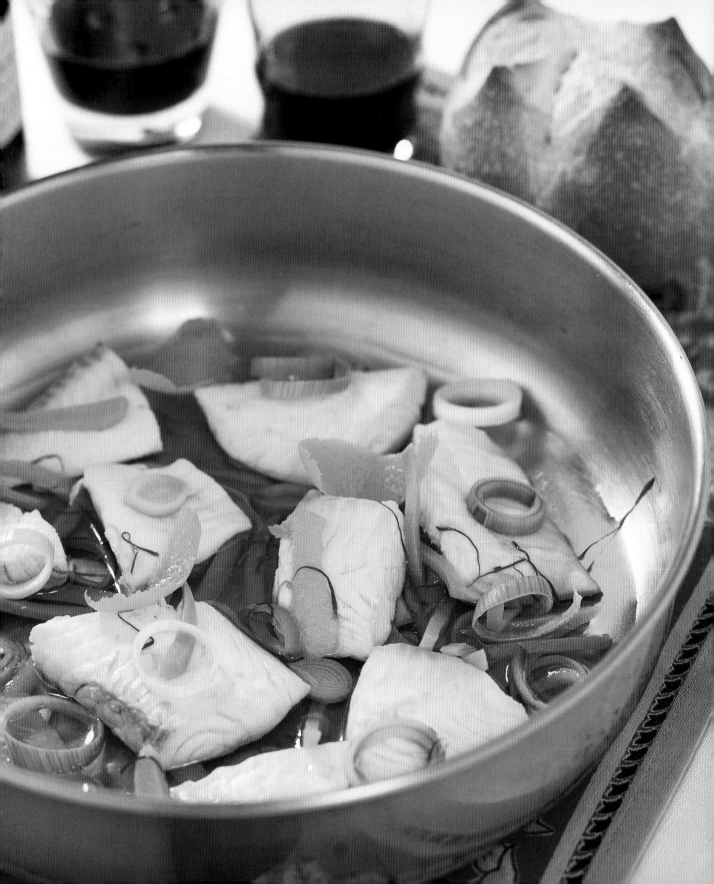

Spanish "Quarter-Hour" Seafood Soup

PREP TIME: 15 minutes
COOK TIME: 40 minutes

Makes 6 servings

Sofrito is a flavoring base composed of Spanish and Italian roots, usually including onion, garlic, tomato and some kind of pork. It is used in bean and rice mixtures, stews, soups, braises, and many other dishes. The exact ingredient mix is region-specific.

5 cups water
8 medium hard-shelled clams, scrubbed
3 tablespoons Spanish extravirgin olive oil
2 medium onions, finely chopped
2 garlic cloves, minced
1 small bay leaf
1 can (14 ounces) petite-diced tomatoes, drained
⅓ cup finely diced serrano ham or prosciutto di Parma (about 1 ounce)
2 tablespoons finely chopped fresh Italian parsley
⅛ teaspoon Spanish saffron threads
⅛ teaspoon smoky Spanish paprika (Pimentón de la Vera)
1 cup shelled fresh peas
¼ cup raw medium- or long-grain white rice (not parboiled or quick-cooking) or Spanish or Italian short-grain rice
½ teaspoon salt or more to taste
¼ teaspoon freshly ground pepper or to taste
8 medium raw shrimp, shelled and deveined
12 ounces cod or halibut fillet
fresh lemon juice to taste
1 hard-cooked egg, shelled, finely chopped, for serving

1. Bring 1 cup water to a boil in a 3-quart saucepan. Add the clams, spread them out, and cover. Cook over medium-high heat until the clams open, about 5 minutes. Discard any unopened clams. Pour the clams and liquid into a bowl. When the clams are cool enough to handle, remove the meat and coarsely chop. Reserve the cooking liquid. Clean the saucepan.

2. Make the sofrito: Heat the oil in the clean saucepan over medium heat until hot. Add the onions and sauté until soft, about 7 minutes. Add the garlic and bay leaf and sauté 1 minute. Add the tomatoes, ham, and parsley; increase the heat to medium-high. Cook, stirring, until slightly thickened, about 5 minutes. Stir in the saffron and paprika and sauté 1 minute.

3. Strain the clam-cooking liquid into the sofrito and stir until mixed. Stir in the remaining 4 cups water, the peas, rice, salt, and pepper; heat to boiling. Cover, reduce the heat to low, and simmer 10 minutes. Add the shrimp and cod; cover and simmer until the cod breaks up and the shrimp are cooked, 5 minutes. Season to taste with lemon juice. Ladle the soup into warmed soup bowls and top with the chopped egg.

Each serving: About 200 calories, 16 g protein, 14 g carbohydrate, 9 g total fat (2 g saturated), 72 mg cholesterol, 586 mg sodium.

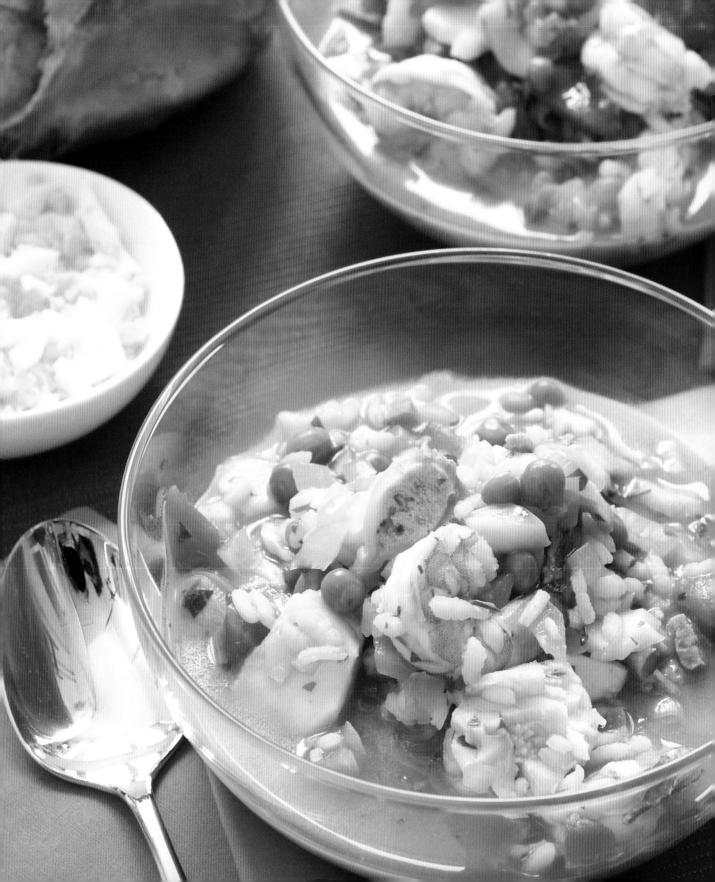

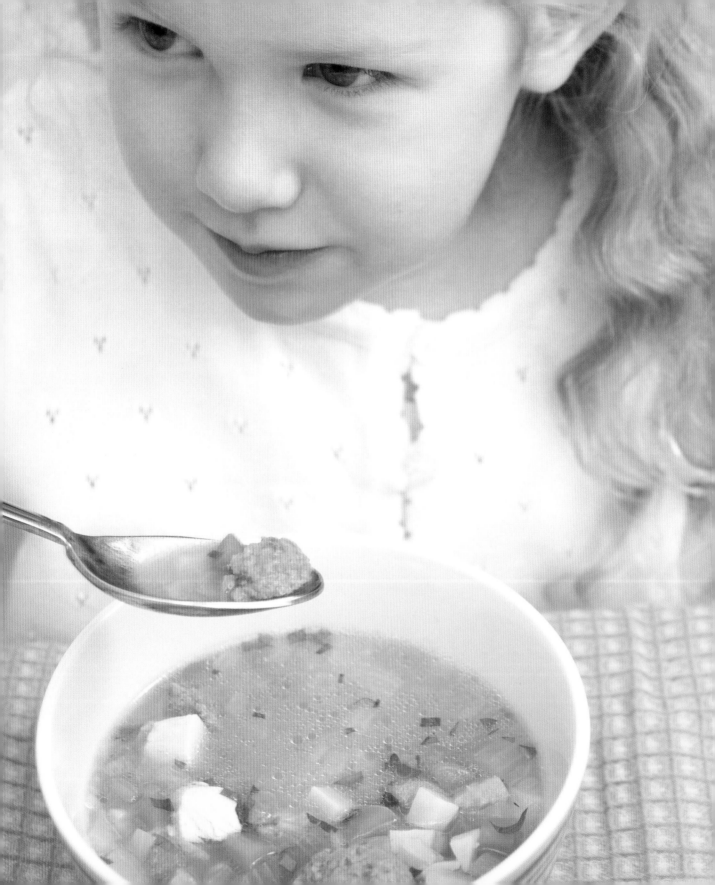

POULTRY SOUPS ⁸

Chicken Noodle Soup with Fresh Tomatoes

PREP TIME: 10 minutes
COOK TIME: 25 minutes

Makes 4 servings

Carrots reign in many traditional chicken-noodle soups; here, tomatoes rule. For directions on peeling and seeding tomatoes, see the tip at Chunky Cream of Tomato Soup with Tarragon (page 118).

2 pounds ripe tomatoes
1 teaspoon olive oil
12 ounces skinless boneless chicken breasts, cut into ½-inch chunks
¼ teaspoon white pepper
1 teaspoon thyme leaves
4 garlic cloves, crushed through a press
1¾ cups Chicken Stock (page 14)
1 teaspoon white wine vinegar
1 cup medium egg noodles
1 cup frozen peas
salt to taste

1. Peel and seed the tomatoes, reserving the juice. Cut the tomatoes into small chunks.

2. Heat the oil in a 6-quart pot over medium-high heat. Coat the chicken with the pepper, thyme, and garlic. Add the chicken to the pot and sauté until lightly browned, about 5 minutes.

3. Stir in the tomatoes, stock, and vinegar. Cover and bring to a boil. Reduce the heat and simmer 10 minutes. Add the reserved tomato juice if the soup is too thick.

4. Stir in the noodles and peas and cook until the noodles are al dente and the peas are tender, about 5 minutes. Taste and season with salt if needed.

Each serving: About 212 calories, 25 g protein, 21 g carbohydrate, 3 g total fat (1 g saturated), 58 mg cholesterol, 388 mg sodium.

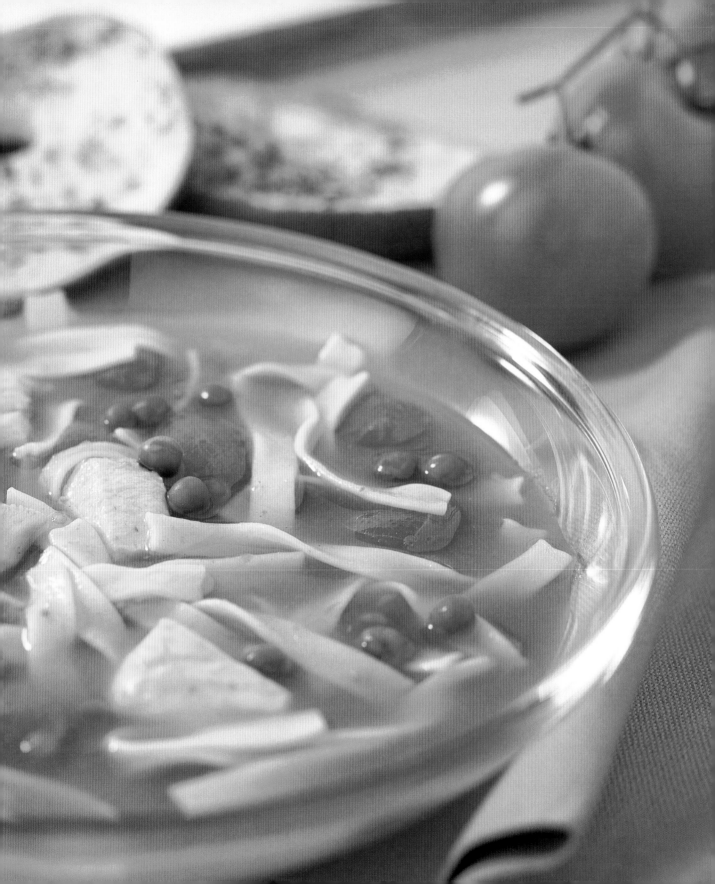

Chicken-Ditalini Soup with Cannellini Beans

PREP TIME: 5 minutes
COOK TIME: 30 minutes

Makes 4 servings

Here's a change-of-pace chicken soup, using ditalini instead of the usual noodles and adding beans for extra fiber and flavor. Can't find fresh lemon thyme? Use regular thyme and add ¼ teaspoon lemon zest.

1 teaspoon olive oil
8 ounces skinless boneless chicken breasts, cut into ½-inch cubes
¼ teaspoon freshly ground black pepper
4 garlic cloves, chopped
1 shallot, chopped
1 quart Chicken Stock (page 14)
1 can (15 ounces) cannellini beans, rinsed and drained
2 carrots, peeled and thinly sliced
1 celery stalk, thinly sliced
2 bay leaves
1 sprig fresh lemon thyme
¾ cup ditalini (tube pasta)
salt to taste

1. Heat the oil in a 6-quart pot over medium-high heat for 1 minute. Sprinkle the chicken with the pepper. Add the chicken, garlic, and shallot to the pot, and sauté until the chicken is lightly browned, about 5 minutes.

2. Stir in the stock, beans, carrots, celery, bay leaves, and lemon thyme. Cover and bring to a boil. Reduce the heat and simmer 10 minutes. Stir in the ditalini and cook until the pasta is al dente, 10 to 12 minutes. Taste and season with salt if needed. Discard the bay leaves.

Each serving: About 283 calories, 27 g protein, 35 g carbohydrate, 3 g total fat (trace saturated), 33 mg cholesterol, 448 mg sodium.

Easy Tortilla Soup with Chicken

PREP TIME: 5 minutes
COOK TIME: 30 minutes

Makes 4 servings

1 teaspoon olive oil
1 pound skinless boneless chicken breasts, cut
    into ½-inch cubes
2 medium onions, finely chopped
4 garlic cloves, minced
4 cups canned crushed tomatoes
3 cups Chicken Stock (page 14)
1 yellow chile pepper, seeded and minced (use
    rubber gloves when handling hot peppers)
2 tablespoons chopped fresh parsley
salt and freshly ground black pepper to taste
8 baked tortilla chips, crushed, for serving
¾ cup shredded Monterey Jack cheese for serving

1. Heat the oil in a 6-quart pot over medium-high heat
   for 1 minute. Add the chicken, onions, and garlic and
   sauté until the chicken is browned and the onions are
   translucent, 5 to 6 minutes.

2. Stir in the tomatoes, stock, chile, and parsley. Cover
   and bring to a boil. Reduce the heat and simmer
   20 minutes. Taste and season with salt and black
   pepper if needed. Top each serving with the tortilla
   chips and Monterey Jack cheese.

Each serving: About 446 calories, 49 g protein, 29 g carbohydrate, 15 g total fat (6 g saturated), 127 mg cholesterol,
1,462 mg sodium.

Chicken Soup with Pistou

PREP TIME: 10 minutes
COOK TIME: 25 minutes

Makes 6 servings

True to its Provençale heritage, this vegetable-packed
chicken soup gets its wonderful garlic flavor from
pistou, the French version of Italian pesto.

3½ cups Chicken Stock (page 14)
12 ounces skinless boneless chicken breasts, cut
    into ½-inch cubes
1 large potato, cut into ½-inch cubes
2 carrots, peeled and diced
1 leek, white part only, thinly sliced, rinsed well
¼ teaspoon white pepper
1 tomato, quartered and sliced
1 medium zucchini, quartered and sliced
2 tablespoons Pistou (page 47) plus more for serving
salt and pepper to taste
¼ cup grated Romano cheese for serving

Combine the stock, chicken, potato, carrots, leek,
and pepper in a 6-quart pot. Cover and bring to a
boil. Reduce the heat and simmer 12 minutes. Add
the tomato and zucchini and simmer 10 minutes. Stir
in the pistou. Taste and season with salt and pepper
if needed. Top each serving with the Romano cheese
and pass additional pistou at the table.

Each serving: About 186 calories, 22 g protein, 16 g carbohydrate, 3 g total fat (2 g saturated), 43 mg cholesterol, 291 mg
sodium.

Chicken Soup Monterey

PREP TIME: 5 minutes
COOK TIME: 20 minutes

Makes 4 servings

Definitely not your run-of-the-mill chicken soup. This version is spiked with smoky mesquite flavoring, and it has a noticeably rich broth thanks to Monterey Jack cheese.

    3½ cups Chicken Stock (page 14)
    2 large potatoes, peeled and cubed
    1 celery stalk, sliced
    2 carrots, peeled and sliced
    1 medium onion, chopped
    2 ounces deli smoked chicken breast, diced
    ½ cup chopped fresh parsley
    ½ teaspoon dried marjoram leaves
    ½ teaspoon freshly ground black pepper
    ⅔ cup shredded reduced-fat Monterey Jack cheese
    1 teaspoon mesquite smoke flavoring
    salt to taste

1. Combine the stock, potatoes, celery, carrots, onion, chicken, parsley, marjoram, and pepper in a 6-quart pot. Cover and bring to a boil. Reduce the heat and simmer until the vegetables are tender, about 15 minutes.

2. Remove from the heat and stir in the cheese and smoke flavoring. Taste and season with salt if needed.

Each serving: About 263 calories, 17 g protein, 39 g carbohydrate, 4 g total fat (2 g saturated), 18 mg cholesterol, 451 mg sodium.

Thai Peanut-Chicken Soup

PREP TIME: 10 minutes
COOK TIME: 15 minutes

Makes 6 to 8 servings

This recipe is based on *Gai Tom Ka*, a Thai chicken soup with coconut. The addition of peanut butter is not traditional—but the earthy aroma and flavor complement the other ingredients well. Try using cashew butter for another unorthodox, but tasty, variation.

2 tablespoons peanut or vegetable oil
6 large garlic cloves, crushed through a press
3 to 4 Thai chiles, seeded and finely chopped
3 (double) fresh kaffir lime leaves, stem and main vein removed, finely chopped
4-inch middle piece fresh lemongrass, thinly sliced
2 shallots, peeled and finely chopped
1 quart Chicken Stock (page 14) or water
2 tablespoons fresh lime juice
2 slices (¼-inch-thick) fresh or frozen peeled galangal (optional)
¼ cup smooth peanut butter
1 can (about 14 ounces) unsweetened coconut milk
1½ pounds chicken cutlets, cut into 1" by ½" strips
6 tablespoons Thai or Vietnamese fish sauce (nam pla or nuoc mam)
2 tablespoons finely chopped fresh basil leaves (preferably Asian basil)
2 tablespoons finely chopped fresh cilantro
3 cups cooked jasmine rice for serving

1. Heat the oil in a 2-quart saucepan over medium heat. Add the garlic, chiles, lime leaves, lemongrass and shallots and sauté until very fragrant, about 5 minutes. Add the stock, lime juice, and galangal (if using) and heat until gently simmering.

2. Blend the peanut butter and 2 tablespoons coconut milk in a small bowl and whisk into the soup until blended. Add the chicken and remaining coconut milk and simmer gently until the chicken is cooked through, about 2 minutes. Stir in the fish sauce, basil, and cilantro and simmer 2 minutes longer. Serve immediately in hot bowls, with rice added to taste.

Each of 6 servings: About 516 calories, 37 g protein, 33 g carbohydrate, 27 g total fat (15 g saturated), 66 mg cholesterol, 1,268 mg sodium.

Chicken and Asparagus in Lemon-Cream Broth

PREP TIME: 25 minutes
COOK TIME: 40 minutes

Makes 4 to 6 servings

1 quart water
2 whole skinless bone-in chicken breasts (about
   1¾ pounds total)
2 large celery stalks, quartered
1 medium onion, quartered
½ teaspoons salt or more to taste
¼ teaspoon freshly ground white pepper or more
   to taste
1½ pounds asparagus, tough ends snapped off
1 cup peeled baby carrots, cut into thin rounds
4 egg yolks
1 cup heavy cream
1 tablespoon fresh lemon juice or more to taste
2 tablespoons chopped fresh Italian parsley

1. Combine the water, chicken, celery, onion, salt, and
   pepper in a 3-quart saucepan and heat to boiling
   over medium-high heat. Reduce the heat to low and
   simmer gently until the chicken is almost cooked
   through, about 20 minutes. Allow the chicken to cool
   in the broth 30 minutes. Transfer the chicken to a
   bowl. Cool completely, then remove the meat from
   the bones and cut into thin strips; set aside.

2. Strain the broth into a clean 3-quart saucepan. Peel
   the asparagus stalks starting 2 inches from the tips.
   Cut the asparagus into 2-inch lengths starting from
   the tips; keep the tips separate from the stalk pieces.

3. Transfer 2 cups broth to a 1-quart saucepan and heat
   to boiling over medium-high heat. Have ready a small
   bowl of ice and water. Add the asparagus tips and carrots to the broth in the smaller pan and cook 5 minutes. Drain the asparagus and carrots through a sieve
   set over the larger pan of broth. Transfer the asparagus tips and carrots to the ice water to cool quickly and
   completely and retain their bright colors. Set aside.

4. Transfer 2 cups broth to the same 1-quart saucepan
   and heat to boiling over medium-high heat. Add the
   asparagus stalks and cook until tender, 5 to 10 minutes. Transfer the stalks with broth to a blender and,
   holding a folded kitchen towel over the top to keep the
   lid in place, carefully puree. Pour the puree through a
   coarse sieve into the broth and heat to boiling over
   medium-high heat. Add the chicken, asparagus tips,
   and carrots; reduce the heat to medium-low.

5. In a medium bowl, whisk the egg yolks with the
   cream until blended. Whisk in a ladleful of hot soup,
   and then whisk it back into the soup. Heat the soup
   but do not let it boil or the egg yolks will curdle.
   Whisk in the lemon juice, taste for seasoning, and add
   more lemon juice, salt, and pepper as needed. Stir in
   the parsley.

Each of 4 servings: About 334 calories, 37 g protein,
17 g carbohydrate, 14 g total fat (6 g saturated), 303 mg
cholesterol, 430 mg sodium.

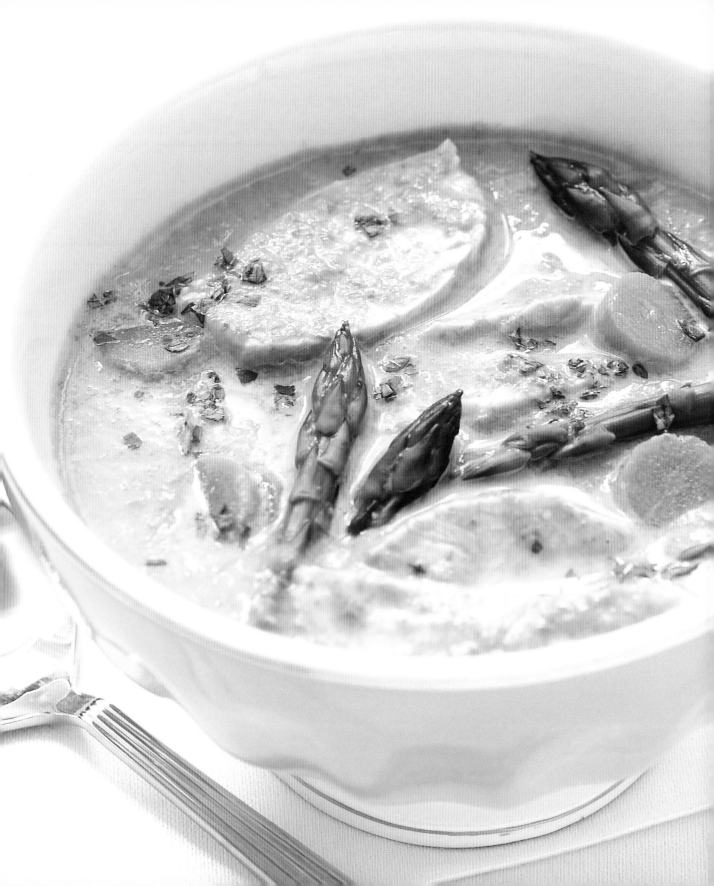

Creamy Chicken-Vegetable Soup with Puff-Pastry Croutons

PREP TIME: 15 minutes
COOK TIME: 30 minutes

Makes 6 to 8 servings

With all the elements of an old-fashioned potpie, this is a nostalgic treat without the soggy crust. Puff-pastry croutons provide the crunchy interlude between bites of juicy chicken breasts and vegetables.

1 quart strong Chicken Stock (page 14) plus more if needed
1½ pounds skinless boneless chicken breasts, cut into 1-inch cubes
1 stick unsalted butter plus more for greasing parchment
1 large red onion, diced
1 pound baby carrots, cut in half diagonally
1 celery heart, cut diagonally and crosswise into ½-inch slices
8 ounces mushrooms, quartered
½ cup all-purpose flour
1½ cups half-and-half
2 tablespoons dry sherry
1 tablespoon chopped fresh thyme leaves (no stems)
1 tablespoon chopped fresh Italian parsley
1 teaspoon chopped fresh rosemary leaves plus sprigs for garnish
salt and freshly ground black pepper to taste
3 tablespoons fresh lemon juice
Puff Pastry Croutons (page 25) for serving

1. In a 2-quart saucepan over medium heat, bring the stock to a boil. Add the chicken, cover, and cook until white but not cooked through, about 3 minutes. Transfer the chicken to a bowl with a slotted spoon.

2. Melt 2 tablespoons butter in a 3-quart saucepan over medium-high heat. Add the onion, carrots, celery, and mushrooms and sauté until soft, about 5 minutes. Transfer to the bowl with the chicken. Clean the saucepan.

3. Heat the stock to boiling. Melt the remaining 6 tablespoons butter in the clean saucepan over medium heat. Whisk in the flour and cook, whisking, until pale gold color, 2 minutes. Whisk in the hot stock, half-and-half, sherry, thyme, parsley, and rosemary and heat to boiling. Taste and season with salt and pepper. Reduce the heat to medium and simmer 5 minutes. (If the soup is not thick enough for desired consistency, reduce by simmering a little longer. If the soup is too thick, add a little more stock.) Stir in the lemon juice, the chicken and vegetables and heat until simmering. Ladle into bowls and top with croutons.

Each of 6 servings without croutons: About 463 calories, 35 g protein, 23 g carbohydrate, 25 g total fat (15 g saturated), 130 mg cholesterol, 489 mg sodium.

Chicken Soup with Bacon, Apples, and Barley

PREP TIME: 20 minutes plus chilling
COOK TIME: 2 hours 10 minutes

Makes 6 to 8 servings

Along with a classic cold-weather combination of bacon, apples, cabbage, and barley, chunks of dark-meat chicken make this a perfect fireside soup. In spite of the long cooking, the chicken thighs remain flavorful and firm enough to be the meat support of this soup.

2 quarts Chicken Stock (page 14) or water
2 pounds skinless bone-in chicken thighs
1 celery stalk, coarsely chopped
4 sprigs fresh parsley
1 teaspoon salt or more to taste
4 ounces thickly sliced bacon, cut crosswise into thin strips
3 medium leeks, cut crosswise into thin rings, rinsed well
2 large carrots, peeled and chopped
2 large Granny Smith apples, peeled, cored and coarsely chopped
1 small head cabbage (Savoy is nice), about 1 pound, coarsely shredded
¼ cup uncooked pearl barley
¼ teaspoon freshly ground pepper or more to taste

1. Combine the stock, chicken, celery, and parsley in a 3-quart saucepan and heat to boiling over medium heat, skimming off any scum from the surface. Stir in the salt, reduce the heat to medium-low, and simmer, partially covered, until the chicken is falling off the bone, about 1½ hours. With a slotted spoon, transfer the chicken to a bowl. Strain the cooking liquid through a colander set over a 2-quart heat-safe glass measure. When the chicken stock is cooled to room temperature, cover and refrigerate overnight or until the fat hardens on the top.

2. Hours later or the next day, discard the fat from the stock. Cut the chicken off the bone into bite-size pieces. Sauté the bacon in a 3-quart saucepan over medium heat until the fat renders and the bacon is crisp but not hard, about 5 minutes. With a slotted spoon, transfer the bacon to a paper towel–lined plate.

3. Discard all but 2 tablespoons bacon drippings from the saucepan. Heat the drippings in the saucepan over medium-high heat. Add the leeks, carrots, apples, and cabbage and sauté until tender, about 10 minutes. Add the stock, chicken, barley, and pepper. Heat to boiling over medium-high heat and simmer until the barley is tender, about 20 minutes. Taste and add salt and pepper if necessary. Ladle the soup into warmed soup bowls and sprinkle with the bacon.

Each of 6 servings: About 334 calories, 26 g protein, 30 g carbohydrate, 13 g total fat (4 g saturated), 71 mg cholesterol, 580 mg sodium.

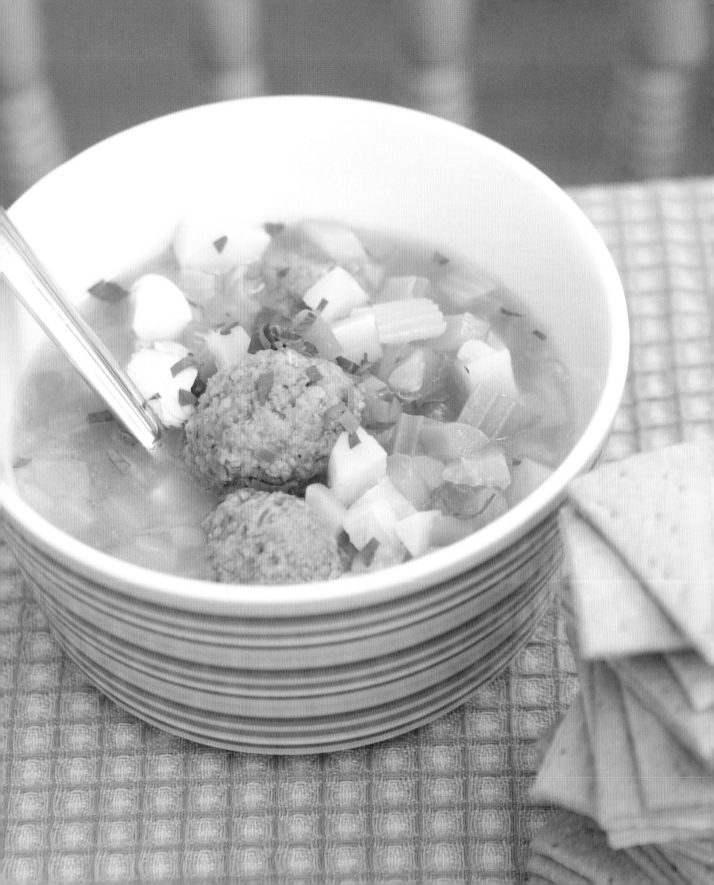

Chicken Soup with Liver Dumplings

PREP TIME: 20 minutes
COOK TIME: about 35 minutes

Makes 6 to 8 servings

Liver dumplings are a classic Middle and Eastern European addition to soups. Serve with Matzoh (page 34).

4 tablespoons unsalted butter
1 small onion, chopped
1 small carrot, peeled and cut into ¼-inch dice
1 inner celery stalk, cut into ¼-inch dice
1 small parsnip, peeled and cut into ¼-inch dice
2 tablespoons all-purpose flour
2 quarts hot Chicken Stock (page 14)

Dumplings
2 slices stale white bread with crusts
¼ cup milk
4 ounces chicken livers, rinsed and trimmed
1 tablespoon unsalted butter
¼ cup finely chopped onion
2 egg whites
1 teaspoon finely chopped fresh Italian parsley leaves
½ teaspoon salt
⅛ teaspoon freshly ground pepper
½ cup dried bread crumbs or more if needed
flour for dusting your hands

3 cups diced cooked chicken
salt and pepper to taste
3 tablespoons chopped fresh Italian parsley leaves for garnish

1. Melt the butter in a 4-quart saucepan over medium-high heat and sauté the onion 2 minutes. Add the carrot, celery, and parsnip and sauté until crisp-tender, about 4 minutes. Remove the pan from the heat and stir in the flour until blended. Stir in 2 cups hot stock until blended; heat to boiling. Boil, stirring, 1 minute. Stir in the remaining stock and simmer over low heat while making the dumplings.

2. Make the dumplings: Soak the bread in the milk in a medium bowl. Squeeze out the milk and place the bread in a food processor; add the chicken livers. Process until finely chopped and transfer to a medium bowl. Melt the butter in an 8-inch skillet over medium heat and sauté the onion until soft and golden, about 7 minutes. Add the onion to the bread mixture. Stir in the egg whites, parsley, salt, and pepper and mix well. Add the bread crumbs and mix well. Shape the mixture into a 1-inch ball, adding more bread crumbs, 1 table-spoon at a time, if the mixture is too wet to shape. When the mixture is satisfactory, shape the whole batch into balls, flouring your hands lightly to keep the dumplings from sticking, and place on a plate.

3. Heat the soup to boiling, add the chicken, and reduce the heat to a gentle simmer. Add the dumplings and gently boil until the dumplings rise to the surface, then simmer gently until cooked through, about 2 minutes longer. To serve: Taste and season with salt and pepper if needed. Ladle the soup into warmed shallow soup bowls and sprinkle with the parsley.

Each of 6 servings: About 377 calories, 35 g protein, 23 g carbohydrate, 16 g total fat (8 g saturated), 164 mg cholesterol, 509 mg sodium.

Soothing Ginger Chicken Soup with Ramen Noodles

PREP TIME: 10 minutes
COOK TIME: 15 minutes

Makes 4 servings

You can use Gingered Chicken Stock (page 14) instead of plain stock for an even more vibrant flavor that is especially appreciated when you're feeling under the weather. This soup is quick to make so your spirits should lift in a jiffy.

1 tablespoon vegetable oil
4 scallions, thinly sliced
1 garlic clove, crushed through a press
3 tablespoons finely grated peeled fresh gingerroot
¼ teaspoon crushed red-pepper flakes
1 quart Chicken Stock (page 14)
2 tablespoons low-sodium soy sauce
2 packages (3 ounces each) ramen noodles (discard seasoning packets)
1 pound chicken cutlets, cut into ¼-inch-wide strips
1 (4-inch) square firm tofu, cut into bite-size cubes
2 tablespoons rice wine or sake
2 tablespoons dark sesame oil
4 radishes, thinly sliced, for serving

1. Heat the oil in a 2-quart saucepan over medium heat. Add three-fourths of the scallions and sauté 1 minute. Add the garlic and sauté 1 minute. Add the ginger and pepper flakes and sauté 30 seconds. Add the stock and soy sauce and heat to boiling over medium-high heat.

2. Add the noodles to the soup and cook, stirring to separate the noodles, 3 minutes. Add the chicken and tofu and reduce the heat to medium. Simmer gently until the chicken is cooked through, about 4 minutes. Stir in the rice wine and sesame oil. Ladle the soup into bowls and sprinkle with the remaining scallions and the radishes.

Each serving: About 489 calories, 38 g protein, 33 g carbohydrate, 22 g total fat (5 g saturated), 66 mg cholesterol, 346 mg sodium.

Chicken and Rice Soup with Quenelles

PREP TIME: 30 minutes
COOK TIME: about 40 minutes

Makes 6 servings

Quenelles are oval, tender, mousse-like dumplings made from ground fish, chicken, meat, or vegetables.

4 tablespoons unsalted butter
8 ounces escarole or spinach, trimmed, and torn into 3-inch pieces
1 small leek, thinly sliced crosswise and rinsed
1 small yellow bell pepper, seeded and diced
6 cups Chicken Stock (page 14)
¼ cup Arborio or other imported short-grain rice
¾ teaspoon salt or more to taste
¼ teaspoon freshly ground pepper or more to taste
6 ounces skinless boneless chicken breast, cut into 1-inch pieces
1 large egg, lightly beaten
½ cup fine dried bread crumbs
2 tablespoons chopped fresh Italian parsley
1 tablespoon milk
1 teaspoon lemon juice
1 teaspoon grated onion
¾ teaspoon anchovy paste (optional)
pinch freshly grated nutmeg
freshly grated Pecorino-Romano cheese for serving

1. Melt the butter in a 3-quart saucepan over medium heat. Add the escarole, leek, and bell pepper and sauté until tender, about 5 minutes. Add the stock, rice, ½ teaspoon salt, and the pepper and heat to boiling over medium-high heat. Reduce the heat to medium-low and simmer, covered, until the rice is al dente, about 20 minutes.

2. Meanwhile, make the quenelles: Place the chicken in a food processor and finely chop. Add the remaining ¼ teaspoon salt, the egg, bread crumbs, parsley, milk, lemon juice, onion, anchovy paste (if using) and nutmeg and pulse to mix. Process just until the ingredients are blended and the mixture is smooth. Scrape the mixture into a bowl.

3. Shape the quenelles: Have ready a small bowl of cold water. With a spoon in each hand, take a spoonful of the quenelle mixture and take it off into the other spoon with the long side of the spoon. Repeat one or two times more to make an oval dumpling and place on a baking sheet. Dip the spoons into the cold water. Repeat with the remaining quenelle mixture.

4. Taste the soup and season with salt and pepper if needed. Increase the heat so the soup is gently boiling. Drop the quenelles into the soup and simmer until they are cooked through, about 5 minutes. Ladle the soup into warmed shallow soup bowls. Pass the cheese at the table.

Each serving: About 253 calories, 17 g protein, 20 g carbohydrate, 12 g total fat (6 g saturated), 76 mg cholesterol, 576 mg sodium.

Harvest Turkey Soup

PREP TIME: 5 minutes
COOK TIME: 20 minutes

Makes 4 servings

When only a classic, home-style soup will do, give this one a try.
Butternut squash and cloves give it a new twist. A dab of butter adds
unexpected richness.

  1 teaspoon olive oil
  1 pound turkey breast cutlets, cut into ½-inch pieces
  3 shallots, sliced
  3½ cups Chicken Stock (page 14)
  1 cup water
  2 medium red potatoes, cut into ½-inch cubes
  1 pound butternut squash, peeled and cut into ½-inch cubes
  ½ teaspoon fresh thyme leaves plus thyme sprigs for garnish
  2 whole cloves
  1 teaspoon butter
  salt and pepper to taste

1. Heat the oil in a 6-quart pot over medium-high heat for 1 minute. Add
   the turkey and shallots and sauté until the turkey is lightly browned.

2. Stir in the stock, water, potatoes, squash, and thyme. Place the cloves in
   a mesh tea ball or tie them up in cheesecloth; add to the pot. Cover and
   bring to a boil. Reduce the heat and simmer until the turkey is cooked
   through and the potatoes and squash are tender, about 15 minutes.
   Discard the cloves. Stir in the butter. Taste and season with salt and
   pepper if needed. Garnish with thyme sprigs.

Each serving: About 354 calories, 31 g protein, 35 g carbohydrate, 10 g total fat
(3 g saturated), 68 mg cholesterol, 351 mg sodium.

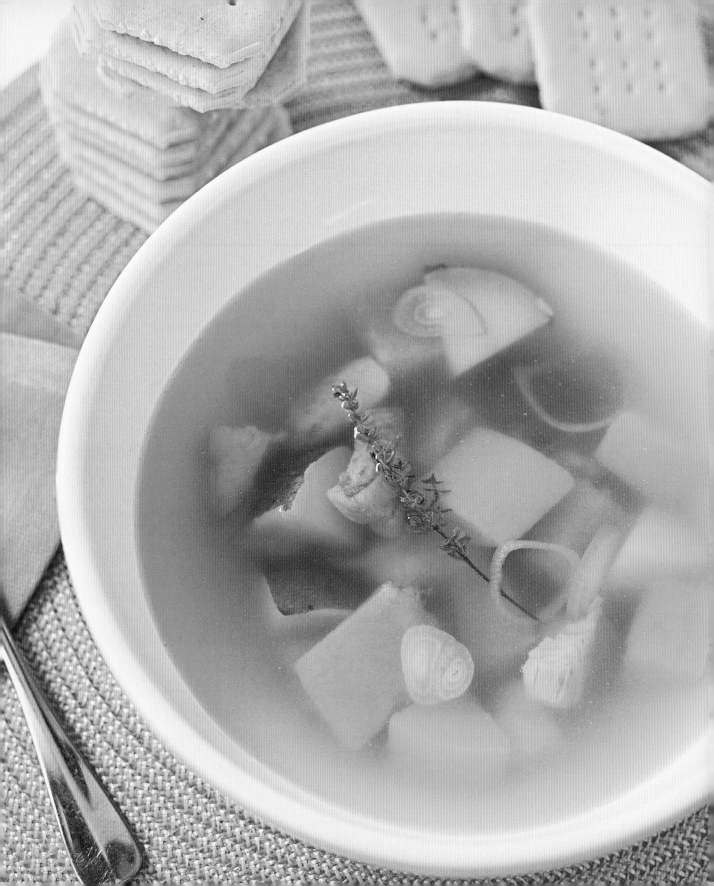

Smoky Turkey Soup

PREP TIME: 5 minutes
COOK TIME: 25 minutes

Makes 4 servings

Impress family and friends with this fast, no-hassle soup of turkey, tomatoes, and beans. Its flavors are delightfully smoky and complex, thanks to hickory smoke flavoring.

2 teaspoons canola oil
1 pound turkey tenderloin, cut into short strips
1 medium red onion, chopped
3½ cups Chicken Stock (page 14)
1 can (15 ounces) Great Northern beans, rinsed and drained
1 can (15 ounces) diced tomatoes
2 celery stalks, sliced
2 teaspoons white wine vinegar
¼ teaspoon white pepper
1 teaspoon hickory smoke flavoring
salt and pepper to taste
½ cup chopped fresh cilantro for garnish

1. Heat the oil in a 6-quart pot over medium-high heat for 1 minute. Add the turkey and onion and sauté until the turkey is lightly browned, about 5 minutes.

2. Stir in the stock, beans, tomatoes, celery, vinegar, and pepper. Cover and bring to a boil. Reduce the heat and simmer until the vegetables are tender and the turkey is cooked through, about 15 minutes.

3. Stir in the smoke flavoring. Taste and season with salt and pepper if needed. Top each serving with cilantro.

Each serving: About 418 calories, 50 g protein, 42 g carbohydrate, 9 g total fat (trace saturated), 80 mg cholesterol, 674 mg sodium.

Turkey and Lentil Soup

PREP TIME: 10 minutes
COOK TIME: 45 minutes

Makes 6 servings

This is a good year-round soup, but it's also another place to put Thanksgiving leftovers to good use. If you have cooked turkey, just cut it into bite-size pieces and forget about the cutlets. Smoked turkey is delicious with lentils, so if you went that route for the holidays, all the better. And if you have sweet potatoes left over, dice some up to use in place of the yellow squash. If it's early autumn, chop up those amazing fresh tomatoes to use instead of the canned counterparts, and add sliced fresh basil leaves.

    1 tablespoon vegetable oil
    1 medium onion, chopped
    2 carrots, peeled and chopped into ¼-inch dice
    ¾ cup dried yellow lentils or split peas
    5 cups Turkey or Chicken Stock (Chapter 1)
      or water
    1 can (about 14 ounces) diced tomatoes with garlic
    1 yellow summer squash, diced
    2 pounds turkey cutlets, cut into thin strips
    Classic Pesto (page 47) for serving

1. Heat the oil in a 3-quart saucepan over medium-high heat. Add the onion and sauté until softened but not browned, about 5 minutes. Add the carrots and sauté 2 minutes. Add the lentils and stock and heat to boiling. Reduce the heat to medium-low and simmer, covered, 20 minutes.

2. Add the tomatoes with their juice, the squash, and turkey and mix well. Heat to boiling over medium-high heat. Simmer over medium heat until the turkey is cooked through, about 10 minutes. Ladle the soup into bowls. Add a dollop of pesto to each bowl.

Each serving: About 356 calories, 45 g protein, 24 g carbohydrate, 8 g total fat (2 g saturated), 98 mg cholesterol, 222 mg sodium.

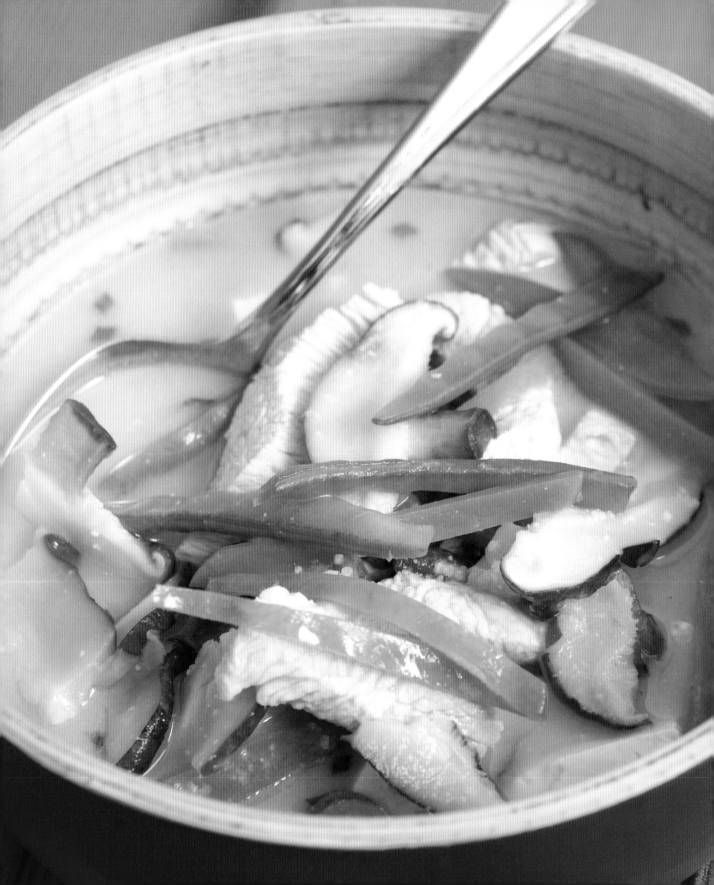

Miso Soup with Turkey and Tofu

PREP TIME: 20 minutes plus standing
COOK TIME: about 20 minutes

Makes 6 servings

Japanese cuisine is based on several items and miso, a flavorful soybean paste, is used as much as soy sauce. Miso is rich in B vitamins and proteins and has a concentrated flavor of grain, so even a dollop of it dissolved in a pot of broth has a strong flavor. Try this soup with Rice-Paper Crisps (page 32).

12 dried shiitake mushrooms
3 cups boiling water
3 cups cold water
8 ounces turkey cutlets, cut into thin strips about
   ¼ inch thick and 1½ inches long
½ cup yellow miso (shinsu ichi or yamabuki shiro)
¾ cup snow peas, stems and strings removed,
   pods slivered lengthwise
1 pound firm tofu, cut into thin slices about
   ¼ inch thick and 1½ inches long
snipped fresh chives for garnish

1. Soak the mushrooms in the boiling water in a heat-safe glass measure until the caps are soft, at least 20 minutes or overnight. Squeeze out the liquid from the mushrooms and place the mushrooms on a cutting board. Cut or tear off the tough stems and sliver the caps.

2. Pour the mushroom liquid through a sieve lined with a double thickness of cheesecloth into a 3-quart saucepan. Add the cold water and heat to boiling over medium-high heat. Add the turkey, and simmer over medium heat until tender and cooked through, about 6 minutes.

3. Mix ½ cup of the soup with the miso in a small bowl until blended. Heat the remaining soup to boiling. Add the slivered mushrooms and snow peas and simmer 3 minutes. Add the tofu and heat through. Stir the miso mixture into the sop and heat until almost boiling. Ladle the soup into warmed soup bowls and sprinkle with chives.

Each serving: About 241 calories, 21 g protein, 32 g carbohydrate, 6 g total fat (1 g saturated), 23 mg cholesterol, 870 mg sodium.

Winter-White Turkey Vegetable Soup

PREP TIME: 5 minutes
COOK TIME: 30 minutes

Makes 6 servings

1 teaspoon olive oil
1 medium onion, chopped
4 garlic cloves, chopped
3½ cups Chicken Stock (page 14)
2 potatoes, peeled and cut into ½-inch cubes
1 white turnip, peeled and cut into ½-inch cubes
1 small yellow squash, quartered lengthwise and sliced
1 can (15 ounces) cannellini beans, rinsed and drained
4 ounces cooked turkey breast, cut into 1-inch cubes
1 teaspoon dried basil leaves
¼ teaspoon white pepper
salt to taste
chopped fresh parsley for garnish

1. Heat the oil in a 6-quart pot over medium-high heat for 1 minute. Add the
   onion and garlic and sauté until the onion begins to brown. Stir in the stock,
   potatoes, turnip, squash, beans, turkey, basil, and pepper. Cover and bring to
   a boil. Reduce the heat and simmer until the vegetables are tender, 15 to 18
   minutes.

2. Remove the pot from the heat. Using a slotted spoon, transfer half the vegetables and turkey to a bowl. Using a handheld immersion blender, puree the
   vegetables and turkey in the pot. Return the reserved vegetables and turkey
   to the pot. Taste and season with salt if needed. Serve the soup garnished
   with parsley.

Each serving: About 185 calories, 14 g protein, 28 g carbohydrate, 3 g total fat (trace
saturated), 13 mg cholesterol, 274 mg sodium.

Zucchini Soup with Turkey-Ricotta Meatballs

PREP TIME: 20 minutes
COOK TIME: 30 to 35 minutes

Makes 6 to 8 servings

16 ounces whole-milk ricotta cheese
2 eggs
1 pound ground turkey
1 cup freshly grated Parmigiano-Reggiano cheese plus more for serving
½ cup packed fresh Italian parsley leaves
1 medium garlic clove, crushed through a press
¼ teaspoon freshly grated nutmeg
¼ teaspoon kosher salt or more to taste
¼ teaspoon freshly ground pepper or more to taste
flour for dusting your hands
½ cup olive oil
1 medium red onion, chopped
1 medium yellow zucchini or summer squash, quartered lengthwise, and cut crosswise in ½-inch chunks
1 medium green zucchini, quartered lengthwise and cut crosswise in ½-inch chunks
¼ cup tomato paste
1 can (about 14 ounces) diced tomatoes with zesty green chilies
½ teaspoon dried oregano leaves
1 quart Turkey Stock (page 18)

1. Place the ricotta in a fine strainer set over a bowl and drain overnight in the refrigerator.

2. The next day, beat the eggs in a medium bowl. Add the drained ricotta, turkey, 1 cup Parmigiano-Reggiano, parsley, garlic, nutmeg, salt, and pepper. Lightly but thoroughly, work the mixture together with your hands to mix. With lightly floured hands, shape the mixture into ¾-inch balls.

3. Heat the oil in a deep 10-inch skillet over medium-high heat. Add the meatballs, in batches if necessary, and cook until evenly browned, not turning the meatballs until the bottoms are browned and release easily from the pan. Transfer the meatballs to a 3-quart saucepan with a slotted spoon and set aside.

4. Add the onion to the drippings in the pan and sauté over medium-high heat until softened, about 7 minutes. Transfer the onion to the pan with the meatballs. Add the zucchini to the skillet and sauté until softened, about 5 minutes. Transfer the zucchini to the pan with the meatballs. Pour off all but 2 tablespoons drippings. Add the tomato paste to the pan and cook over medium-high heat, stirring, until rust-colored, about 1 minute. Add the tomatoes with their juice and the oregano and heat to boiling, stirring and scraping up the browned bits on the bottom of the pan. Pour the mixture into the saucepan.

5. Add the stock to the saucepan, cover, and heat the soup to boiling over medium heat. Taste and season with salt and pepper if needed. Ladle the soup into warmed bowls and sprinkle with cheese.

Each serving: About 569 calories, 36 g protein, 12 g carbohydrate, 42 g total fat (14 g saturated), 182 mg cholesterol, 919 mg sodium.

Sweet Italian Sausage Soup with Peppers

PREP TIME: 5 minutes
COOK TIME: 25 minutes

Makes 6 servings

Can't decide whether to have a sausage and pepper sandwich or a heartwarming soup? Have the best of each.

8 ounces sweet Italian turkey sausage, sliced
1 large onion, chopped
2 garlic cloves, minced
3½ cups Chicken or Vegetable Stock (Chapter 1)
½ pound red potatoes, chopped
½ teaspoon fennel seeds
¼ teaspoon freshly ground black pepper
1 can (14 ounces) stewed tomatoes, cut up
½ green bell pepper, seeded and chopped
½ yellow bell pepper, seeded and chopped
salt and freshly ground black pepper to taste

1. Heat a nonstick skillet over medium-high heat. Add the sausage and cook 10 minutes. Add the onion and garlic and sauté until the onions are translucent, about 3 minutes. Transfer to a 6-quart pot.

2. Stir in the stock, potatoes, fennel seeds, and black pepper. Cover and bring to a boil. Reduce the heat and simmer 15 minutes. Stir in the tomatoes, green pepper, and yellow pepper. Simmer 5 minutes. Taste and season with salt and black pepper if needed.

Each serving: About 190 calories, 10 g protein, 15 g carbohydrate, 11 g total fat (3 g saturated), 20 mg cholesterol, 447 mg sodium.

Crispy Duck Soup

PREP TIME: 25 minutes
COOK TIME: 2 hours 20 minutes

Makes 4 servings

You can crisp the breasts of pheasants, quail, dove, or guinea hen and use them in this soup instead of duck.

2 boneless duck breast halves
2 tablespoons soy sauce
2 medium Yukon Gold potatoes, peeled and cut into ¼-inch dice
1 slender carrot, peeled and cut into ¼-inch-thick slices
salt and freshly ground pepper to taste
1 scallion, cut into ¼-inch wide pieces
6 cups Game-Bird Stock (page 18) made with duck bones and giblets or 1 quart Chicken Stock (page 14)
2 tablespoons Calvados or other apple brandy
1 cup slivered red cabbage
1 cup slivered green cabbage

1. With a sharp knife, score the duck skin ¼ inch deep in a ½-inch crisscross pattern. Rub the soy sauce over the duck flesh and skin. Heat a heavy, deep skillet over medium heat and place the duck breasts skin side down in the pan. Cook, basting the meat with hot fat to cook from the top and adjusting the heat so the skin doesn't burn, until the fat is rendered and the skin is browned, about 10 minutes. Turn the breasts over and cook 4 minutes longer. Transfer to a cutting board and let rest 15 minutes.

2. While the duck rests, heat the drippings in the pan over medium-high heat and sauté the potatoes and carrot until tender, about 10 minutes. Transfer to a paper towel–lined plate to drain and sprinkle lightly with salt and pepper. Add the scallion and sauté until tender, about 3 minutes. Transfer to another paper towel–lined plate to drain. Pour off the fat and wipe the pan with a paper towel. Return the sautéed vegetables to the pan and keep warm over medium heat.

3. Heat the stock and Calvados to boiling in a 3-quart saucepan over medium-high heat and season with salt and pepper. Add the cabbage and cook until tender, about 3 minutes.

4. To serve: Thinly slice the duck in diagonal slices across the grain. Pour any juices into the stock. Ladle the stock and cabbage into 4 warmed shallow soup bowls. Fan out one-fourth of the duck slices in the center of each and surround with one-fourth of the vegetables.

Each serving: About 252 calories, 23 g protein, 16 g carbohydrate, 8 g total fat (2 g saturated), 76 mg cholesterol, 728 mg sodium.

Duck Soup with Cherries and Frizzled Leeks

PREP TIME: 15 minutes
COOK TIME: 25 minutes

Makes 4 to 6 servings

To make the duck fat to fry the leeks, cut the duck skin and fat from the breasts and poke holes with a fork into the fat on the skin side. Place the skin and fat in a skillet over low heat and slowly render the fat. (For a decadent treat, make duck cracklings: Cut the skin into small tidbits, sprinkle with salt, and serve as cocktail bites, or add them to the soup just before serving.)

6 cups Game-Bird Stock (page 18) made with
    duck bones and giblets or 1 quart Chicken Stock
    (page 14)
2 (¼-inch-thick) slices peeled celeriac, julienned
1 tablespoon julienned orange peel
2 boneless duck breast halves, skin removed
2 medium leeks
1 cup duck fat or olive oil
½ cup dried cherries
¼ cup dry Madeira or red wine
sea salt and freshly ground pepper to taste
freshly grated nutmeg to taste

1. Place the stock, celeriac, and orange peel in a 2-quart saucepan and heat to boiling over medium-high heat. Reduce the heat to medium-low, add the duck, and simmer gently until barely cooked through, about 5 minutes. Transfer the duck to a bowl with a slotted spoon and let cool. Simmer the stock over low heat.

2. While the duck cools, trim the leeks and split lengthwise. Rinse very well and julienne. Pat the pieces dry with paper towels. Heat the duck fat in a small skillet over medium-high heat until hot. Add the leeks and sauté until browned, crisp, and frizzled, about 3 minutes. Drain on paper towels and sprinkle with salt while hot. Keep warm but do not cover or the leeks will get soggy.

3. To serve: Add the cherries and Madeira to the simmering stock. Season with salt, pepper, and nutmeg. Cut the duck into thin strips, add to the soup, and heat through. Ladle the soup into warmed soup bowls and sprinkle each bowl generously with leeks.

Each of 4 servings: About 229 calories, 21 g protein, 16 g carbohydrate, 7 g total fat (2 g saturated), 66 mg cholesterol, 220 mg sodium.

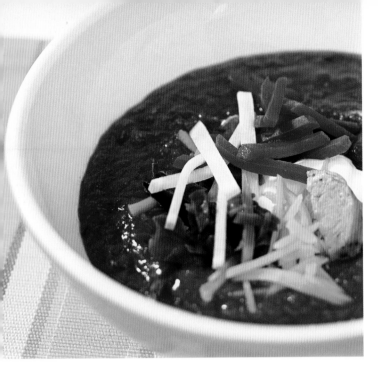

9

MEAT SOUPS

A Big Pot of Old-Fashioned Vegetable-Beef Soup

PREP TIME: 20 minutes plus chilling
COOK TIME: 3 hours 40 minutes

Makes 10 to 12 servings

This is a weekend project, requiring overnight chilling of the stock and another night for the finished soup to mellow. Freeze it in batches and your labors will pay tasty, quick dividends.

4 quarts water
2-pound beef shank, cut crosswise into 2-inch pieces
1 pound meaty soup bones or short ribs, rinsed
1 large onion, quartered
4 medium carrots
2 celery stalks, chopped
4 whole sprigs fresh parsley plus 2 tablespoons chopped
1 tablespoon salt or more to taste
1 medium potato
2 cups shredded cabbage
1 cup fresh or thawed frozen lima beans
1 cup fresh or thawed frozen corn kernels
1 cup fresh or thawed frozen cut green beans
1 cup fresh or thawed frozen peas
1 can (about 14 ounces) diced tomatoes
½ teaspoon freshly ground pepper or more to taste

1. Combine the water, beef, bones, onion, 2 carrots, half the celery, the parsley sprigs, and salt in a very large stockpot. Heat to boiling over medium heat, skimming off any foam that forms on the surface. Reduce the heat to medium-low and simmer, uncovered, for 3 hours. Strain the stock through a colander placed over another large pot. Discard all the solids except the meat. When the meat is cool enough to handle, cut into bite-size pieces. Place the meat in a bowl, cover, and refrigerate overnight. Cool the stock to room temperature and refrigerate overnight.

2. The next day, discard the hardened fat on top of the stock. Peel the remaining carrots and the potato and dice. Add the diced vegetables to the stock and heat to boiling over medium-high heat. Add the meat, cabbage, lima beans, corn, green beans, peas, and tomatoes with their juice. Gently boil over medium heat, partially covered, until the vegetables are tender, about 30 minutes. Stir in the chopped parsley and pepper. Taste for seasoning and add more salt and pepper if needed.

Each of 10 servings: About 258 calories, 30 g protein, 14 g carbohydrate, 9 g total fat (3 g saturated), 68 mg cholesterol, 68 mg sodium.

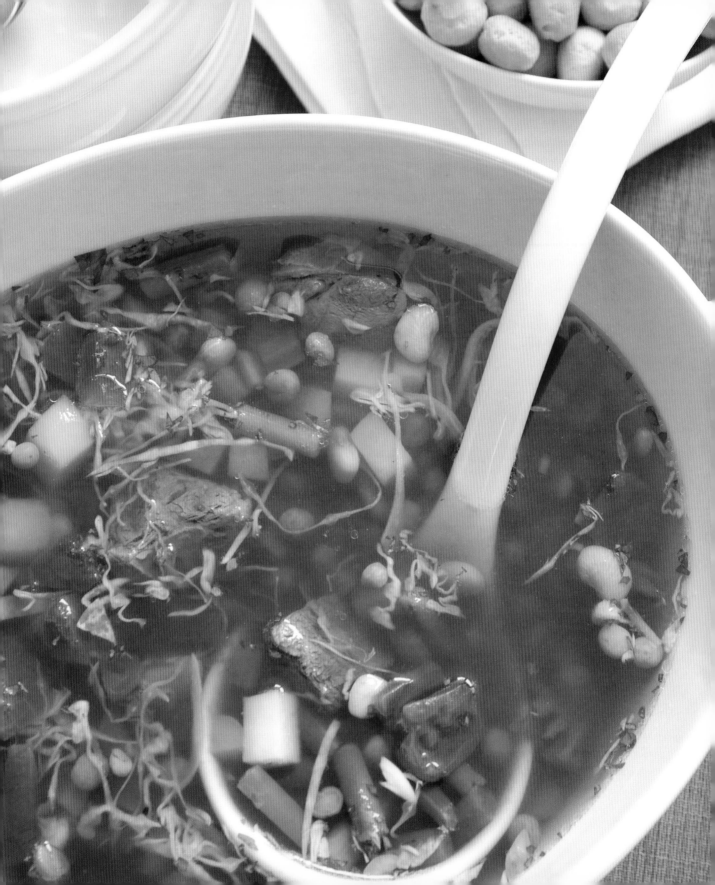

Hearty Oxtail Soup

PREP TIME: 35 minutes plus chilling
COOK TIME: 13 hours

Makes 12 servings

Because this soup takes a long time to prepare, it's best
to make a lot of it and freeze the leftovers in 1-quart
amounts. Many cookbooks call for cooking oxtails three,
four, or five hours, but there is still a tremendous
amount of flavor and substance still left on the bones
after that amount of time. So here's one version that is
an all-day simmer, hours to cool, and an overnight in
the refrigerator to allow the fat to harden on top. All the
time and energy invested will result in one of the most
delicious soups you'll ever taste.

The Soup

   4 pounds oxtails, cut crosswise into 2-inch chunks
   2 large carrots, peeled, halved lengthwise, cut
     crosswise into 2-inch chunks
   1 large Spanish onion, cut into 6 wedges through
     the root so the wedges stay together
   1 large celery rib, cut crosswise into 2-inch chunks
   3 large garlic cloves, unpeeled
   2 tablespoons olive oil
   1 tablespoon soy sauce
   1 teaspoon fennel seeds, crushed
   1 teaspoon dried oregano leaves, crumbled
   1 teaspoon dried thyme leaves, crushed
   1 teaspoon salt plus more to taste
   1 teaspoon freshly ground pepper plus more to taste
  cold water

To Finish the Soup

   3 large carrots, peeled and cut into ¼-inch dice

   3 small turnips, peeled and cut into ¼-inch dice
   ½ cup port wine, amontillado sherry, rice wine,
     or sake
   ¼ cup finely chopped fresh Italian parsley
   2 tablespoons grated peeled fresh gingerroot or
     more to taste

1. Preheat the oven to 500 degrees. Rinse the oxtails
   well with cold water, pat dry with paper towels, and
   place in a very large, heavy roasting pan. Add the
   carrots, onion, celery, and garlic. Mix the olive oil, soy
   sauce, fennel seeds, oregano, thyme, salt, and pepper
   together in a small bowl; rub over the oxtails and
   vegetables. Roast the meat and vegetables on the
   center oven rack until browned, about 20 minutes,
   turning the pieces to brown on all sides.

2. Remove the pan from the oven and transfer the contents to a 6-quart stockpot. Place the roasting pan on
   the stovetop over a burner and heat over medium-
   high heat. Add 2 cups of water and stir constantly to
   loosen the browned bits on the bottom of the pot.
   Pour the liquid into the pot and fill with enough cold
   water to cover the oxtails by at least 3 inches.

3. Heat the soup to boiling over medium heat,
   skimming off any foam that forms on the surface.
   Simmer over medium-low heat until the meat is
   falling off the bones, about 12 hours, checking the
   soup frequently and adding enough water (about

every 2 hours) to keep the contents covered by 3 inches. Cool the soup completely, about 4 hours.

4. Ladle the stock into a sieve lined with a double-thickness of cheesecloth set over another large pot. Transfer the solids to a colander placed over a bowl. Discard all the solids in the colander except the meat. Shred the meat and place in a bowl. Pour the stock in the bowl through the cheesecloth-lined sieve into the large pot. Cover the stock and the meat and refrigerate overnight.

5. The next day: Discard the layer of fat from the top of the stock. At this point you can divide the stock among 1-quart containers, add portions of meat to each, and freeze. Then, reheat a batch of soup when you want, adding vegetables of your choice. Or, you can heat the pot of stock to boiling over medium-high heat. While the stock heats, transfer about 2 cups to a small saucepan and add the diced carrots and turnips. Heat to boiling over medium heat and simmer until tender, about 15 minutes. Add the vegetables and their liquid to the big pot, along with the meat, wine, parsley, and ginger. Taste and season with salt, pepper, and ginger if needed. Serve the soup in warmed soup bowls.

Each serving: About 222 calories, 34 g protein, 5 g carbohydrate, 6 g total fat (2 g saturated), 59 mg cholesterol, 339 mg sodium.

Ginger-Garlic Beef Soup

PREP TIME: 15 minutes
COOK TIME: 1 hour 40 minutes

Makes 6 servings

2 quarts Vietnamese Spicy Stock (page 21)
8 scallions, cut crosswise into ½-inch slices, plus ¼ cup minced scallions for serving
4 large garlic cloves, crushed through a press
¼ cup low-sodium soy sauce
2 pounds well-trimmed chuck or beef stew meat, trimmed, cut into ½-inch pieces
1 pound baby spinach leaves, washed and drained
¼ cup rice wine or sake
2 tablespoons grated peeled fresh gingerroot
ground cinnamon for dusting

1. Combine the stock, sliced scallions, garlic, and soy sauce in a 4-quart saucepan over medium-high heat and heat to boiling. Add the beef, reduce the heat to medium-low, cover, and cook until the beef is tender, about 1½ hours, frequently skimming the foam from the surface.

2. Add the spinach, rice wine, and ginger to the soup, increase the heat to medium-high, and heat to boiling. Ladle the soup into warmed soup bowls, sprinkle with the minced scallions and dust with the cinnamon.

Each serving: About 226 calories, 33 g protein, 7 g carbohydrate, 7 g total fat (2 g saturated), 71 mg cholesterol, 1,014 mg sodium.

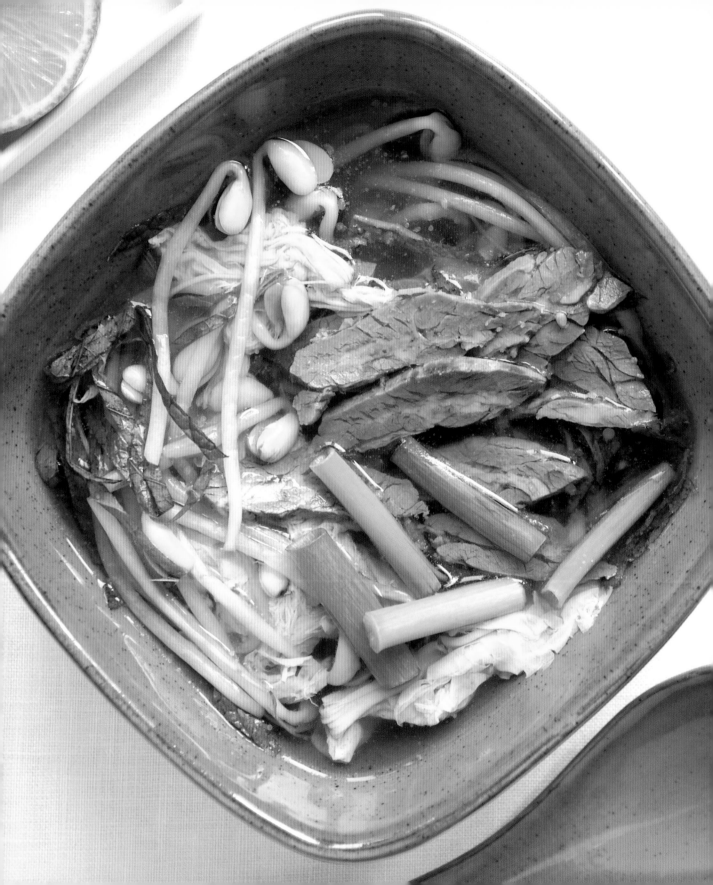

Beef Soup with Eggs and Mint

PREP TIME: 20 minutes
COOK TIME: 2 hours 10 minutes

Makes 6 servings

This main-course soup is complete with Rice-Paper Crisps (page 32) and a fresh-fruit compote.

    1 pound flank steak
    3 quarts water
    12 scallions, 6 cut crosswise into 1-inch pieces
       and 6 cut crosswise into thin slices
    2 star anise
    3-inch cinnamon stick
    2-inch piece fresh gingerroot (unpeeled is OK),
       thinly sliced and crushed
    6 garlic cloves, minced
    2 tablespoons nam plah (Thai fish sauce) or more
       to taste
    1 tablespoon soy sauce or more to taste
    1 teaspoon sugar
    ½ teaspoon freshly ground pepper
    3 cups fresh bean sprouts, rinsed, roots and
       pods removed
    1 cup mint leaves, shredded
    2 eggs beaten with 2 tablespoons water

1. Cut the meat into 6 large pieces and place in a 4-quart saucepan. Add the water, 1-inch pieces of scallions, the star anise, cinnamon, and ginger. Heat to boiling over medium heat; reduce the heat and simmer until the beef is tender, about 2 hours, frequently skimming off the foam that forms on the surface.

2. Strain the soup through a fine sieve into a 3-quart saucepan. Discard all the solids except the meat. When the meat is cool enough to handle, cut into thin slices across the grain. Add the meat to the stock and stir in the garlic, nam plah, soy sauce, sugar, and pepper. Add the bean sprouts and mint and heat over medium-high heat, stirring, until almost boiling. Remove the pan from the heat and, with chopsticks, slowly stir in the eggs in a circle near the side of the pan. Stir once or twice more in a circular motion so the eggs form streamers as they cook. Taste and add more nam plah and soy sauce if needed. Ladle into warm soup bowls and sprinkle with the sliced scallions.

Each serving: About 198 calories, 20 g protein, 8 g carbohydrate, 10 g total fat (4 g saturated), 110 mg cholesterol, 719 mg sodium.

Savory Steak and Sweet Potato Soup

PREP TIME: 10 minutes
COOK TIME: 25 minutes

Makes 4 servings

Instead of the usual potatoes and carrots, this scrumptious beef soup relies on sweet potatoes for body, flavor, and color. Use the moist, red (deep orange) variety of sweet potato.

    2 tablespoons chopped fresh sage
    ½ teaspoon freshly ground black pepper
    ½ pound round steak, cut into ½-inch cubes
    2 teaspoons olive oil
    1 medium Spanish onion, chopped
    3½ cups Beef Stock (page 15)
    2 cups shredded peeled sweet potato
    ¼ cup dry red wine
    1 cup frozen peas
    salt to taste
    ½ teaspoon paprika for garnish

1. Combine the sage and pepper. Coat the beef cubes with 1 teaspoon olive oil. Rub the pepper-sage mixture into the beef. Heat the remaining 1 teaspoon oil in a 6-quart pot. Add the beef and onions and sauté until the beef is lightly browned, about 5 minutes.

2. Stir in the stock, sweet potato, and wine. Cover and bring to a boil. Reduce the heat and simmer 15 minutes. Stir in the peas and simmer for 5 minutes. Taste and season with salt if needed. Top each serving with paprika.

Each serving: About 272 calories, 26 g protein, 21 g carbohydrate, 8 g total fat (2 g saturated), 56 mg cholesterol, 319 mg sodium.

Chinese Hot and Sour Soup

PREP TIME: 50 minutes
COOK TIME: about 25 minutes

Makes 4 to 6 servings

It's not traditional, but a little ham in the soup is nice with the pork and other ingredients. A handful of strips of thinly sliced Smithfield or baked ham is all you need.

4 dried Chinese mushrooms

¼ cup dried tree-ear mushrooms

30 dried day lily buds

1 (4-inch) square tofu, cut into ½-inch cubes

1¼ teaspoons salt or more to taste

2 tablespoons cornstarch

1 quart Chicken Stock or Gingered Chicken Stock (page 14)

1 tablespoon soy sauce

4 to 8 ounces boneless pork (from chops or tenderloin), julienned or ground

2 tablespoons Chinese rice wine vinegar or aged sherry vinegar or more to taste

¼ teaspoon ground white pepper or more to taste

1 egg, lightly beaten

2 scallions, cut into thin rounds

1 teaspoon dark sesame oil

1. Soak the Chinese mushrooms and tree-ear mushrooms in a bowl with ½ cup hot water and the day lily buds in a separate bowl with ½ cup hot water until softened, 30 minutes. Handling the tofu gently, place it on a cutting board and cut into ¼-inch-wide strips. Cut the strips crosswise in half and place in a bowl. Sprinkle with ¼ teaspoon salt; set aside.

2. Remove the mushrooms and day lily buds from their soaking liquids, squeezing them to extract the liquid. Discard the day lily bud soaking liquid. Strain the mushroom soaking liquid through a fine sieve into a bowl and stir in the cornstarch. Set aside. Tear or cut off the hard stems of the Chinese mushrooms and cut the caps into thin slices. Tear the tree-ear mushrooms into bite-size pieces. Tear or cut off the hard stem ends of the day lily buds. Stack the buds, slice lengthwise, and cut crosswise in half.

3. Combine the stock, soy sauce, and remaining 1 teaspoon salt in a 3-quart saucepan and heat to boiling. Add the pork, stirring to separate the pieces. Skim any scum that forms on the surface. Add the mushrooms and day lily buds. Cook over medium heat 2 to 3 minutes. Drain the tofu if necessary and gently add to the soup. Stir in the vinegar and pepper. Stir the mushroom liquid and cornstarch to recombine and stir into the soup. Cook, stirring, until the soup is clear and thickened.

4. Remove the pan from the heat and stir in the egg. Let stand until the egg is cooked but still soft, about 2 minutes. Taste and add more vinegar and pepper if needed. Stir in the scallions and sesame oil and serve.

Each serving, using 4 ounces of pork: About 208 calories, 18 g protein, 21 g carbohydrate, 7 g total fat (2 g saturated), 72 mg cholesterol, 296 mg sodium.

Goulash Soup

PREP TIME: 10 minutes
COOK TIME: 40 minutes

Makes 6 servings

In this robust noodle and beef soup, cocoa and a generous spoonful of paprika give a tomato-beef broth a rich depth of flavor and color.

12 ounces beef round roast
1 teaspoon olive oil
1 large onion, cut into rings
2 cups sliced white mushrooms
5 cups Beef Stock (page 15)
1 can (15 ounces) stewed tomatoes, chopped
1 teaspoon cocoa
4 ounces Hungarian egg noodles (kluski) or thin egg noodles
1 tablespoon paprika
salt and pepper to taste
2 teaspoons caraway seeds for garnish

1. Trim visible fat from the round roast and tenderize the meat with a mallet. Cut into ½-inch cubes.

2. Heat the oil in a 6-quart pot over medium-high heat for 1 minute. Add the beef and sauté until lightly browned, about 6 minutes. Add the onion and mushrooms and sauté until the onion is translucent, about 3 minutes.

3. Stir in the stock, tomatoes, and cocoa. Cover and bring to a boil. Reduce the heat and simmer 10 minutes. Stir in the noodles and paprika and simmer 18 minutes. Taste and season with salt and pepper if needed. Top each serving with caraway seeds.

Each serving: About 255 calories, 24 g protein, 22 g carbohydrate, 7 g total fat (2 g saturated), 57 mg cholesterol, 309 mg sodium.

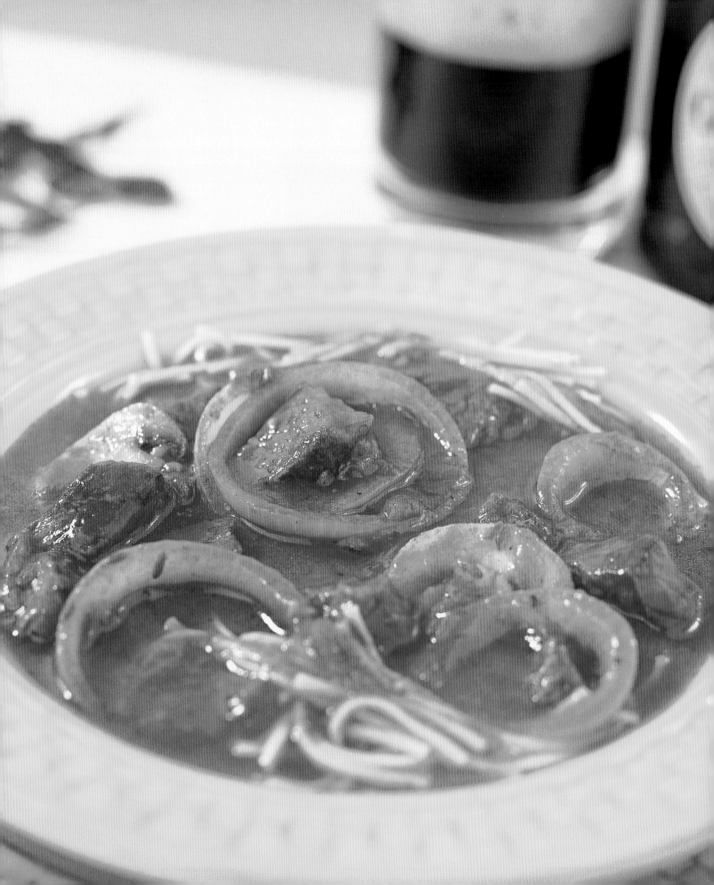

Pho Bo (VIETNAMESE SPICY SOUP WITH RICE NOODLES)

PREP TIME: 35 minutes
COOK TIME: 10 minutes

Makes 6 to 8 servings

You can make this soup using any kind of stock and the cooked meat or poultry used to make it. In the warm, southern part of Vietnam, chicken is used, but in the colder north the soup is made with beef. Serve soup bowls of just the noodles and soup and allow guests to add the seasonings as they wish.

16 ounces banh pho (Vietnamese rice noodles)
water for soaking and cooking the noodles
2 quarts Vietnamese Spicy Stock made with beef
  stock (page 21)
2 cups fresh bean sprouts, rinsed, roots and
  pods removed
3 cups shredded cooked beef
¼ cup nuoc mam (Vietnamese fish sauce) plus
  more for serving
1 cup fresh Thai purple or holy basil leaves or
  regular basil leaves, stemmed and shredded,
  for serving
¼ cup minced scallions for serving
¼ cup minced fresh cilantro leaves for serving
¼ cup minced fresh mint leaves for serving
2 hot fresh chiles, thinly sliced, for serving
1 lime, cut into wedges, for serving

1. Place the noodles in a large bowl and cover with cold water. Let soak 30 minutes.

2. Heat 4 quarts of water to simmering in a 4-quart pot. Heat the stock to boiling in a 3-quart saucepan over high heat. Add the bean sprouts to the stock and cook 1 minute. Reduce the heat to simmering, add the beef and nuoc mam, and keep the soup warm over medium heat.

3. Add the noodles to the simmering water and stir to untangle. Let stand until tender, about 30 seconds; drain immediately in a colander. Rinse under running warm water and drain again.

4. To serve: Place piles of noodles in warmed soup bowls and ladle the soup on top. Serve the soup and pass additional nuoc mam, the basil, scallions, cilantro, mint, chiles, and lime wedges at the table for guests to season to taste.

Each serving: About 508 calories, 28 g protein, 68 g carbohydrate, 13 g total fat (5 g saturated), 51 mg cholesterol, 1,158 mg sodium.

Noodle Soup Bolognese

PREP TIME: 5 minutes
COOK TIME: 25 minutes

Makes 4 servings

Traditional Bolognese, named after the rich culinary style of Bologna, Italy, refers to a flavorful meat and vegetable sauce that's often served over pasta. This dish simmers the noodles right along with the beef, prosciutto, mushrooms, and tomatoes.

  1 tablespoon unsalted butter
  1 tablespoon olive oil
  1 large onion, chopped
  2 ounces prosciutto, chopped
  ¾ pound ground sirloin
  1 cup white mushrooms, chopped
  4 cups Beef Stock (page 15)
  1 can (15 ounces) diced tomatoes
  4 ounces wide egg noodles
  2 teaspoons no-salt-added tomato paste
  ½ teaspoon freshly ground black pepper
  salt to taste
  1 cup Garlic Croutons (page 22) for serving

1. Melt the butter in the oil in a 6-quart pot. Add the onion and prosciutto and cook until the onion is golden, about 5 minutes. Add the sirloin and mushrooms and cook, stirring occasionally, until the meat is browned and crumbly, about 8 minutes. Drain off excess liquid.

2. Stir in the stock, tomatoes, noodles, tomato paste, and pepper. Cover and bring to a boil. Reduce the heat and simmer until the noodles are al dente, 8 to 10 minutes. Taste and season with salt if needed. Top each serving with croutons.

Each serving: About 477 calories, 39 g protein, 40 g carbohydrate, 18 g total fat (6 g saturated), 105 mg cholesterol, 1,622 mg sodium.

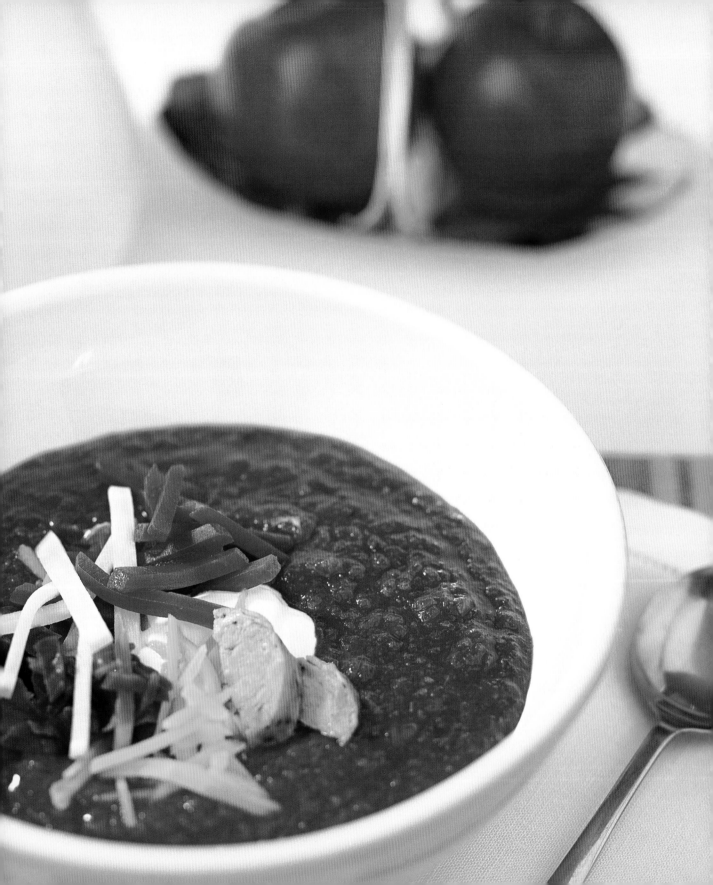

Borscht with Veal Sausage

PREP TIME: 5 minutes
COOK TIME: 20 minutes

Makes 4 servings

Spicy veal sausage brings zip to this fast version of a traditional Russian beet soup. Serve it hot with a dollop of sour cream.

  2 cups canned diced beets with liquid
  3½ cups Beef Stock (page 15)
  1 cup shredded peeled carrots
  1 cup coarsely chopped red cabbage
  1 medium onion, chopped
  4 ounces cooked veal sausage, chopped
  ½ cup shredded white turnip
  1 tablespoon tomato paste
  2 teaspoons red wine vinegar
  ½ teaspoon sugar
  ½ teaspoon freshly ground black pepper
  ½ cup nonfat or reduced-fat sour cream for serving
  salt to taste

1. Combine the beets, stock, carrots, cabbage, onion, sausage, turnip, tomato paste, vinegar, sugar, and pepper in a 6-quart pot. Cover and bring to a boil. Reduce the heat and simmer 15 minutes.

2. Remove the pot from the heat. Using a handheld immersion blender, process the mixture until partially pureed. Taste and season with salt if needed. Top each serving with a swirl of sour cream.

Each serving: About 119 calories, 7 g protein, 22 g carbohydrate, 1 g total fat (trace saturated), 3 mg cholesterol, 460 mg sodium.

Veal Scaloppini and Mushroom Soup

PREP TIME: 5 minutes
COOK TIME: 20 minutes

Makes 4 servings

The traditional ingredients that make up an elegant Veal Scaloppini—
veal scallops, shallots, white wine, mushrooms—are terrific in a soup!
If veal scallops are hard to find, substitute very thin slices of veal.

2 teaspoons olive oil
1 pound veal scallops, about ⅛-inch thick, cut into bite-size pieces
4 ounces mushroom caps, quartered if large
2 shallots, thinly sliced
2 garlic cloves, chopped
3½ cups Chicken Stock (page 14)
½ cup Chardonnay or other dry white wine
½ teaspoon white pepper
½ teaspoon marjoram leaves
salt to taste
¼ cup roasted red peppers, chopped, for serving
¼ cup chopped fresh parsley for serving

1. Heat the oil in a 6-quart pot over medium-high heat for 1 minute. Add
   the veal, mushrooms, shallots, and garlic and sauté until the veal is no
   longer pink, 3 to 7 minutes.

2. Stir in the stock, wine, and white pepper. Cover and bring to a boil.
   Reduce the heat and simmer 10 minutes. Stir in the marjoram.
   Taste and season with salt if needed. Top each serving with the red
   peppers and parsley.

Each serving: About 298 calories, 22 g protein, 5 g carbohydrate, 19 g total fat
(6 saturated), 84 mg cholesterol, 388 mg sodium.

Chinese Pork Noodle Soup

PREP TIME: 10 minutes
COOK TIME: 20 minutes

Makes 4 servings

Bok choy, pork, Chinese noodles, sesame oil, and soy sauce all add up to a captivating soup with tons of Asian-style flavor. Can't find any Chinese noodles? Substitute angel hair pasta.

   8 ounces center-cut pork loin
   1 teaspoon sesame oil
   6 mushroom caps, sliced
   4 cups Chicken Stock (page 14)
   1 tablespoon dry sherry
   2 teaspoons reduced-sodium soy sauce
   1 cup sliced bok choy
   2 cups torn spinach leaves
   2 scallions, sliced
   4 ounces Chinese wheat noodles
   2 cups bean sprouts
   salt and pepper to taste

1. Using a meat mallet, pound the pork to tenderize it. Cut the pork into thin 1-inch-long strips. Heat the oil in a skillet over medium-high heat for 1 minute. Add the pork and mushrooms, and sauté until the pork is lightly browned.

2. Transfer the mixture to a 6-quart pot and add the stock, sherry, soy sauce, bok choy, spinach, and scallions. Cover and bring to a boil. Reduce the heat and simmer 4 minutes.

3. Stir in the noodles and sprouts and cook 3 minutes more. Taste and season with salt and pepper if needed.

Each serving: About 387 calories, 30 g protein, 23 g carbohydrate, 18 g total fat (5 g saturated), 49 mg cholesterol, 832 mg sodium.

Chinese Vegetable Soup with Pork Meatballs

PREP TIME: 20 minutes
COOK TIME: 15 minutes

Makes 4 servings

If you want more vegetables in the soup, add a big handful of coarsely shredded fresh spinach or napa cabbage and a grated carrot with the snow peas.

½ pound lean ground pork
1 medium garlic clove, crushed through a press
1½ teaspoons minced peeled fresh gingerroot
2 teaspoons dry sherry
2 teaspoons soy sauce
1 teaspoon cornstarch
½ teaspoon sugar
½ teaspoon salt
big pinch cayenne pepper
1 tablespoon canola oil
½ cup finely chopped scallions
2 plum tomatoes, skinned, seeded, and diced
1 quart Gingered Chicken Stock (page 14)
8 ounces snow peas, strings removed

1. In a medium bowl, mix the pork, garlic, ginger, sherry, soy sauce, cornstarch, sugar, salt, and cayenne pepper until blended. Form into marble-sized balls.

2. Heat the oil in a 2-quart saucepan over medium heat. Add half the scallions and sauté until softened, about 3 minutes. Add the tomatoes and sauté 1 minute. Add the stock and heat to boiling.

3. Add the snow peas and meatballs and reduce the heat to medium. After the meatballs rise to the surface (about 4 minutes), cook another 2 minutes. Ladle the soup into warmed soup bowls. Sprinkle with the remaining scallions.

Each serving: About 225 calories, 12 g protein, 9 g carbohydrate, 16 g total fat (5 g saturated), 41 mg cholesterol, 500 mg sodium.

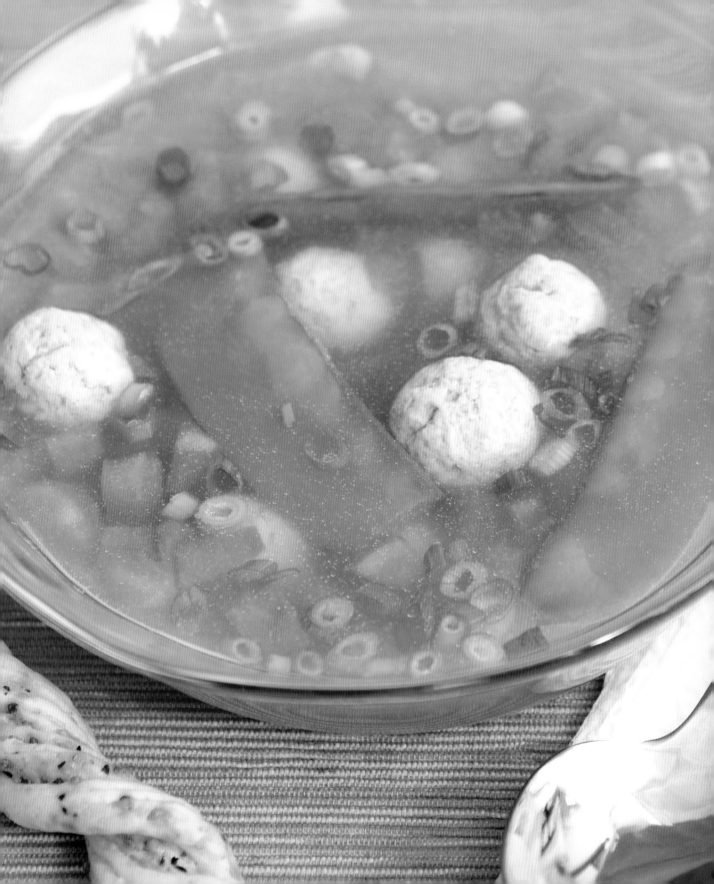

Asian Pork and Vegetable Soup

PREP TIME: 15 minutes
COOK TIME: about 20 minutes

Makes 8 servings

It's a time-consuming labor of love to trim the hairy roots and often-soggy pods from fresh bean sprouts, but maybe by the third time you've done it, you'll be convinced that it's a worthwhile task. If you'd like to tackle the task ahead of time, rinse the cleaned sprouts and spread them out in a single layer on paper towels; roll up and store in the crisper (the idea is to keep the sprouts hydrated but dry on the outside). Scallion Pancakes (page 32) would be an amazing accompaniment to this easy soup.

1½ teaspoons canola oil
4 scallions, julienned
1 garlic clove, minced
pinch crushed red pepper flakes
2 quarts Chicken Stock (page 14)
1 pound pork tenderloin, halved lengthwise and sliced crosswise into ¼-inch-thick strips
¼ cup oyster sauce
1 can (14 ounces) baby corn, rinsed
1 cup sugar snap peas, trimmed
1 cup thinly sliced shiitake mushrooms
2 cups sliced baby bok choy
2 cups fresh bean sprouts, rinsed, roots and pods trimmed
2 tablespoons rice wine, dry sherry, or sake
2 tablespoons cornstarch
2 tablespoons dark sesame oil for serving
2 tablespoons finely chopped cilantro leaves for serving

1. Heat the oil in a 4-quart saucepan over medium heat and sauté the scallions, garlic, and pepper flakes until fragrant, about 3 minutes. Add the stock and heat to boiling over medium-high heat. Add the pork and stir to separate the pieces. Stir in the oyster sauce and corn.

2. Bring the soup to a boil and add the sugar snap peas and mushrooms. Bring to a boil and add the bok choy and bean sprouts. Stir the rice wine with the cornstarch until blended, then stir into the soup. Simmer just until the soup is clear. Ladle into warmed shallow soup bowls, drizzle with the sesame oil and sprinkle with the cilantro.

Each serving: About 221 calories, 20 g protein, 17 g carbohydrate, 8 g total fat (2 g saturated), 37 mg cholesterol, 107 mg sodium.

Pork and Clam Soup

PREP TIME: 10 minutes
COOK TIME: 35 minutes

Makes 4 servings

The unexpected combination of pork and clams is a staple in Portuguese cuisine. If you want a more dramatic presentation, leave the clams in their shells. Slightly sweet store-bought Portuguese bread is a delicious and obvious serve-with; or bake up some French Peasant Flat Bread (page 28) with Portuguese olive oil.

1½ cups dry white wine
24 small clams, scrubbed
3 tablespoons extravirgin olive oil (preferably Portuguese or Spanish)
2 medium onions, thinly sliced
1 large red bell pepper, seeded and cut into ½-inch squares
1 pound pork tenderloin, cut into ½-inch cubes
2 medium garlic cloves, minced
1 tablespoon sweet paprika
⅛ teaspoon crushed pepper flakes
2 medium tomatoes, skinned, seeded, and diced
3 cups tomato juice cocktail (Clamato juice)
¼ teaspoon salt or more to taste
¼ teaspoon freshly ground black pepper or more to taste
¼ cup finely chopped fresh cilantro leaves for garnish
lemon wedges for serving
sliced French bread for dunking in the broth

1. Heat the wine in a 3-quart saucepan over medium-high heat to boiling. Add the clams and cover. Steam, stirring once or twice to make sure all the clams have room to open, until the clams open, about 8 minutes. Discard any unopened clams. Drain the clams through a colander lined with a double-thickness of cheesecloth set over a bowl. Set aside the cooking liquid. Remove the clams from the shells and set aside. Clean the pan.

2. Heat the oil in the cleaned pan set over medium-high heat. Add the onions and bell pepper and sauté until softened, about 5 minutes. Add the pork, garlic, paprika, and pepper flakes and sauté until the pork is lightly browned, about 5 minutes. Add the clam cooking liquid, tomatoes, tomato juice cocktail, salt, and black pepper and heat to simmering. Simmer, partially covered, 10 minutes to blend the flavors. Stir in the clams and heat through.

3. To serve: Ladle the soup into warmed shallow soup bowls. Sprinkle with cilantro and serve with lemon wedges to squeeze as desired; set out bread for dunking.

Each serving without lemon or bread: About 494 calories, 38 g protein, 36 g carbohydrate, 16 g total fat (3 g saturated), 99 mg cholesterol, 915 mg sodium.

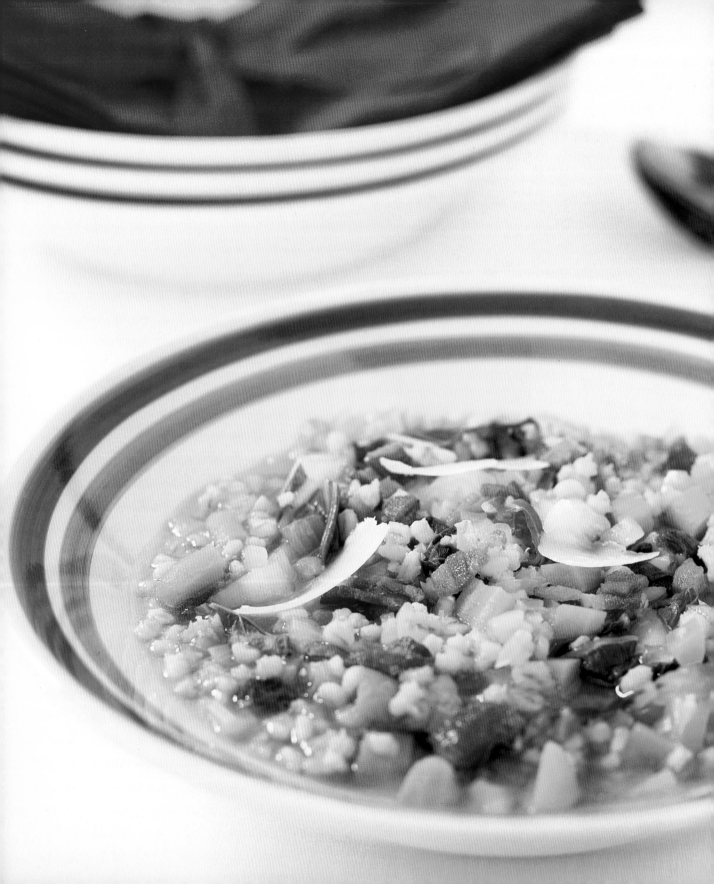

Porcini, Pancetta, and Barley Soup

PREP TIME: 10 minutes
COOK TIME: 50 minutes

Makes 6 servings

If you want to prepare this soup one day ahead, cook through step 2 and let cool slightly. Refrigerate uncovered until cold, then cover. To serve, bring to a simmer before adding the Swiss chard.

4 ounces pancetta or thick bacon slices, cut into ½-inch-wide strips
½ cup chopped shallots
½ cup finely chopped carrots
½ cup finely chopped celery
2 garlic cloves, minced
2 cups water
2 cups Beef Stock (page 15)
1½ cups Chicken Stock (page 14)
½ cup pearl barley
½ ounce dried porcini mushrooms, brushed clean of grit
2 large Swiss chard leaves, thinly sliced crosswise (about 2 packed cups)
salt and pepper to taste
extravirgin olive oil for serving
shaved Romano cheese for serving

1. Cook the pancetta or bacon in a 6-quart pot over medium-high heat until crisp, about 6 minutes (if using bacon, drain off excess drippings). Add the shallots, carrots, celery, and garlic and cook until soft, about 5 minutes. Add the water, beef stock, chicken stock, barley, and porcini mushrooms and bring to a boil. Reduce the heat and simmer, stirring occasionally, until the barley is tender, about 40 minutes.

2. Add the chard and cook until wilted, about 1 minute. Taste and season with salt and pepper if needed. Ladle the soup into bowls, drizzle with oil, and top with cheese.

Each serving: About 116 calories, 8 g protein, 19 g carbohydrate, 2 g total fat (1 g saturated), 10 mg cholesterol, 596 mg sodium.

Baked Chinese Cabbage Soup

PREP TIME: 35 minutes
COOK TIME: 1 hour 50 minutes

Makes 4 servings

1 tablespoon unsalted butter
¼ cup finely chopped onion
¾ cup water
¼ cup long-grain white rice (not converted)
½ teaspoon salt
¼ teaspoon finely chopped fresh thyme leaves (no stems)
¾ teaspoon freshly ground black pepper
1 medium head (about 8 ounces) Napa cabbage
8 ounces lean ground pork
8 ounces lean ground veal
1 egg, lightly beaten
3 teaspoons canola oil
2 tablespoons minced scallions, white part only
1½ tablespoons minced peeled fresh gingerroot
1 large garlic clove, crushed through a press
2 tablespoons rice wine or sake
5 cups Chicken Stock (page 14)
2 tablespoons soy sauce
1½ teaspoons dark sesame oil
salt to taste

1. Melt the butter in a Dutch oven over medium-high heat. Add the onion and sauté until soft, about 5 minutes. Add the water, rice, salt, thyme, and ¼ teaspoon pepper and mix well. Cover and simmer over low heat until the rice is partially cooked, about 10 minutes. Transfer the mixture to a large heat-safe bowl and toss until cooled. Wash and dry the pan and set aside.

2. Meanwhile, separate the leaves of the cabbage, rinse, and drain. Cut out the hard stems. Select and set aside 4 leaves and cut the remainder into 2-inch squares.

3. Add the pork and veal to the rice mixture and toss to mix. Knead with both hands until mixed thoroughly. Add the egg and stir with a wooden spoon until combined. Shape the mixture into 4 oval balls, dipping your hands in cold water frequently.

4. Heat 2 teaspoons canola oil in an 8-inch skillet over medium-high heat and brown the meatballs well on one side. Turn them over and brown on the other side. (Do not turn the meatballs until browned or they will break up.) Place the meatballs on a plate.

5. Preheat the oven to 350 degrees. Heat the remaining 1 teaspoon oil in the Dutch oven over medium heat. Add the scallions, ginger, and garlic and sauté until fragrant, about 2 minutes. Add the rice wine and cook 30 seconds. Add the cabbage squares and sauté 2 minutes. Add the stock, soy sauce, sesame oil, and remaining ½ teaspoon pepper; heat to boiling, partially covered. Uncover and simmer until the soup has thickened, about 30 minutes.

6. Place the meatballs in the center of the pan and cover each with a reserved cabbage leaf; cover the pan. Bake 45 minutes. Season with salt. Ladle the soup into warmed bowls, including one cabbage-covered meatball in each serving.

Each serving: About 437 calories, 31 g protein, 15 g carbohydrate, 27 g total fat (9 g saturated), 148 mg cholesterol, 938 mg sodium.

White Bean and Ham Soup

PREP TIME: 5 minutes
COOK TIME: 20 minutes

Makes 6 servings

A little white cheddar cheese smoothes out the earthiness of this singular soup. Serve it with Basic Croutons (page 22) or crusty bread to sop up the flavorful broth.

    3½ cups Chicken Stock (page 14)
    1 can (15 ounces) Great Northern beans, rinsed and drained
    2 large potatoes, peeled and cubed
    1 turnip, peeled and cubed
    1 celery stalk, sliced
    1 small onion, chopped
    2 ounces cooked lean deli ham, chopped
    2 garlic cloves, chopped
    1 teaspoon white wine vinegar
    ¼ teaspoon white pepper
    ¼ teaspoon ground dried savory
    ½ cup reduced-fat white cheddar cheese
    salt to taste
    paprika for garnish

1. Combine the stock, beans, potatoes, turnip, celery, onion, ham, garlic, vinegar, pepper, and savory in a 6-quart pot. Cover and bring to a boil. Reduce the heat and simmer until the vegetables are tender, about 15 minutes.

2. Remove the soup from the heat. Using a handheld immersion blender, coarsely puree the vegetables. Stir in the cheddar. Taste and season with salt if needed. Serve the soup garnished with the paprika.

Each serving: About 212 calories, 14 g protein, 35 g carbohydrate, 1 g total fat (1 g saturated), 5 mg cholesterol, 527 mg sodium.

Ham and Cheese Soup

PREP TIME: 15 minutes
COOK TIME: about 20 minutes

Makes 6 servings

Serve this hearty main-dish soup with Brittle Bread (page 35) and a mixed green salad.

4 tablespoons unsalted butter
1 medium onion, thinly sliced
1 medium carrot, peeled and cut into thin rounds
1 celery stalk with some leaves, cut crosswise into thin pieces
1 small red bell pepper, seeded and chopped
1 package (10 ounces) frozen peas, thawed
1 jalapeño pepper, minced (use rubber gloves when handling hot peppers)
8 ounces smoked, boiled, or baked ham, cut into bite-size chunks
2 tablespoons all-purpose flour
½ teaspoon baking soda
3 cups Chicken Stock (page 14), preferably unsalted or low-salt, or more if needed
3 cups milk, at room temperature
8 ounces shredded extra-sharp Cheddar cheese
freshly ground white pepper
chopped toasted hazelnuts for garnish (optional)
chopped fresh parsley leaves for garnish

1. Melt the butter in a 3-quart saucepan over medium heat. Add the onion, carrot, celery, bell pepper, peas, jalapeño, and ham and sauté until the onion is softened, about 7 minutes. Add the flour and cook, stirring, until bubbly, about 2 minutes.

2. Whisk in the baking soda. Whisk in a little stock, and then the remaining stock and the milk. Add the cheese and cook, stirring with a wooden spoon in one direction only until the cheese melts and blends into the liquid. Stir in a little more stock if the soup is too thick. Season with white pepper and garnish with hazelnuts (if using) and parsley.

Each serving without nuts: About 457 calories, 27 g protein, 22 g carbohydrate, 30 g total fat (17 g saturated), 99 mg cholesterol, 915 mg sodium.

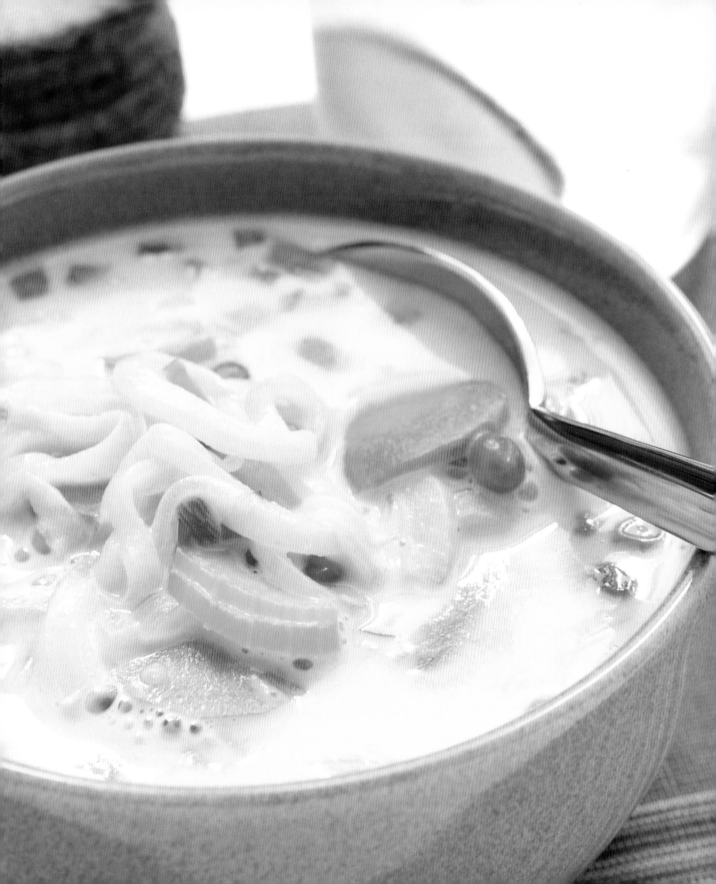

Caldo Verde (PORTUGUESE KALE AND POTATO SOUP WITH SPICY SAUSAGE)

PREP TIME: 25 minutes
COOK TIME: about 35 minutes

Makes 6 to 8 servings

Oh boy, get ready to enlarge your list of food favorites! This Portuguese national dish is peasant cuisine, but the stuff explorers are made of. Two things are important to this soup: It's worth searching for Portuguese olive oil and chouriço to add authentic flavor, and the thinner your slivers of kale are, the more sensuous the result.

2 quarts water
1 teaspoon salt or more to taste
1 pound kale or collard greens, washed, trimmed of coarse stems and veins
5 medium baking potatoes, peeled and cut into ¼-inch-thick rounds
6 ounces chouriço or linguiça (spicy, garlicky Portuguese sausages), chorizo (spicy Spanish sausage), pepperoni, or any other dry smoked garlicky sausage, skinned and thinly sliced
½ cup extravirgin olive oil (preferably Portuguese)

1. Heat the water with the salt to boiling in a 4-quart saucepan over medium-high heat. While the water heats, stack 6 to 8 leaves of kale on a cutting board and cut crosswise into fine shreds and place in a bowl; repeat with the remaining kale.

2. Add the potatoes to the water and cook, covered, until they start to fall apart, about 20 minutes. While the potatoes cook, sauté the chouriço in a medium skillet over medium-low heat until the fat has rendered, about 10 minutes. Transfer the chouriço to a plate with a slotted spoon; discard the fat in the pan.

3. When the potatoes are cooked, mash them in the pan with a potato masher or the back of a wooden spoon. Return the pan to the stove and heat to simmering over medium heat. Add the chouriço and olive oil and simmer, covered, 5 minutes. Increase the heat to medium-high and when boiling, add the kale. Cook, uncovered, until tender, about 2 minutes. Taste and adjust the salt if necessary. Ladle into wide soup bowls and serve.

Each of 6 servings: About 386 calories, 11 g protein, 22 g carbohydrate, 29 g total fat (7 g saturated), 25 mg cholesterol, 772 mg sodium.

Kielbasa with Roasted Pepper Soup

PREP TIME: 5 minutes
COOK TIME: 25 minutes

Makes 4 servings

To reduce prep time, replace freshly roasted red peppers with the variety
from a jar.

    1 teaspoon olive oil
    ¼ pound cooked kielbasa, halved lengthwise and sliced
    1 large onion, chopped
    3½ cups Chicken Stock (page 14)
    1 large potato, peeled and diced
    1 celery stalk, sliced
    1 teaspoon white wine vinegar
    ½ teaspoon dried thyme leaves
    ¼ teaspoon lemon pepper
    salt to taste
    ¼ cup diced roasted red peppers for garnish

1. Heat the oil in a 6-quart pot over medium-high heat for 1 minute. Add
   the kielbasa and onion and sauté until the onion begins to brown, about
   6 minutes. Add the stock, potato, celery, vinegar, thyme, and lemon pepper.

2. Cover and bring to a boil. Reduce the heat and simmer until the vegetables are tender, about 15 minutes. Taste and season with salt if needed.
   Top each serving with red peppers.

Each serving: About 186 calories, 12 g protein, 20 g carbohydrate, 6 g total fat
(20 g saturated), 25 mg cholesterol, 378 mg sodium.

Bratwurst and Beer Soup

PREP TIME: 5 minutes
COOK TIME: 20 minutes

Makes 2 servings

1 teaspoon olive oil
4 ounces cooked bratwurst, halved lengthwise and sliced
2 cups Beef Stock (page 15)
2 leeks, white part only, sliced, rinsed well
1 large potato, peeled and cut into ½-inch cubes
¼ teaspoon white pepper
1 red bell pepper, seeded and chopped
1 cup nonalcoholic beer
salt to taste
¼ cup snipped fresh chives for garnish

1. Heat the oil in a 6-quart pot over medium-high heat for 1 minute. Add the bratwurst and sauté until lightly browned. Transfer to a bowl.

2. Combine the stock, leeks, potato, and pepper in the same 6-quart pot. Cover and bring to a boil. Reduce the heat and simmer until the potatoes are tender, about 15 minutes. Transfer half the mixture to a bowl.

3. Using a potato masher, mash the vegetables remaining in the pot. Stir in the bratwurst and reserved vegetables. Stir in the bell pepper and beer and simmer 5 minutes. Taste and season with salt if needed. Top each serving with the chives.

Each serving: About 360 calories, 22 g protein, 50 g carbohydrate, 8 g total fat (6 g saturated), 40 mg cholesterol, 228 mg sodium.

Venison-Vegetable Soup

PREP TIME: 15 minutes
COOK TIME: 45 minutes to 1 hour 30 minutes

Makes 6 to 8 servings

If you only have the venison meat and not the stock, you can use beef, chicken, or even vegetable stock with delicious results. If using uncooked venison, first brown it in 2 tablespoons of the oil, breaking it into bite-size chunks with a wooden spoon. Remove it from the pan, and then proceed with the remaining oil and vegetables in step 1.

¼ cup extravirgin olive oil or canola oil
3 large carrots, peeled and diced
3 medium waxy potatoes (Yukon Gold adds great color and flavor), peeled and diced
1 onion, diced
1 inner celery stalk with leaves, chopped
shank meat from making the stock (page 19) or 2 pounds ground or diced venison, browned
2 quarts Venison Stock (page 19)
1 can (about 15 ounces) diced tomatoes with garlic and basil
½ teaspoon dried thyme leaves, crushed
salt and freshly ground pepper to taste

1. Heat the oil in a 4-quart saucepan over medium-high heat. Add the carrots, potatoes, onion, and celery and sauté until softened but not browned, about 7 minutes. Cover the pan, reduce the heat to medium, and sweat the vegetables until tender, about 10 minutes.

2. Add the venison, stock, tomatoes, and thyme to the vegetables. Taste the soup and season with salt and pepper. Heat the soup to simmering over medium-high heat, skimming off any foam that forms on the surface. Reduce the heat to medium and simmer, partially covered, 20 minutes to 1 hour. Taste the soup again and adjust seasoning if necessary.

Each of 6 servings: About 221 calories, 24 g protein, 25 g carbohydrate, 3 g total fat (1 g saturated), 64 mg cholesterol, 357 mg sodium.

Lamb Soup with Orzo and Lentils

PREP TIME: 10 minutes
COOK TIME: 3 hours 30 minutes

Makes 8 servings

Pass some Olive Pesto (page 46) at the table to stir in at will; you will be surprised at the way all the ingredients respond.

2 tablespoons olive oil
1½ pounds lean lamb, cut into ¾-inch cubes
2 large onions, sliced
2 large garlic cloves, crushed through a press
2 quarts water
2 teaspoons grated orange zest
1 teaspoon salt or more to taste
½ teaspoon dried oregano leaves
¼ teaspoon freshly ground pepper or more
   to taste
1 cup dried lentils, rinsed
1 large carrot, peeled and cut into ½-inch cubes
1 cup uncooked orzo pasta
2 tablespoons chopped fresh Italian parsley

1. Heat the oil in a 4-quart saucepan over medium-high heat; add the lamb, and sauté until browned on all sides. Add the onions and sauté until softened, about 5 minutes. Add the garlic and sauté 2 minutes. Add the water, 1 teaspoon orange zest, the salt, oregano, and pepper. Heat to boiling, reduce the heat, cover, and simmer over medium-low heat until the lamb is tender, about 2½ hours. Add the lentils and carrot; cover, and simmer 15 minutes.

2. Add the orzo to the soup and simmer, uncovered, until tender, about 7 minutes. Stir in the remaining 1 teaspoon orange zest and the parsley. (The soup should be thick.) Taste the soup and season with additional salt and pepper if necessary. Ladle into warmed soup bowls and serve immediately.

Each serving: About 405 calories, 28 g protein, 28 g carbohydrate, 20 g total fat (7 g saturated), 74 mg cholesterol, 356 mg sodium.

Curried Lamb and Rice Soup

PREP TIME: 15 minutes
COOK TIME: 1 hour 15 minutes

Makes 4 servings

If your curry powder has been sitting on the shelf for over 3 months, consider upping the amount or buying a new batch. Give the soup a little extra kick by stirring in some Skordalia (page 45).

2 tablespoons extravirgin olive oil
8 ounces lean boneless lamb shoulder, trimmed of fat, sliced into 1-inch-long slivers
1 tablespoon grated peeled fresh gingerroot
¼ teaspoon hot curry powder
5 cups water
2 ripe tomatoes, skinned, seeded, and cut into 1-inch chunks
½ cup finely chopped onions
1½ teaspoons salt
1 teaspoon freshly ground pepper
1 cup cooked long-grain white rice
2 eggs, lightly beaten
1 tablespoon fresh lemon juice
2 tablespoons finely chopped cilantro for garnish
ground cinnamon for dusting

1. Heat the oil in a 2-quart saucepan over medium-high heat. Add the lamb and sauté until browned well, about 5 minutes. Add the ginger and curry and sauté 1 minute. Add the water, tomatoes, onion, salt, and pepper. Heat to boiling and simmer over medium heat, partially covered, for 1 hour.

2. Add the rice and heat through. Remove the pan from the heat and gradually pour the eggs in a circle near the side of the pan, not just in the middle. Stir once in a circular motion to allow the egg to set in strands. Let stand 3 minutes, or until the egg is firm but not hard. Stir in the lemon juice. Ladle the soup into warmed soup bowls, sprinkle with cilantro, and dust with cinnamon.

Each serving: About 313 calories, 15 g protein, 17 g carbohydrate, 21 g total fat (6 g saturated), 147 mg cholesterol, 942 mg sodium.

Rustic Lamb Soup with Adzuki Beans

PREP TIME: 5 minutes
COOK TIME: 20 minutes

Makes 4 servings

Enjoy the classic pairing of rosemary and lamb in this 30-minute soup. To bring out rosemary's delightful piney essence, crush the leaves between your fingers before using them.

2 teaspoons dried rosemary
½ teaspoon freshly ground black pepper
8 ounces lean lamb shoulder, cut into
    ½-inch cubes
1 teaspoon olive oil
1 medium onion, thinly sliced
2½ cups Beef Stock (page 15)
1 turnip, cut into ½-inch cubes
1 medium red potato, cut into ½-inch cubes
¾ cup rinsed canned adzuki beans
1 cup torn sorrel leaves
salt and pepper to taste

1. Combine the rosemary and pepper and sprinkle over the lamb.

2. Heat the oil in a 6-quart pot over medium-high heat for 1 minute. Add the lamb and onion and sauté until the lamb is lightly browned, about 5 minutes.

3. Stir in the stock, turnip, potato, and beans. Cover and bring to a boil. Reduce the heat and simmer until the vegetables are tender, about 15 minutes. Stir in the sorrel. Taste and season with salt and pepper if needed.

Each serving: About 340 calories, 32 g protein, 38 g carbohydrate, 6 g total fat (2 g saturated), 61 mg cholesterol, 168 mg sodium.

Scotch Broth

PREP TIME: 15 minutes
COOK TIME: 2 hours 30 minutes

Makes 10 to 12 servings

Though this may have been considered somewhat of a bore of a soup a generation ago, the concept of lamb and barley survives and prevails. It's a classic example of ethnic (Celtic) ingredients bound together in a thera-peutic counterpoint to cold winters. Who would dare say it is too much of an indulgence to serve some Sweet Onion Focaccia (page 30) on the side?

2 pounds lamb shoulder or stew meat, cut into ½-inch cubes

3 sprigs fresh thyme

3 sprigs fresh Italian parsley plus ¼ cup chopped parsley for serving

1 bay leaf

⅓ cup pearl barley, soaked overnight in 2 cups water

1 teaspoon salt or more to taste

3 large leeks, cut crosswise into ¼-inch-thick rings and rinsed well

2 large slender carrots, peeled and cut into ¼-inch rounds

2 small turnips, peeled and cut into ½-inch dice

1 inner celery rib with some leaves, finely chopped

1 shallot, finely chopped

¼ teaspoon freshly ground pepper or more to taste

1. Place the meat in a 6-quart stockpot and add enough cold water to cover by 3 inches. Heat slowly to boiling over medium heat, skimming off any foam that forms on the surface.

2. Tie the thyme, parsley, and bay leaf together in several places with cotton kitchen string. Add the herb bundle to the soup along with the barley and salt. Simmer slowly over medium-low heat 1½ hours, skimming the foam frequently and adding enough water to keep the contents covered by 3 inches.

3. Add the leeks, carrots, turnips, celery, shallot, and pepper. Cover the soup and simmer 1 hour. Taste and add more salt and pepper if needed. Stir in the chopped parsley, ladle the soup into warmed soup bowls, and serve.

Each of 10 servings: About 275 calories, 17 g protein, 12 g carbohydrate, 17 g total fat (7 g saturated), 64 mg cholesterol, 312 mg sodium.

Quick Steak and Onion Soup

PREP TIME: 15 minutes
COOK TIME: 50 minutes

Makes 6 servings

This is a good Saturday-night supper or whenever you need a quick, hearty dinner.

    1 pound thin round steak
    2 large yellow onions, thinly sliced
    1 can (28 ounces) crushed tomatoes
    1 can (about 15 ounces) diced tomatoes with garlic and basil
    1 tablespoon vegetable shortening or oil
    salt and freshly ground pepper to taste
    2 cups hot mashed potatoes

1. Thinly slice the steak into 1-inch pieces. Combine the steak, onions, tomatoes, and shortening in a 2-quart saucepan over medium heat and cook, covered, until the onions are tender, about 50 minutes. Taste and season with salt and pepper.

2. To serve, ladle the soup into warmed soup bowls and add a dollop of potatoes to each serving.

Each serving: About 240 calories, 19 g protein, 26 g carbohydrate, 7 g total fat (2 g saturated), 43 mg cholesterol, 612 mg sodium.

INDEX